DIAGNOSIS AND MANAGEMENT OF POLYCYSTIC OVARY SYNDROME

Nadir R. Farid · Evanthia Diamanti-Kandarakis
Editors

DIAGNOSIS AND MANAGEMENT OF POLYCYSTIC OVARY SYNDROME

Springer

Editors
Nadir R. Farid
The London Endocrine Clinic
21 Wimpole Street
London WIG 8GG
farid@thelondonendocrineclinic.com

Evanthia Diamanti-Kandarakis
University of Athens Medical School
Athens, Greece
akandara@otenet.gr

ISBN 978-1-4419-3523-6 e-ISBN 978-0-387-09718-3
DOI 10.1007/978-0-387-09718-3

Printed on acid-free paper

springer.com

Preface

Consulting citation trends in PubMed for key words or phrases is instructive as to the interest of the scientific community in the subject and by inference its currency and likely importance. In the 5 years between 1985 and 1989 there were 91 papers on PCOS. The rate escalated rapidly in the next half-decades to 727, 1642, and 4355, 2005–July 2008. Insulin resistance was more topical and references reference to the term increased rapidly: 1995–1999, 8517, 2000–2004, 21,828 and in 2005–July 2008 only rose to 48,914.

The observation that most women with PCOS are insulin resistant has been an important turning point. From being predominantly the domain of gynaecologists as an ovarian disorder, PCOS was thereafter recognized as a heterogeneous metabolic disorder with polycystic ovaries as part of its manifestations. We have since learnt that not all women with PCOS are insulin resistant, apparently this predominates in those who suffer from both hyperandrogenism and anovultion. Some women with PCOS who have apparently normal serum insulin levels are nevertheless show increased ovarian androgens secretion at those levels of insulin.

With the mounting epidemic of insulin resistance, many doctors in practice encounter women who are symptomatic, have more or less regular cycles, are sub-fertile, are at most slightly hyperandrogenemic and without PCOS ovarian morphology . There is no consensus on how to manage these women. We also do not know the rate at which untreated mild PCOS becomes more severe or that at which women satisfying the criteria of The Androgen Excess Society (AES) who are not anovulatory become so and apparently acquire insulin resistance.

PCOS, a complex multigenic disorder, can have major impact on quality of life with depressive tendencies, infertility, obesity, manifestations of hyperandrogenism as well as long term increased risks for diabetes, the metabolic syndrome non-alcoholic fatty liver and cardiovascular disease. These and other issues are expertly laid out in the pages of this book, as is their management. The intuitive expectation that PCOS is associated with increased risk for cardiovascular disease is supported by strong surrogate evidence, although outcome studies are lacking. And for now at least an increased risk for women who had PCOS and have entered the menopause is tentative.

The authors, all international experts in their areas of contribution, clear lay out the problem, offer practical advice in the management of various aspects of the syndrome and raise question where current knowledge is incomplete or new data is necessary.

The idea of this book arose out of a consensus among the contributing authors and many others we consulted with that knowledge about the diagnosis, health implications and up-to-date management of PCOS among community doctors and trainees is at best incomplete and at most spotty. This book is an effort to redress that deficit.

That this book has materialized at all is thanks to the efforts of Ms Laura Walsh who worked hard to find a niche for this book in the ranks of what now become one of the largest publishing houses in the world. Mrs Maureen Tobin kept us all on track, and has done a wonderful organizational job...all very quietly.

It was an immense pleasure for me to work again with Maureen and Laura on a new successful project.

Nadir R. Farid

Contents

Contributors

Jean-Patrice Baillargeon
Associate Professor, Departments of Medicine and Physiology/Biophysics, Director, Program of Endocrinology and Metabolism, University of Sherbrooke, Sherbrooke, QC J1H 5N4, Canada, Jean-Patrice.Baillargeon@USherbrooke.ca

Thomas M. Barber, MA (Hons), MBBS, MRCP (UK)
Research Fellow and Specialist Registrar, Department of Endocrinology, Oxford Centre for Diabetes, Endocrinology and Metabolism, University of Oxford, Oxford, UK, tom.barber@drl.ox.ac.uk

Susan J. Barter, MBBS, MRCP, DMRD, FRCR
Consultant Radiologist, Addenbrookes Hospital University Trust, Hills Road, Cambridge CB2 2QQ, UK, suebarter@btinternet.com

Salvatore Benvenga, MD
Master on Childhood, Adolescent and Women's Endocrine Health, University of Messina, Programma di Endocrinologia Molecolare Clinica, A.O.U. Policlinico G. Martino, Padiglione H, 4 piano, 98125 Messina, Italy, s.benvenga@me.nettuno.it

Susan Calhoun, PhD
Sleep Research and Treatment Center, Department of Psychiatry, Pennsylvania State University College of Medicine, Hershey, PA, USA, scalhoun@hmc.psu.edu

Enrico Carmina, MD, PhD
Professor of Medicine, Professor of Endocrinology and Head of Endocrine Unit, Department of Clinical Medicine, University of Palermo, Via delle Croci 47 90139 Palermo, Italy, enricocarmina@libero.it

Charikleia D. Christakou, MD
Endocrine Section of the 1st Department of Medicine, University of Athens, Medical School, Athens, Greece, cchristak@med.uoa.gr

Colin J Davis
Consultant Obstetrician and Gynaecologist, St Bartholomews Hospital London, London, UK, cdavisobgyn@aol.com

Evanthia Diamanti-Kandarakis, MD
Endocrine Section of the 1st Department of Medicine, University of Athens, Medical School, Athens, Greece, akandara@otenet.gr

Brad Eilerman, MD
Division of Endocrinology, Department of Medicine, University of Cincinnati College of Medicine, The Vontz Center for Molecular Studies, Cincinnati, OH 45267, USA

Nadir R. Farid, MD
The London Endocrine Clinic, 21 Wimpole Street, London WIG 8GG, farid@thelondonendocrineclinic.com

Neoklis A. Georgopoulos, MD
Department of Obstetrics and Gynecology, Division of Reproductive Endocrinology, Patras Medical School, Greece, neoklisg@hol.gr

Sabrina Gill, MD
Division of Endocrinology & Metabolism, St. Paul's Hospital and University of British Columbia, Vancouver, BC, Canada, SGill@providencehealth.bc.ca

Ettore Guastella
Department of Obstetrics and Gynecology, University of Palermo, Palermo, Italy, ettore_guastella@libero.it

Janet E. Hall, MD
Reproductive Endocrine Unit, Massachusetts General Hospital and Harvard Medical School, Boston, MA, USA, jehall@partners.org

Robert A. Hegele, MD
Director, Blackburn Cardiovascular Genetics Laboratory, Scientist, Vascular Biology Research Group, Robarts Research Institute, 406 - 100 Perth Drive, London, Ontario, Canada N6A 5K8, hegele@robarts.ca

Melissa J. Himelein, PhD
Professor of Psychology, University of North Carolina at Asheville, Licensed Psychologist, Center for Applied Reproductive Science, Johnson City, TN, & Asheville, NC, USA, himelein@unca.edu

Roy Homburg, FRCOG
Professor of Reproductive Medicine, VU University Medical Centre, 1007MB Amsterdam, the Netherlands; IVF, Department of Obstetrics and Gynecology, Barzilai Medical Center, Ashkelon, Israel, r.homburg@vumc.nl

Tisha R. Joy
Robarts Research Institute, 406 – 100 Perth Drive, London, Ontario, Canada N6A 5K8, tjoy@uwo.ca

Eleni Kandaraki, MD
Second Department of Obstetrics and Gynecology, Division of Human Reproduction, Aristotle University of Thessaloniki, Greece, akandara@otenet.gr

Heather A. Kenna, MA
Department of Psychiatry and Behavioral Sciences, Stanford University, School of Medicine, Stanford, CA, USA, hkenna@stanford.edu

Alexandra Lawrence, MD, MRCOG
Subspeciality Trainee in Gynaecological Oncology, Hammersmith Hospital, Du Cane Road, London, W12 0HS, UK, AlexandraC.Lawrence@imperial.nhs.uk

Kate Marsh, BSc, M Nutr Diet, Grad Cert Diab Edn & Mgt
Advanced Accredited Practising Dietitian (AdvAPD) and Credentialled Diabetes Educator (CDE), The PCOS Health & Nutrition Centre, Sydney, Australia, kate@nnd.com.au

W. Peter Mason, MD
Gynaecological Oncologist, Chairman North West London Network, Hammersmith Hospital NHS Trust, London, UK, wpetermason@aol.com

John E. Nestler, MD
Division of Endocrinology and Metabolism, Virginia Commonwealth University, Richmond, VA 23298-0111, USA, nestler@hsc.vcu.edu

Dimitrios Panidis
Second Department of Obstetrics and Gynecology, Division of Human Reproduction, Aristotle University of Thessaloniki, Greece, panidisd@med.auth.gr

Natalie L. Rasgon, MD, PhD
Department of Psychiatry and Behavioral Sciences Stanford University, School of Medicine, Stanford, CA, USA, nrasgon@stanford.edu

Pasquali Renato
Division of Endocrinology, Department of Internal Medicine, S. Orsola-Malpighi Hospital, University Alma Mater Studiorum, Via Massarenti 9, 40138, Bologna, Italy, renato.pasquali@aosp.bo.it

Manfredi Rizzo
Department of Clinical Medicine, University of Palermo, Via delle Croci 47, 90139 Palermo, Italy, mrizzo@unipa.it

Marzieh Salehi, MD
Division of Endocrinology, Department of Medicine, University of Cincinnati College of Medicine, Cincinnati, OH, USA, Marzieh.Salehi@uc.edu

Rehan Salim, MD, MRCOG
Assisted Conception Unit, University College London, London, UK, Rehan.Salim@uclh.nhs.uk

Paul Serhal, MBBS, MRCOG
Assisted Conception Unit, University College London, London WC1X 8LD, Paul.serhal@uclh.nhs.uk

Susmeeta T. Sharma, MBBS
Department of Internal Medicine, University of Florida, Gainesville, FL, USA, susmeetasharma@yahoo.com

Pascale G. Stemmle, BS
Department of Psychiatry and Behavioral Sciences, Stanford University, School of Medicine, Stanford, CA, USA, pascale@stanford.edu

Emma Stevenson, MD
School of Psychology and Sports Sciences, Northumbria University, Newcastle Upon Tyne, NE1 8ST, UK, e.stevenson@unn.ac.uk

Samuel S. Thatcher, MD, PhD
Director, Center for Applied Reproductive Science, Johnson City, TN and Asheville, NC, USA

Yaron Tomer, MD, FACP
Division of Endocrinology, University of Cincinnati College of Medicine, The Vontz Center for Molecular Studies, Cincinnati, OH 45267, USA, tomery@UCMAIL.UC.EDU

Agathocles Tsatsoulis, MD, PhD, FRCP
Professor of Medicine/Endocrinology, Department of Endocrinology, University of Ioannina, Ioannina, 45110, Greece, atsatsou@uoi.gr

Evert JP van Santbrink, MD, PhD
Senior consultant in Reproductive Medicine, Division of Reproductive Medicine , Department of Obstetrics and Gynecology, Erasmus Medical Center, Rotterdam, the Netherlands, e.vansantbrink@erasmusmc.nl

Alexandros N. Vgontzas, MD
Sleep Research and Treatment Center, Department of Psychiatry, Pennsylvania State University College of Medicine, Hershey, PA 17033, USA, avgontzas@hmc.psu.edu

Nectaria Xita, MD
Department of Endocrinology, University of Ioannina, Ioannina, 45110, Greece, nxita@yahoo.com

Part I
The Syndrome

Chapter 1
Clinical Manifestations of PCOS

Pasquali Renato

1.1 Introduction

The PCOS is the commonest hyperandrogenic disorder in women and one of the most common causes of ovulatory infertility, with an estimated prevalence of 4–7% worldwide [1]. Over the years, after the first description by Stein and Leventhal in 1935 [2], its definition has been re-addressed several times. In 1990 the National Institutes of Health (NIH) established new diagnostic criteria, based on the presence of hyperandrogenism and chronic oligo-anovulation, with the exclusion of other causes of hyperandrogenism such as adult-onset congenital adrenal hyperplasia, hyperprolactinemia and androgen-secreting neoplasms [3]. The inclusion of ultrasound morphology of the ovaries as a further potential criterion to define PCOS was proposed by the Rotterdam consensus conference, which established that at least two of the following criteria – oligo- and/or anovulation, clinical and/or biochemical signs of hyperandrogenism and polycystic ovaries (PCO) at ultrasound – are sufficient for the diagnosis [4]. More recently, the fundamental role of hyperandrogenism has been pointed out [5]. However, PCOS compromises other pathological conditions that strongly modify the phenotype and play a dominant role in the pathophysiology of the disorder, including insulin resistance and hyperinsulinemia, obesity and metabolic disorders, all favouring, together with androgen excess, an increased susceptibility to develop type 2 diabetes mellitus (T2DM) and, possibly, cardiovascular diseases (CVD). PCOS by itself may also have some genetic component as documented by familial aggregation and recent genetic studies [1]. All the clinical features may however change throughout the lifespan, starting from adolescence to postmenopausal age. Therefore, PCOS should be considered as a lifespan disorder, although the specific phenotype of PCOS in postmenopausal women is still poorly defined [6]

1.2 How to Approach the Patient

Most patients do not know anything about the definition of PCOS, with some exceptions. They go to the doctor because of their health problems, which are sometimes relevant only for cosmetic reasons, particularly in young women. Major concerns in asking for the doctor's help are represented by (i) clinical signs of androgen excess, particularly hirsutism; (ii) menses irregularities, including amenorrhea; (iii) unexplained infertility; or (iv) obesity and related features. Doctors should be aware that all these problems are often differently perceived on an individual basis, and that the patient may be greatly involved in the solution of one of them and relatively disinterested in the others, depending on age, cultural background and perceived importance of clinical features. Accordingly, affected women may refer to different specialists, such as dermatologists, gynaecologists or endocrinologists. Nonetheless, each doctor should try to evaluate all the signs and symptom of the patient in a holistic clinical approach, in order to make a diagnosis and select appropriate treatment, when needed.

P. Renato (✉)
Division of Endocrinology, Department of Internal Medicine, S. Orsola-Malpighi Hospital, University Alma Mater Studiorum, Via Massarenti 9, 40138, Bologna, Italy
e-mail: renato.pasquali@unibo.it

N.R. Farid, E. Diamanti-Kandarakis (eds.), *Diagnosis and Management of Polycystic Ovary Syndrome*,
DOI 10.1007/978-0-387-09718-3_1,

1.3 Clinical Picture of PCOS

The clinical evaluation should include a complete medical history and physical examination, and consideration of differential diagnosis. Although diagnostic criteria for PCOS for research studies have been proposed, it should be remembered that many patients may not meet the strict criteria reported above, therefore requiring blood testing and other diagnostic procedures. In addition, the definition does not cover all features of PCOS, with particular emphasis on excess body weight and metabolic disorders. Therefore, in an individual patient, the history should always naturally begin with the symptoms and signs that are causing most concern to the patient. Fundamental methodological aspects to consider should be

(a) if a patient has signs of androgen excess (such as hirsutism), does she have irregular menses and anovulation?
(b) if a patient has irregular menses, particularly during adolescence, does she have hyperandrogenic signs, or should these alterations be related to androgen excess, if necessary investigated by blood tests?
(c) if a patient is infertile, should androgen excess conditions (clinically evident or biochemically defined) be investigated?
(d) how to define the frequent presence of excess body weight in relation to the previously reported problems?
(e) how to frame metabolic alterations from a pathophysiological and therapeutic perspective?
(f) given the potential genetic background of PCOS, how useful is the family history to define the diagnosis?

If these aspects are appropriately taken into consideration, the clinical diagnosis of PCOS is not complex and does not require extensive laboratory evaluation, provided a differential diagnosis with other overlapping conditions responsible for androgen excess, menses irregularities, infertility, obesity and metabolic disturbances is performed.

Past medical history should also include a knowledge of prior ovarian surgery that could impact current hormonal and menstrual status, and prior records of an abdominal procedure may provide information as to the appearance of the uterus and/or ovaries. A complete history of prior therapies must be documented, including topical treatments for acne and hirsutism that are likely to influence the appearance of the skin over time. In some cases, it may be apparent that the symptoms of PCOS merely became evident because a woman has recently discontinued oral contraceptive pills that had masked the symptoms. At the other extreme, new onset androgenic symptoms could also be explained by the recent use of topical testosterone creams for the treatment of low libido or vulvar dermopathies. The medication list may also reveal prior treated conditions that the patient had not recognized which might be related to variability in their menstrual cycles or weight profiles. Finally, acne is known to be caused by certain medications, including azathioprine, barbiturates, corticosteroids, cyclosporine, disulfiram, halogens, iodides, isoniazid, lithium, phenytoin, psoralens, thiourea and vitamins [7]. Finally, a list of all cosmetic therapies is necessary for the interpretation of physical findings; topical and other treatments of hirsutism and acne will in fact influence the clinical manifestations of these conditions.

1.4 Family History

Several studies have documented an increased risk of PCOS in sisters and daughters of women with PCOS, so the history provides an opportunity to identify new cases of PCOS. Hirsutism, acne, menstrual irregularity, early cardiovascular disease, obesity and T2DM are all potential indicators of a familial tendency towards the PCOS [8]. A family history of infertility and/or hirsutism may also indicate disorders such as non-classic congenital adrenal hyperplasia. The presence of symptoms that are very different from those of other family members may increase the level of concern for a more pathologic explanation for the menstrual defects or the androgenic symptoms. The family history of metabolic defects and CVD is also an opportunity to quantify the risk of the patient.

1.5 Evaluation of Clinical Hyperandrogenism

Hyperandrogenic signs and symptoms are the hallmark characteristic of PCOS. Most women with PCOS have clinical evidence of hyperandrogenism, which includes hirsutism, acne, oily skin and, sometimes, male pattern balding or alopecia. Rarely, virilizing symptoms may be present, such as increased muscle mass, deepening of the voice, or clitoromegaly, although these findings should prompt a search for an underlying ovarian or adrenal neoplasm, or classic form of previously undiagnosed congenital adrenal hyperplasia. The age at onset, the rate of progression and any change with any treatment or with fluctuations in weight or skin problems should be determined.

In general, hirsutism is the most representative sign of clinical hyperandrogenism. It is defined as excess terminal (thick, pigmented) body hair in a male distribution, which usually starts during pubertal development or right after it, although not infrequently it may manifest in the adult age. It can also be expressed earlier, even during mid-childhood, where it can be associated in a mild form with a premature adrenarche characterized by the appearance and progressive development of pubic and/or axillary hair [9]. Typical areas of androgen-dependent terminal hair are face (particularly upper lip and chin); around the nipples and the breast area; and the abdomen, along the linea alba. Rapid and progressive worsening of hirsutism, or a later age of onset, suggest the possibility of ovarian or adrenal tumour, although they could even follow suspension of previous treatments or changes in weight.

Acne is typically the first manifestation of hyperandrogenism after menarche, in the teenage years. The typical acne lesions vary in increasing order of severity (see: *Physical examination*), which are highly dependent on previous topical, systemic and cosmetic treatments. A familiar prevalence of acne may be present.

Androgenic alopecia may also occur. Terminal hair growth is age dependent, and it may not be apparent until the early twenties after several years of exposure to excess androgens. Male pattern hair loss tends to present even later, in the later twenties and beyond. Androgenic alopecia may be graded by well-known subjective methods (see: *Physical examination*).

1.6 Evaluation of Menstrual Irregularity and Chronic Anovulation

Anovulation is undetectable in childhood, whereas in the perimenarcheal phase, adolescent women exhibit a transient state of anovulation, characterized by accentuated 24-hour LH levels [10]. However, making a correct clinical diagnosis of ovarian dysfunction at this age represents a difficult task and another 2 or 3 years may be needed. In fact, the menstrual cycle is rather long and variable during the first few years after menarche, and the establishment of regular ovulatory cycles is a slow process in physiological conditions. Using sequential progesterone measurements, it has been shown that more than 80% of the cycles are anovulatory during the first year after menarche, 60% during the third year and 25% after the sixth year are still anovulatory [10]. On the other hand, there are data supporting the finding that anovulatory pubertal or post-pubertal girls may have higher testosterone, androstenedione and LH levels than their ovulatory counterparts [10]. These young girls therefore appear to be characterized by endocrinological features resembling PCOS, although it cannot be excluded that even "physiological" anovulation during and after puberty may be associated with transient hyperactivity of the hypothalamic-pituitary-gonadal axis leading, in turn, to increased androgen production. Moreover, in early puberty, ovarian hyperandrogenism is rarely detected, but it becomes more common after the age of 14–15 years. On the other hand, the persistence of the high LH level profile in hyperandrogenic adolescent girls may be responsible for anovulation and therefore for irregular menses [11]. This should be appropriately considered in clinical practice. In fact, the typical clinical manifestations of PCOS occurring at puberty and adolescent age include irregular menses, particularly oligomenorrhea, increased LH levels and signs of androgen excess, such as hirsutism or acne.

The menstrual irregularity of PCOS typically manifests in the peripubertal period, although some women may apparently have regular cycles at first and subsequently develop menstrual irregularity in association with weight gain. Menses irregularities include mild or severe oligomenorrhea (cycle length more than 35–40 days) or amenorrhea (no cycles for 6 or more consecutive months).

In addition, anovulation is very common in the presence of mild oligomenorrhea, but also when normal cycles are present [12]. Some cycles may be associated with dysfunctional bleeding. Endometrial atrophy may be present in some women with PCOS who have prolonged amenorrhea, which may be related to androgen excess.

Chronic anovulation is one of the most important criteria in the diagnosis of PCOS. Some women with hyperandrogenic symptoms appear to have regular menstrual cycles, which necessarily require at least one or two assessments to document ovulation, at least in adult women. In the majority of women with severe oligomenorrhea or amenorrhea, chronic anovulation is usually present. However, occasional ovulation may occur, particularly in women with less severe oligomenorrhea. Ovulation can be easily detected by measuring progesterone levels in the luteal phase, at approximately days 20–22 after cycle onset. Appropriate hormone levels suggesting an adequate luteal phase are 6–8 ng/mL.

Additional information in a young or adult woman suspected to have PCOS should be obtained: age of menarche, presence of symptoms of ovulation or of premenstrual symptoms (ovulatory pain, premenstrual discomfort, breast tenderness), previous pregnancies or abortion and particularly oral contraceptive (OC) use [12]. Most young women, in fact, have a history of long-term OC use, often with different preparations, and this may have masked or delayed the recognition of menstrual dysfunction or hyperandrogenic symptoms [6]. In women presenting while taking OC, blood testing or pelvic ultrasounds should not be performed until they have discontinued OC use for at least three months. Notably, a sudden onset of menstrual dysfunction should raise the consideration of other aetiologies. Obviously, in the presence of recent unexplained amenorrhea, pregnancy should be excluded by appropriate testing. Moreover, weight- and exercise-related causes, hyperprolactinemia, subclinical or overt thyroid dysfunction, particularly in young women, should be investigated. Premature ovarian failure should also be suspected in adult women with unexplained amenorrhea.

1.7 Evaluation of Infertility

PCOS is a common cause of counselling in infertility clinics. Infertility was already included in the original description of PCOS by Stein and Leventhal [2]. Infertility related to PCOS is typically not difficult to diagnose due to the associated menstrual irregularity and anovulation. The primary cause is chronically irregular ovulation, leading to a reduced number of ovulations and unpredictable timing. However, some women do not receive the diagnosis of PCOS until they are being evaluated for infertility. The presence of PCOS does not rule out other abnormalities, so that male factor infertility and tubal patency must still be assessed. If the patient is at risk for metabolic defects, these must be screened for and treated as appropriate, to minimize pregnancy complications related to diabetes in particular. An increased rate of early pregnancy loss in PCOS may be an additional cause of infertility, but the mechanism of this is poorly understood [13]. A reduced rate of conception relative to the rate of ovulation after therapy with clomiphene citrate and exogenous gonadotropins is also well known; by contrast there are data suggesting that women diagnosed with polycystic ovaries (PCO) at ultrasound may be more likely to hyperstimulate in response to ovulation-inducing medications [7]

1.8 Evaluation of Overweight and Obesity

From the earliest descriptions of PCOS, obesity has been a prominently recognized clinical feature. Thus, some clinicians mistakenly fail to consider the PCOS diagnosis in lean women. However, several recent population-based studies of PCOS indicate that obesity is not a universal feature, with 30–70% of women with menstrual dysfunction and evidence of hyperandrogenism not being obese, depending on geographical areas and ethnicities [1]. Some recent data support the evidence that prevalence of PCOS may increase with increasing BMI [14].

Overweight and obesity, as well as different patterns of body fat distribution, can be easily assessed by anthropometric measures (see *Physical examination*). In adolescent girls, weight gain often precedes the onset of menses abnormalities [6]. In addition, a careful weight history should be performed, focusing on factors influencing weight gain, and on changes in clinical hyperandrogenic signs (hirsutism, etc.), menses and ovulation and, if pertinent, on fertility in relation to previous weight fluctuations. Major stressful events should also be investigated, since they may precede weigh loss or gain. Finally, previous dietary treatments or eating disorders should be investigated. Birthweight and subsequent catch-up should also be recorded, when data are available (particularly in adolescent and young women), with the help of parents and obstetric charts. This information can in fact help to understand the pathophysiological development of PCOS.

Obesity has profound effects on the clinical, hormonal and metabolic features of PCOS, which largely depend on the degree of excess body fat and on the pattern of fat distribution [15]. In massively obese women, the prevalence of PCOS may be much higher than expected [16]. A higher proportion of obese PCOS women complain of hirsutism and other androgen-dependent disorders, such as acne and androgenic alopecia, in comparison to normal-weight women. Moreover, obese PCOS women are characterized by significantly lower sex hormone binding globulin (SHBG) plasma levels and worsened hyperandrogemia (particularly total and free testosterone, and androstenedione) in comparison with their normal-weight counterparts. The androgen profile can be further negatively affected in PCOS women by the presence of abdominal body fat distribution with respect to those with the peripheral phenotype, regardless of BMI values [15].

Menstrual abnormalities can also be more frequent in obese than normal-weight PCOS women. Reduced incidence of pregnancy and blunted responsiveness to pharmacological treatments to induce ovulation may also be more common in obese PCOS women [17]. A decreased efficiency of assisted reproductive technologies (ART) has also been demonstrated, with the consequence that in some countries, e.g., the United Kingdom, obese women with a BMI greater than 35 are not entitled to ART through the National Health System until they have reduced their body weight by appropriate therapeutic strategies [18].

Lipodystrophic states are rare disorders in which PCOS should also be ruled out [19].

1.9 Additional Information: Insulin Resistance, Metabolic Syndrome, T2DM and Risk for CVD

Metabolic abnormalities are very common in PCOS [20,21] and should always be investigated. Other than PCOS status per se, a positive family history for T2DM, obesity, dyslipidaemia and CVD is common. Second, the presence of the abdominal pattern of fat distribution should be considered, this condition being a clinical sign of dysmetabolic disorders and cardiovascular risk. Insulin resistance can also be present in otherwise normal weight PCOS women, and most of them tend to have an android shape. Acanthosis nigricans may be a valuable sign of insulin resistance.

Most patients consult the doctor after they have *undergone* laboratory *tests* or other diagnostic procedures; therefore, their careful evaluation should be part of the first clinical approach. Confirmation of insulin resistance can be obtained by simple biochemical tests, based on the ratio between glucose and insulin blood concentration, in both fasting and glucose-stimulated condition. However, they are relatively inaccurate on *an* individual basis [22]; reference tests, such as the euglycemic hyperinsulinemic clamp technique and the frequent-sampling intravenous glucose tolerance *test,* are reserved *for* research purposes. In the presence of normal fasting glucose values, fasting insulin levels can however predict in by approximately 80% insulin resistance measured by the clamp tech*n*ique [23].

Approximately half of PCOS patients have the metabolic syndrome, which can be clinically suspected in the presence of abdominal obesity, although an abdominal fatness pattern can be present even in normal weight women [23]. According to the National Cholesterol Education Program Expert Panel (NECP/ATPIII) criteria [24], the threshold values for waist circumference should be 88 cm in women, whereas the International Diabetes Federation (IDF) more recently adjusted the threshold according to the different ethnicities, and in Europeans it should be 80 cm [25]. A relatively but significantly small increase of arterial blood pressure can be found in PCOS women, particularly if they are overweight or obese. Values of systolic and diastolic blood pressure higher than 130 mmHg and 80 mmHg, respectively, can further suggest the metabolic syndrome. A biochemical evaluation of fasting glucose, triglyceride and HDL-cholesterol blood levels are however needed to confirm the diagnosis.

Because women with PCOS have an increased risk of insulin resistance and T2DM [26], it is important to assess the specific risk factors in each patient. In addition to weight, which is a major factor that increases the risk of diabetes, a history of glucose intolerance during pregnancy also increases the risk of later diabetes. The risk can be increased especially in women with a first-degree relative with T2DM [26].

The prevalence of non-alcoholic fatty liver disease (NAFLD), a benign condition of ectopic fat deposition and non-alcoholic steatohepatitis (NASH), is increased not only in obesity or the metabolic syndrome, but also probably in women with PCOS [27]. It appears reasonable to inquire about symptoms and risk factors for liver disease, including family history and alcohol ingestion. Liver dimensions are usually increased in these conditions and can be determined by physical examination.

There is a great debate as to whether women with PCOS are susceptible to a significant risk for CVDs [28]. In the last few years, a growing amount of data has been published showing that states of insulin resistance such as T2DM, obesity (particularly the abdominal phenotype) and PCOS are characterized, among other well-defined factors, including hormonal and metabolic alterations, by impaired coagulation and fibrinolysis, anatomical and functional endothelial injury and vascular dysfunctions, and a state of subclinical inflammation, which overall represent independent risk factors for CVDs. Retrospective studies have however not confirmed a higher prevalence of myocardial infarction or stroke in PCOS [29]. Nevertheless, a careful clinical examination of the cardiovascular system should be always performed, particularly in adult premenopausal and particularly postmenopausal women with previously diagnosed PCOS.

1.10 The Impact of Obesity on Insulin Resistance, Metabolic Syndrome, T2DM and Risk for CVD

Obese PCOS women are invariably more insulin resistant than their insulin resistant normal weight counterparts, and they may have more severe fasting and glucose-stimulated hyperinsulinemia. Although it is commonly accepted that both obesity and PCOS status (i.e. androgen excess) have an additional deleterious effect on insulin sensitivity, specific mechanisms have still not been adequately defined and could even be different among obese and non-obese PCOS women [15,30]. In the presence of obesity, studies performed to investigate insulin secretion in relation to the magnitude of ambient insulin resistance have however shown that there is a subset of PCOS women exhibiting a significant impairment of β-cell function. Interestingly, β-cell dysfunction has been particularly found in those women who had a first-degree relative with T2DM, so that a heritable component of β-cell secretion in families of women with PCOS has been suggested [31].

Worsening insulin resistance in the long term may represent an important factor in the development of glucose intolerance states (including impaired glucose tolerance and T2DM) in PCOS women, particularly in the presence of obesity [30]. This rarely occurs in those with normal weight [20], which suggests that obesity may represent a indispensable prerequisite.

Although PCOS per se may be associated with alterations of both lipid and lipoprotein metabolism, the coexistence of obesity usually leads to a more atherogenetic lipoprotein pattern, characterized by lower HDL cholesterol and higher triglyceride blood concentrations. Therefore, it is not surprising that the prevalence of the metabolic syndrome is significantly more common in obese PCOS women. It is, however, still unclear whether the increased prevalence of other risk factors for CVD reported in PCOS women may depend on the presence of obesity.

1.11 Sleep Disorders

Recent studies have shown that PCOS women may have an increased risk of the obstructive sleep apnoea syndrome (OSAS), diagnosed either by questionnaire or by overnight polysomnography [32]. This sleeping disorder is much more common in the presence of obesity. Thus, women with PCOS should be questioned about signs and symptoms of OSAS. Such symptoms include habitual snoring, nocturnal restlessness and daytime sleepiness.

1.12 Diet History and Food Intake

Dietary habits and history should be helpfully used in every patient with hyperandrogenism, infertility and metabolic disorders, such as obesity, and particularly in those with PCOS. These can be obtained with the help of dieticians or using standardized questionnaires. Excess energy and fat intake can be found in PCOS patients, although contradictory data have been reported [15]. Notably, a potential role of advanced glycation end-products (AGEs), known to be implicated in the atherosclerotic process and correlated with molecular damage, oxidative stress and endothelial cell activation, has been recently emphasized in the pathophysiology of insulin resistance associated with PCOS [33]. Since AGEs are present in many foods, it is expected that this will be extensively investigated in future research. Although a clear role of dietary factors has not yet clearly been defined in the pathophysiology of PCOS, it has been clearly demonstrated that changes in lifestyle towards a healthy diet may significantly improve not only body weight and fat distribution in otherwise affected obese women, but also menses and fertility, besides metabolic disturbances [15].

1.13 Psychological Aspects and Quality of Life

A few recent studies have evaluated the quality of life in women with PCOS and have begun to document the adverse psychological and health impacts of this condition. This can be performed using specific questionnaires adapted to PCOS and investigating different domains, such as emotions, body hair, weight, infertility and menstrual problems [34]. Moreover, studies using psychological questionnaires to investigate obsessive-compulsive behaviour, interpersonal sensitivity, depression, anxiety, aggression and psychoticism have shown a significant prevalence of these problems [35]. The extensive use of these questionnaires could improve the clinical assessment of patients with PCOS and provide effective treatment based on personal complaints rather than on a doctor's targets. This is particularly relevant in improving patient compliance and avoiding over-treatment in otherwise healthy women.

1.14 PCOS After Menopause

PCOS after menopause still represents an undefined endocrinological entity. In normal women, the transition to postmenopause involves not only a decrease in ovarian oestrogen formation but also a reduction of ovarian androgens [6]. Little is known about what happens to ovarian morphology and androgen production in women with PCOS after menopause. In one study analyzing a group of postmenopausal women, it was found that 42–44% of them had morphological ultrasound features consistent with PCO, and the comparison between the two groups showed that postmenopausal women with PCO had higher serum concentrations of testosterone and triglycerides than postmenopausal women with normal ovaries [36]. These findings strongly resemble PCOS features and indicate that this disorder is probably higher than expected in postmenopausal women. On the other hand, it should also be considered that hyperandrogenism appears to partly resolve before the menopause in women with PCOS [6]. In fact, one study found that total and non-SHBG-bound testosterone levels were reduced by approximately 50% among women aged 42–47 years with respect to 20–42 years of age and remained stable in women older than 47 years of age [37]. When PCOS women were compared to controls, testosterone levels were similar between the two groups in the age range of 42–47 years, whereas they were significantly higher in PCOS women than controls under or above this range. The assumption that hyperandrogenism tends to improve during late fertile age in PCOS women may explain the tendency of women with PCOS to cycle regularly as they grow older. These preliminary studies emphasize the need for further research, with particular emphasis on the role of androgen excess in the pathophysiology of metabolic and cardiovascular diseases [38], which are dramatically increasing in postmenopausal women. In a recent study [39] aimed at evaluating the risk of CV events in 390 postmenopausal women enrolled in the NIH–NHLBI sponsored Women's Ischemia Syndrome Evaluation (WISE) study, it was found that a total of 104 women had clinical features of PCOS defined by a premenopausal history of irregular menses and current biochemical evidence of hyperandrogenemia. These women were found to be more often diabetic ($p<0.0001$), obese ($p=0.005$), more frequently had the metabolic syndrome ($p<0.0001$) and more angiographic coronary artery disease (CAD, $p=0.04$) compared to women without clinical features of PCOS. These data emphasize that identification of postmenopausal women with clinical features of PCOS may provide an opportunity for prevention of CVD events.

1.15 Physical Examination

1.15.1 Anthropometry

It is important to measure height (metres) and weight (kilograms), calculate body mass index (BMI) (kg/m^2) and assess body fat distribution by waist, hip and the waist-to-hip ratio (WHR) [40] at baseline and during follow-up. Waist circumference may add additional information as to the cardiovascular risk profile for individual women. In addition to truncal obesity, a buffalo hump and supraclavicular fat deposition may suggest the presence of Cushing's syndrome.

1.15.2 Skin

Hirsutism is defined as excess terminal (thick pigmented) body hair in a male distribution, and it is commonly noted on the upper lip, chin, periareolar area of the breast, in the midsternum and along the linea alba of the lower abdomen. There is substantial ethnic variability in hirsutism; Asian women, for example, often have a lesser degree of hirsutism [7]. Hirsutism should be distinguished from hypertrichosis, the excessive growth of androgen-independent hair which is vellus, prominent in non-sexual areas, and most commonly familial or caused by systemic disorders (hypothyroidism, anorexia nervosa, malnutrition, porphyria and dermatomyositis) or medications (phenytoin, penicillamine, diazoxide, minoxidil or cyclosporine). The most widely used semi-quantitative method for estimating hirsutism is the Ferriman and Gallway score [41]. However, recent studies support the concept that hair growth on the face may be more relevant than in other parts of the body [42]. By means of this score, the efficacy of treatment can be easily quantified and followed-up.

Typical acne lesions include blackheads, whiteheads, inflammatory lesions, severe pustular lesions and scars, in increasing order of severity. Acne can be graded according to different stages [43], which are highly dependent on previous topical, systemic and cosmetic treatments. Obviously, evaluation and monitoring of therapy in women with PCOS is mandatory, although there are no controlled studies.

Androgenic alopecia may be graded by well-known subjective methods, such as the Ludwig score [44]. More sophisticated information can be obtained with the help of dermatologists, who are confident with much more extensive diagnostic methods, including pulling and weighing hairs in a defined region, standardized photographs and assessing hair density in defined regions of the scalp.

Other skin findings that should be sought include seborrhea, acanthosis nigricans, and striae, thin skin, or bruising, which suggests possible Cushing's syndrome. Acanthosis nigricans is particularly relevant in the clinical evaluation of PCOS. As reported above, this is a common finding in women with PCOS, particularly in those with obesity. It can be found on the nape of the neck and in the axillary region, and sometimes in other parts of the body (elbows, folds of the skin, hands, etc.). Its presence may represent a skin marker of insulin resistance and the metabolic syndrome. Its presentation may, however, be poorly defined, and clinical skin examination may be very insensitive for detecting acanthosis nigricans, as documented by a study comparing clinical staging with histological examination [45].

1.15.3 Reproductive System

A complete reproductive system examination should be conducted at the time of diagnosis and in follow-up examinations as appropriate to the initial findings and progression of symptoms. The breast exam should include a specific assessment of atrophy (potential evidence of significant hyperandrogenemia), and galactorrhea, as well as the mandatory assessment for pathologic masses. The external genitalia should be examined for evidence of clitoromegaly, which should prompt a search for androgen-producing neoplasms or undiagnosed class 21-hydroxilase deficiency. The examination should also verify that the internal genitalia (vagina, uterus and ovaries) are present. Otherwise, an evaluation for other rare causes of amenorrhea and hyperandrogenism (ex testicular feminization) must be considered.

Pelvic ultrasound may assist in the physical examination and therefore the diagnosis of PCO should be performed according to the criteria described by the Rotterdam Consensus Conference [4], unless updated.

1.15.4 General

PCOS is a systemic disorder that requires a complete physical investigation, from head to toe in an objective search for abnormalities. Skill in physical diagnosis is acquired with experience, but it is not merely technique that determines success in eliciting signs, and it reflects a way of thinking more than a way of doing. Previous paragraphs have focussed particular attention on anthropometry, signs of androgen excess and a systematic evaluation of the reproductive system. Arterial blood pressure should always be measured, and a careful investigation of the cardiovascular system should be performed. The abdominal examination should include assessment of hepatic size (to evaluate possible hepatic enlargement due to NAFLD), as well as palpation for adrenal and pelvic masses, if possible. Other skills depend on the specific phenotype.

1.15.5 Differential Diagnosis

The diagnosis of PCOS is often a diagnosis of exclusion. Other causes of hyperandrogenism include hyperprolactinemia, drugs (danazol and androgenic progestins, valproate), non-classic congenital adrenal hyperplasia, Cushing's syndrome and androgen secretion (ovarian or adrenal) tumours.

The differential diagnosis of acne includes acne rosacea (which generally responds to antibiotic therapy and is not a typical feature of PCOS), acne fulminans (which is most common in adolescent males and is associated with fever, arthalgias and leukocytosis), the SAPHO syndrome (defined as synovitis, acne, pustulosis, hyperostosis and osteitis and requires referral for systemic therapy).

Other causes of menstrual dysfunction need to be considered, including pregnancy, ovarian failure, outflow track obstruction and hypothalamic amenorrhea, in the appropriate clinical context.

References

1. Ehrmann DA. Polycystic ovary syndrome. N Engl J Med. 2005; 352:1223–1236.
2. Stein I, Leventhal M. Amenorrhea associated with bilateral polycystic ovaries. Am J Obstet Gynecol. 1935; 29:181.
3. Zawadzki JK, Dunaif A. Diagnostic criteria for polycystic ovary syndrome. In Dunaif A, Givens JR, Haseltine FP, Merriam GR eds. Polycystic ovary syndrome. Boston, Blackwell, 1992; 377–384.
4. The Rotterdam ESHRE/ASRM-Sponsored PCOS consensus workshop group. Revised 2003 consensus on diagnostic criteria and long-term health risks related to polycystic ovary syndrome (PCOS). Hum Reprod. 2004; 19:41–47.
5. Azziz R, Carmina E, Dewailly D, Diamanti-Kandarakis E, Escobar-Morreale HF, Futterweit W, Janssen OE, Legro RS, Norman RJ, Taylor AE, Witchel SF; Androgen Excess Society. Positions statement: criteria for defining polycystic ovary syndrome as a predominantly hyperandrogenic syndrome: an Androgen Excess Society guidelines. J Clin Endocrinol Metab. 2006; 91:4237–4245.

6. Pasquali R, Gambineri A. PCOS: a multifaceted disease from adolescence to adult age. Ann NY Acad Sci. 2006; 1092: 158–174.
7. Taylor AE. Clinical evaluation of polycystic ovary syndrome. In: Insulin Resistance and Polycystic Ovarian Syndrome: Pathogenesis, Evaluation, and Treatment. Diamanti-Kandarakis E, Nestler JE, Panidis D, Pasquali R eds. The Humana Press, 2007; 131–143.
8. Escobar-Morreale HF, Luque-Ramírez M, San Millán JL. The molecular-genetic basis of functional hyperandrogenism and the polycystic ovary syndrome. Endocr Rev. 2005; 26:251–282.
9. Bulun SE and Adaghi EY. The physiology and pathology of the females reproductive axis. In: Wlliams Textbook of Endocrinology. Kronemberg HM, Melmed S, Polonsky KS, Larsen PR eds. Saunders Elsevier, Philadelphia, 2008; 541–614.
10. Apter D, Sibila I. Development of children and adolescence: physiological, pathophysiological, and therapeutic aspects. Curr Opin Obstet Gynecol. 1993; 5:764–773.
11. Venturoli S, Porcu E, Fabbri R, Magrini O, Gammi L, Paradisi R, Flamigni C. Longitudinal evaluation of the different gonadotropin pulsatile patterns in anovulatory cycles of young girls. J Clin Endocrinol Metab. 1992; 74:836–841.
12. Chang RJ. The reproductive phenotype in polycystic ovary syndrome. Nat Clin Pract Endocrinol Metab. 2007; 3:688–695.
13. Boomsma CM, Eijkemans MJ, Hughes EG, Visser GH, Fauser BC, Macklon NS. A meta-analysis of pregnancy outcomes in women with polycystic ovary syndrome. Hum Reprod Update. 2006 Nov–Dec; 12(6):673–683.
14. Yildiz BO, Knochenhauer ES, Azziz R. Impact of obesity on the risk for polycystic ovary syndrome. J Clin Endocrinol Metab. 2008 Jan; 93(1):162–168.
15. Gambineri A, Pelusi C, Vicennati V, Pagotto U, Pasquali R. Obesity and the polycystic ovary syndrome. Int J Obes Rel Metab Dis. 2002; 26: 883–896.
16. Escobar-Morreale HF, Botella-Carretero JI, Alvarez-Blasco F, Sancho J, San Millán JL. The polycystic ovary syndrome associated with morbid obesity may resolve after weight loss induced by bariatric surgery. J Clin Endocrinol Metab. 2005; 90: 6364–6369.
17. Kabiru W, Raynor D. Obstetric outcome associated with increase in BMI category during pregnancy. Am J Obstet Gynaecol. 2004; 191, 928–932.
18. Balen AH, Anderson RA. Policy & Practice Committee of the BFS. Impact of obesity on female reproductive health: British Fertility Society, Policy and Practice Guidelines. Hum Fertil (Camb). 2007; 10:195–206.
19. Bloomgarden ZT. Gut hormones, obesity, polycystic ovarian syndrome, malignancy, and lipodystrophy syndromes. Diabetes Care. 2007 Jul; 30(7):1934–1939.
20. Dunaif A. Insulin resistance and the polycystic ovary syndrome: mechanisms and implications for pathogenesis. Endocr Rev. 1997; 18: 774–800.
21. Poretsky L, Cataldo NA, Rosenwaks Z, Giudice LC. The insulin-related ovarian regulatory system in health and disease. Endocr Rev. 1999; 20: 535–582.
22. Diamanti-Kandarakis E, Kouli C, Alexandraki K, and Spina G. Failure of mathematical indices to accurately assess insulin resistance in lean, overweight, or obese women with polycystic ovary syndrome. J Clin Endocrinol Metab. 2004; 89: 1273–1276.
23. Pasquali R, Gambineri A. Insulin resistance. Definition and epidemiology in normal women and polycystic ovary syndrome women. In: Contemporary Endocrinology: Insulin resistance and polycystic ovary syndrome: pathogenesis, evaluation, and treatment. Nestler JE, Diamanti-Kandarakis E, Panidis D, and Pasquali R eds. Humana Press Inc, Towota, NJ, 2007; 385–396.
24. Executive Summary of the Third Report of The National Cholesterol Education Program (NCEP) Expert Panel on Detection, Evaluation, and Treatment of High Blood Cholesterol In Adults (Adult Treatment Panel III). JAMA. 2001; 285: 2486–2497.
25. International Diabetes Federation: the IDF worldwide definition of the metabolic syndrome. Available from http:www.cdc.gov/nchs/about/major/nhanes/nhanes/99-02.htm Accessed 18 May 2005.
26. Salley KE, Wickham EP, Cheang KI, Essah PA, Karjane NW, Nestler JE. Glucose intolerance in polycystic ovary syndrome–a position statement of the Androgen Excess Society. J Clin Endocrinol Metab. 2007; 92:4546–4556. Review.
27. Setji TL, Holland ND, Sanders LL, Pereira KC, Diehl AM, Brown AJ. Nonalcoholic steatohepatitis and nonalcoholic Fatty liver disease in young women with polycystic ovary syndrome. J Clin Endocrinol Metab. 2006; 91:1741–1747.
28. Legro RS. Polycystic ovary syndrome and cardiovascular disease: a premature association? Endocr Rev. 2003; 24:302–312.
29. Pierpoint, T, McKeigue, PM, Isaacs, AJ, et al. Mortality of women with polycystic ovary syndrome at long-term follow-up. J Clin Epidemiol. 1998; 51:581.
30. Pasquali R, Gambineri A, Pagotto U. The impact of obesity on reproduction in women with polycystic ovary syndrome Br J Obstet Gynecol. 2006; 113:1148–59.
31. Dunaif A. Finegood DT. β-cell dysfunction independent of obesity and glucose intolerance in the polycystic ovary syndrome. J Clin Endocrinol Metab. 1996; 81: 942–947.
32. Fogel RB, Malhotra A, Pillar G, Pittman SD, Dunaif A, White DP. Increased prevalence of obstructive sleep apnea syndrome in obese women with polycystic ovary syndrome. J Clin Endocrinol Metab. 2001; 86:1175–80.
33. Diamanti-Kandarakis E. Polycystic ovarian syndrome: pathophysiology, molecular aspects and clinical implications. Expert Rev Mol Med. 2008; 10:e3.
34. Cronin L, Guyatt G, Griffith L, Wong E, Azziz R, Futterweit W, Cook D, Dunaif A. Development of a health-related quality-of-life questionnaire (PCOSQ) for women with polycystic ovary syndrome (PCOS). J Clin Endocrinol Metab. 1998; 83: 1976–1987.

35. Elsenbruch S, Hahn S, Kowalsky D, Offner AH, Schedlowski M, Mann K, Janssen OE. Quality of life, psychosocial well-being, and sexual satisfaction in women with polycystic ovary syndrome. J Clin Endocrinol Metab. 2003; 88:5801–5807.
36. Birdshall MA, Farquhar CM. Polycystic ovary syndrome in pre- and post-menopausal women. Clin Endocrinol (Oxf) 1996; 44:269–276.
37. Winters SJ, Talbott E, Guzick DS, et al. Serum testosterone levels decrease in middle age in women with the polycystic ovary syndrome Fertil Steril 2000; 73:724–729.
38. Wu FC, von Eckardstein A. Androgens and coronary artery disease. Endocr Rev. 2003; 24:183–217.
39. Shaw LJ, Merz CN, Azziz R, Stanczyk FZ, Sopko G, Braunstein GD, Kelsey SF, Kip KE, Cooper-Dehoff RM, Johnson BD, Vaccarino V, Reis SE, Bittner V, Hodgson TK, Rogers W, Pepine CJ. Post-Menopausal Women with a History of Irregular Menses and Elevated Androgen Measurements at High Risk for Worsening Cardiovascular Event-Free Survival: Results from the National Institutes of Health National Heart, Lung, and Blood Institute (NHLBI) Sponsored Women's Ischemia Syndrome Evaluation (WISE). J Clin Endocrinol Metab. 2008; 93:1276–1284.
40. WHO. Measuring obesity-classification and description of anthropometric data. Copenhagen, Denmark: WHO Regional Office for Europe; Eur/ICP/NUT 125-0612v, 1988.
41. Ferriman D, Gallwey JD. Clinical assessment of body hair growth in women. J Clin Endocrinol Metab. 1961; 21:1440.
42. DeUgarte CM, Woods KS, Bartolucci AA, Azziz R. Degree of facial and body terminal hair growth in unselected black and white women: toward a populational definition of hirsutism. J Clin Endocrinol Metab. 2006; 91:1345–50.
43. Pochi PE, Shalita AR, Strauss JS, Webster SB, Cunliffe WJ, Katz HI, Kligman AM, Leyden JJ, Lookingbill DP, Plewing G et al. Report of the consensus conference on acne classification. Washington DC, March 24 and 25, 1990.
44. Ludwig E. Classification of the types of androgenic alopecia (common baldness) occurring in the female sex. Br J Dermatol 1977; 97:247–254.
45. Dunaif A, Green G, Phelps RG, Lebwohl M, Futterweit W, Lewy L. Acanthosis Nigricans, insulin action, and hyperandrogenism: clinical, histological, and biochemical findings. J Clin Endocrinol Metab. 1991; 73:590–595.

Chapter 2
The Menstrual Cycle in PCOS

Sabrina Gill and Janet E. Hall

Polycystic ovary syndrome (PCOS) is defined as a syndrome of ovarian dysfunction along with the cardinal features of hyperandrogenism and polycystic ovary morphology in the absence of other explanatory endocrinopathies [1]. The etiology of PCOS is multifactorial and complex with hyperinsulinemia, abnormal ovarian steroidogenesis, and neuroendocrine abnormalities playing significant interactive roles. The vast majority of patients have menstrual irregularities and recent studies have indicated that those with menstrual cycle dysfunction also tend to be more hyperandrogenic and hyperinsulinemic [2, 3]. This chapter will review the integration of ovarian, hypothalamic and pituitary factors that occur in normal menstrual cycles; will discuss the variable patterns of menstrual dysfunction in patient with PCOS; and will review what is known about the potential etiology of ovarian dysfunction in PCOS.

2.1 The Normal Menstrual Cycle

The normal menstrual cycle is divided into two stages (Fig. 2.1) – the follicular phase begins with day 1 of menses and is noted by the emergence of a cohort of follicles that develop in response to rising levels of FSH. In normal women, a single follicle from this cohort will develop into a dominant follicle and ovulate in response to the mid-cycle LH surge (MCS). The luteal phase begins after ovulation when hormonal events prepare the endometrium for implantation should conception occur.

Neuroendocrine axes regulate and integrate neural and hormonal information and translate these signals to physiological actions that impact the synthesis and secretion of different hormonal systems. Neuroendocrine regulation of the menstrual cycle involves a complex integrated network of feedback mechanisms between the hypothalamus, pituitary, and target organs. The hypothalamic-pituitary-gonadal (HPG) system is comprised of the gonadotropin-releasing hormone (GnRH) producing neurons of the hypothalamus, the pituitary gonadotropes which secrete luteinizing hormone (LH) and follicle-stimulating hormone (FSH), and the ovary which responds to gonadotropin secretion with follicular development and ovulation and with secretion of estradiol, progesterone, and the gonadal peptides, inhibin A and inhibin B. Ovarian steroid and non-steroidal hormones, in turn, modulate the hypothalamic and pituitary components of the reproductive axis [for review see ref. 4].

2.2 Dynamics of Hypothalamic Secretion During the Normal Menstrual Cycle

Frequent blood sampling studies with measurement of LH as a marker of GnRH secretion and the use of pharmacological probes, such as GnRH antagonists, have been utilized to evaluate the physiology of GnRH secretion

S. Gill (✉)
Division of Endocrinology & Metabolism, St. Paul's Hospital and the University of British Columbia, Vancouver, BC, Canada
e-mail: SGill@providencehealth.bc.ca

N.R. Farid, E. Diamanti-Kandarakis (eds.), *Diagnosis and Management of Polycystic Ovary Syndrome*,
DOI 10.1007/978-0-387-09718-3_2, © Springer Science+Business Media, LLC 2009

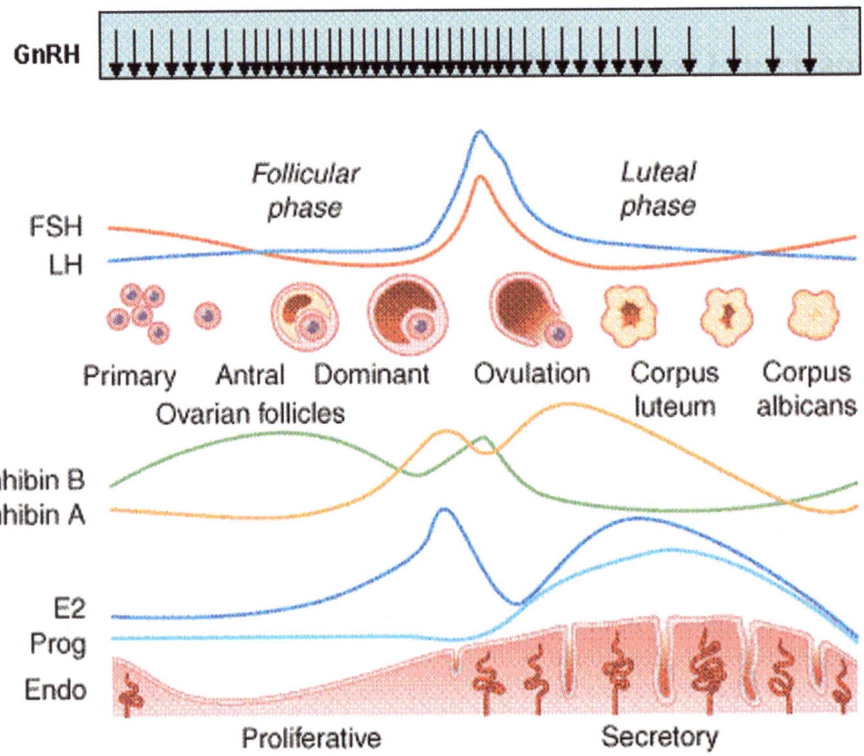

Fig. 2.1 Hormonal dynamics of the normal menstrual cycle. Adapted from [4]

in studies in women with normal menstrual cycles [4] and in women with PCOS [5]. In normal women, the frequency of pulsatile GnRH secretion is dynamically regulated across the menstrual cycle (Fig. 2.1). The transition from the end of one cycle to the beginning of the next is marked by an increase in pulsatile LH/GnRH secretion from the luteal phase frequency of one pulse every four hours to a pulse of every 90 minutes in the early follicular phase. During the mid-follicular phase, LH pulse frequency increases to one pulse per hour, and this frequency is maintained through the MCS. After the MCS and ovulation, the GnRH pulse generator slows down to one pulse every 90 minutes, followed by a further decline to one pulse every four hours during the late luteal phase. The luteal phase decrease in GnRH pulse frequency is secondary to rising progesterone levels in the presence of estrogen. Although gonadal steroid levels fluctuate less dramatically because of prolongation of their half-life due to binding to sex hormone binding globulin (SHBG), progesterone concentrations can fluctuate dramatically in the mid and late luteal phases (from 2.3 to 40.1 ng/mL) in response to the relatively infrequent pulses of LH [6].

Changes in the frequency of pulsatile GnRH secretion across the menstrual cycle are important because of the effect of GnRH pulse frequency on the differential regulation of pituitary LH and FSH synthesis and secretion. At slow GnRH pulse frequencies, GnRH receptor (GnRHR) concentrations on gonadotrope cell surfaces are relatively low with activation of a single signal transduction pathway stimulating expression of α-subunit, LHβ, and FSHβ. Faster GnRH pulse frequencies increase GnRHR concentrations resulting in greater activation of the signal transduction pathway and stimulation of a second signal transduction pathway that specifically inhibits FSHβ gene expression [7]. Thus, slow frequencies of pulsatile GnRH stimulation of the gonadotrope result in increased synthesis of FSH while faster GnRH pulse frequencies favor the synthesis and secretion of LH.

2.3 Feedback During the Normal Menstrual Cycle

FSH levels rise 3-fold in the early follicular phase in response to release from the negative feedback effects of estradiol and probably inhibin A (Fig. 2.1). FSH release is further facilitated by the increase in GnRH pulse frequency that occurs with the late luteal phase decline in progesterone [4]. The luteal-follicular rise in FSH is critical for initiation of folliculogenesis and the beginning of a new cycle of follicle development. With recruitment and early development of a new cohort of follicles, estradiol and inhibin B increase, inhibiting FSH. This mid-follicular phase decrease in FSH is important for ensuring that only a single follicle emerges as dominant and reaches maturity. While the initial increase in estradiol inhibits GnRH, LH, and FSH secretion, the exponential rise in estradiol that subsequently occurs with growth of the dominant follicle exerts a positive feedback effect on gonadotropin secretion and LH levels rise 10-fold. Ovulation occurs within 36 hours after the midcycle LH surge. LH levels subsequently decrease and reach a nadir by the late luteal phase. Progesterone secretion begins with luteinization of the theca-granulosa cells which is induced by the LH surge, reaching peak concentrations in the mid-luteal phase. The corpus luteum also secretes estrogen and inhibin A, which follows a similar pattern to that of progesterone.

2.3.1 Normal Folliculogenesis

At the level of the ovary, growth factors, such as stem cell growth factor, basic fibroblast growth factor, growth differentiation factor-9 (GDF9), and anti-mullerian hormone (AMH or MIS), regulate recruitment of primordial follicles for growth [8]. The selected follicles proliferate in response to the luteal-follicular rise in FSH. FSH also improves survival of granulosa cells and recruitment of a dominant follicle. With selection and development of the follicles, secretions of inhibin B, estradiol, and subsequently inhibin A combine to inhibit FSH secretion. Local positive factors (such as insulin-like growth factor), which promote growth and inhibit apoptosis of follicles, and negative factors (such as AMH), which decreases granulosa cell sensitivity to FSH and inhibits aromatase activity, play roles in selective negative differentiation of the remaining follicles allowing a single dominate follicle to emerge [4, 9]

2.4 Menstrual Dysfunction in PCOS

Normal menstrual cycles range between 25 and 35 days due to variability in the length of the follicular phase in different women. In PCOS, 60–80% of patients present with menstrual irregularities with fewer than nine menstrual periods per year [10]. In some patients, menses occur very infrequently or not at all while in 5–10% of PCOS women, more frequent bleeding and menorrhagia may occur. Importantly, not all episodes of vaginal bleeding follow ovulation. Anovulatory bleeding has been reported in up to 20% of women who report normal menstrual cycles [11], and measurement of progesterone may be required. For this reason, current guidelines for the diagnostic criteria of PCOS specify oligo- or anovulation rather than oligo- or amenorrhea [1]. The pathophysiology of PCOS is multifactorial with dysregulation of gonadal and adrenal steroidogenesis, abnormal neuroendocrine regulation and insulin resistance.

2.5 Gonadal Steroids in PCOS

The polycystic ovary is characterized by an increased number of antral follicles and an increase in the mass of theca cells surrounding each follicle. Serum levels of inhibin B are higher in PCOS reflecting an increase in the number of antral follicles while the reported decrease in dimeric inhibin B production per follicle is consistent with a decrease in the number of granulosa cells per follicle and arrested folliculogenesis [12]. Inhibin does not

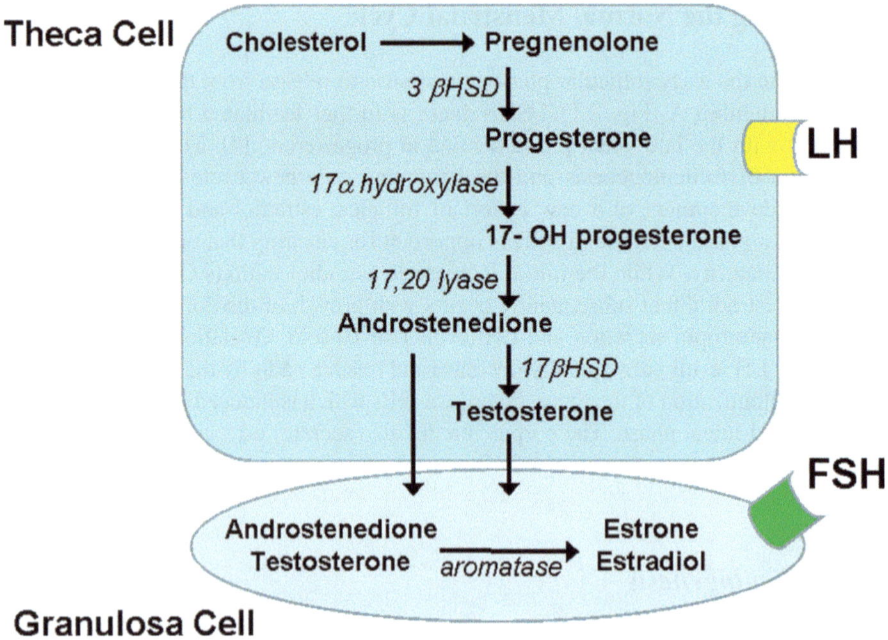

Fig. 2.2 Ovarian steroidogenesis in the theca and granulosa cells

fully account for the relative suppression of FSH compared to LH in women with PCOS, but higher LH levels may suppress inhibin B [13].

Ovarian steroidogenesis requires the coordinated activities of the theca cells, which synthesize androgens from cholesterol under the control of LH and granulosa cells, which aromatize these androgen precursors to synthesize estrogens under the control of FSH (Fig. 2.2). Theca cells in patients with PCOS exhibit defects in a number of enzymes in the steroidogenic pathway, such as 17-hydroxylase and 17,20-lyase, that may contribute to increased ovarian androgen production [14].

Ovarian 17-hydroxyprogesterone hyper-responsiveness to hCG or a GnRH agonist in women with PCOS is indicative of the increased sensitivity of the ovary to LH stimulation [15] and likely reflects the combination of theca cell hyperplasia, the increased number of antral follicles and steroidogenic pathway dysregulation. In addition, studies showing that suppression of LH either acutely using a GnRH antagonist or chronically using a GnRH agonist results in decreased testosterone levels support the importance of the increased LH in the etiology of ovarian hyperandrogenism in PCOS [16].

There is evidence that adrenal hyperandrogenemia may also play a role in biochemical hyperandrogenemia in some patients with PCOS and girls with premature pubarche, and exaggerated adrenarche are at higher risk of development of PCOS in adulthood [17].

2.6 Follicular Development in PCOS

Follicular development in PCOS is abnormal for two reasons. First, in the ovarian hyperandrogenemia environment, there is a 6-fold increase in the number of primary growing follicles (2–5 mm). Androgens promote preantral and antral follicle development by increasing proliferation and sensitivity of theca and granulosa cells to gonadotropins and inhibiting apoptosis [18]. In the theca cells, there is upregulation of steroidogenic enzymes, such as 3β-hydroxysteroid dehydrogenase, and 17α-hydroxylase/17,20 lyase, with increased androgen and progesterone secretion [14]. The inhibins, particularly inhibin A, may also increase LH-induced androgen production in thecal cells [19].

In addition to the increase in follicular development in PCOS, the appropriate process of follicular arrest with selection and development of the dominant follicle is inconsistent. These patients lack the dynamic modulation of FSH that characterizes the normal luteal-follicular transition and is responsible for orderly recruitment of follicles into the growing pool. Serum and follicular fluid AMH levels are also higher in women with PCOS [18] potentially decreasing aromatase activity and inhibiting development of the dominant follicle. Finally, premature exposure of the granulosa cells to LH also leads to inhibition of cell proliferation and follicle growth resulting in poor follicular development [20].

2.7 Neuroendocrine Abnormalities in PCOS

While abnormalities at the level of the ovary itself are clearly important, the neuroendocrine abnormalities in PCOS also contribute to abnormal follicular development. LH levels are elevated in comparison to FSH resulting in 94% of women having an elevated LH/FSH ratio [5]. The LH amplitude response to GnRH is exaggerated and GnRH pulse frequency is increased in PCOS at approximately one pulse per 50–60 min [21]. Furthermore, recent studies have also shown an increase in the overall amount of GnRH secreted that is similar in magnitude to the increase in pulse frequency [21]. As discussed above, this pattern of GnRH secretion favors the synthesis and secretion of LH over FSH. Spontaneous ovulation transiently improves the abnormal LH/FSH ratio in PCOS [5]. However, studies have shown that the sensitivity to progesterone-induced slowing of GnRH pulse frequency in women with PCOS is less than in normal women [22]. There has been considerable controversy regarding whether the neuroendocrine abnormality in PCOS is a primary abnormality or is secondary to other factors. However, reversal of abnormalities in progesterone-induced slowing of pulse frequency by androgen receptor blockade suggests that it is due at, least in part, to secondary mechanisms.

In normal adolescents, menstrual irregularities are not uncommon for several years after menarche. However, irregular menstrual cyclicity may persist ultimately leading to the diagnosis of PCOS. In peripubertal girls with hyperandrogenemia, there is early evidence of neuroendocrine abnormalities, including an increased LH/FSH ratio, and a faster frequency and higher amplitude of LH pulses [22]. It has been hypothesized that hyperandrogenemia in adolescence may lead to reduced sensitivity of the GnRH pulse generator to progesterone-induced slowing resulting in an increase in the LH to FSH ratio, impairment of ovarian folliculogenesis and augmentation of hyperandrogenemia.

In women with PCO morphology and regular ovulatory cycles, gonadotropin dynamics are identical to those in normal ovulatory women [23]. Thus, PCO morphology in an abnormal gonadotropin environment is required for development of menstrual dysfunction in PCOS. Testosterone levels are higher in this population than in women with normal ovarian morphology, independent of any abnormalities in gonadotropin secretion, possibly due to the increased ovarian thecal mass with PCO morphology.

In anovulatory women with PCOS, correction of abnormal FSH dynamics by reducing the negative feedback effect of estrogen using estrogen receptor blockers or aromatase inhibitors or more directly through administration of exogenous gonadotropins or pulsatile GnRH does not universally correct the ovulatory defect. With all treatment modalities, improved ovulation is negatively affected by hyperandrogenemia, high BMI, and insulin resistance [24, 25]. Such factors impact both locally at the ovary and on the neuroendocrine axis.

2.7.1 Impact of Hyperandrogenemia

Androgens appear to influence folliculogenesis through effects both at the hypothalamus and directly at the ovary. Animal studies support the hypothesis described above that the increased GnRH pulse frequency that is characteristic of PCOS is related to hyperandrogenemia [26]. In animal studies, prenatal androgen exposure is associated with increased LH pulsatility and decreased sensitivity to progesterone-induced slowing of GnRH pulses and increased GABAergic drive on GnRH neurons [22]. At the level of the ovary, androgens interrupt ovulation by providing a negative environment for egg release [27].

2.7.2 Impact of BMI

Obesity is prevalent in PCOS, occurring in approximately 30–60% of patients and is negatively associated with the success of ovulation induction. BMI and percent body fat are negatively correlated with LH and in very obese women with PCOS, the LH/FSH ratio may be relatively normal [5]. There is no effect of BMI on either the amount or frequency of GnRH secretion in women with PCOS [21] indicating that obesity does not exert its effect on LH secretion at the hypothalamic level. The decrease in LH responsiveness to GnRH as a function of obesity supports a direct effect of factors relating to BMI at the pituitary level as does the increase in clearance of LH, which is proposed to be due to changes in the isoforms of LH secreted [27]. Leptin, which is secreted by adipocytes and is regulator of appetite and energy homeostasis, is higher in women with PCOS and inversely related to LH levels [28] suggesting that it may mediate the effect of BMI on LH secretion. Other potential mediators include ghrelin which is also inversely related to BMI, and hyperinsulinemia, which is discussed further below. At the level of the ovary, inhibin B is inversely related to BMI [29] suggesting that follicular development is also negatively impacted by obesity.

2.7.3 Impact of Hyperinsulinemia

Insulin resistance to glucose uptake is observed in approximately 50–75% of lean and obese women with PCOS [30]. Hyperinsulinemia is positively associated with anovulation and hyperandrogenemia. Importantly, reduction of insulin resistance and insulin levels with weight loss, metformin or thiazolidenediones improves spontaneous follicular development, ovulation, and hyperandrogenemia [31]. Hyperinsulinemia and/or insulin resistance may play a role at multiple levels.

Hyperinsulinemia secondary to peripheral insulin resistance has important effects at the level of the ovary, synergizing with LH in stimulation of androgen synthesis in the granulose cell [32]. Hyperinsulinemia is associated with lower levels of inhibin B, and there is evidence that high concentrations of insulin result in premature differentiation of granulosa cells and follicular arrest. While the effects of medications that improve insulin resistance and decrease peripheral insulin levels are most obvious in obese women, the significant response of lean women with PCOS to insulin sensitizers is consistent with additional in vitro evidence of a direct effect of insulin-sensitizing agents on ovarian steroidogenesis [33] and supports the hypothesis that abnormalities in insulin signaling [30] may play a role in disordered menstrual cycle dynamics in women with PCOS, independent of BMI.

Insulin receptors are present on the pituitary and hypothalamus. Unlike anti-androgen agents, metformin failed to have a significant impact on the sensitivity of the GnRH pulse generator on gonadal steroid feedback [34]. The role of insulin at the pituitary is controversial. However, recent studies suggest that in women with PCOS, insulin suppresses the LH response to GnRH and may be responsible, at least in part, for the inverse relationship between LH and BMI in PCOS [35]. Finally, insulin decreases hepatic production of sex-hormone biding globulin, resulting in elevated bioavailable androgens [30].

2.8 Summary

Menstrual cycle dysfunction is common in PCOS due to disordered folliculogenesis and anovulation and may present as oligoamenorrhea, amenorrhea, or dysfunctional bleeding. The degree of menstrual dysfunction is highly variable between patients and is generally more marked in association with higher androgen and insulin levels and a higher BMI. Menstrual dysfunction in PCOS is attributed to multiple factors: neuroendocrine abnormalities, ovarian dysregulation of steroidogenesis and insulin resistance, each contributing at various levels to impact folliculogenesis and ovulation. Intervention at various levels has been shown to improve and promote appropriate follicle development and fertility.

References

1. Revised 2003 consensus on diagnostic criteria and long-term health risks related to polycystic ovary syndrome: Rotterdam consensus workshop; Hum Reprod 2004; 19(1):41–7.
2. Welt CK, Gudmundsson JA, Arason G, Adams J, Palsdottir H, Gudlaugsdottir G, Ingadottir G, Crowley WF. Characterizing descrete subsets of polycystic ovary syndrome as defined by the Rotterdam Criteria: The impact of weight on phenotype and metabolic features. J Clin Endocrinol Metab 2006; 91:4842–4848.
3. Dewailly D, Catteau-Jonard S, Reyss A, Leroy M, Pigny P. Oligoanovulation with polycystic ovaries but not overt hyperandrogenism. J Clin Endocrinol Metab 2006; 91:3922–3927.
4. Hall JE. The Ovary, Infertility and Contraception. In: Fauci AS, Kasper DL, Braunwald E, Hauser SL, Longo DL, Jameson JL, Loscalzo J (eds) Harrison's Principles of Internal Medicine, 17th Edition, 2007; pp. 2324–2334.
5. Taylor AE, McCourt B, Martin MA, Anderson EJ, Adams JM, Schoenfeld D and Hall JE; Determinants of abnormal gonadotropin secretion in clinically defined women with polycystic ovary syndrome. J Clin Endocrinol Metab 1997; 82: 2248–2256.
6. Filicori M, Butler JP, Crowley WF, Jr. Neuroendocrine regulation of the corpus luteum in the human. Evidence for pulsatile progesterone secretion. J Clin Invest 1984; 73:1638–1647.
7. Kaiser UB, Sabbagh E, Katzenellenbogen R, Conn PM, Chin WW. A mechanism for the differential regulation of gonadotropin subunit gene expression by gonadotropin-releasing hormone. Proc Natl Acad Sci USA 1995; 92:12280–12284.
8. Matzuk MM, Lamb DJ; Genetic dissection of mammalian fertility pathways. Nat Cell Biol 2002 Oct; 4 Suppl:s41–9.
9. Zeleznik AJ and Fairchild-Benyo DF. Control of follicular development, corpus luteum function, and the recognition of pregnancy in higher primates. In Knobel E and Neill J (eds) The Physiology of Reproduction. Raven Press, New York, 1994: 751–782.
10. Carmina E, Rosato F, Janni A, Rizzo M, Long RA. Relative prevalence of different androgen excess disorders in 950 women referred because of clinical hyperandrogenism. J Clin Endocrinol Metab 2006; 91:2–6.
11. Azziz R, Waggoner WT, Ochoa T, Knochenhauer ES, Boots LR Idiopathic hirsutism: an uncommon cause of hirsutism in Alabama. Fertil Steril 1998 Aug; 70(2):274–278.
12. Welt, CK, Taylor AE, Fox J, Messerlain GM, Adams JM, Schneyer AL. Follicular arrest in polycystic ovary syndrome is associated with deficient inhibin A and inhibin B biosynthesis. J Clin Endocrinol Metab 2005; 90:5582–5587.
13. Welt CK, Taylor AE, Martin KA, Hall JE. Inhibin B in polycystic ovary syndrome: Regulation by insulin and luteinizing hormone. J Clin Endocrinol Metab 2002; 87:5559–5565.
14. Nelson VL, Qin KN, Rosenfield RL, Wood JR, Penning TM, Legro RS, Strausss JF III and McAllister JM. The biochemical basis for increased testosterone production in theca cells propagated from patients with polycystic ovary syndrome. J Clin Endocrinol Metab 2001;86:5925–5933.
15. Ibanez L, Hall JE, Potau N, Carrascosa A, Prat N, Taylor AE. Ovarian 17-hydroxyprogesterone hyperresponsiveness to gonadotropin-releasing hormone agonist challenge in women with polycystic ovary syndrome is not mediated by luteinizing hormone hypersecretion: Evidence from GnRH agonist and human gonadotropin stimulation testing. J Clin Endocrinol Metab 1996; 81:4103–4107.
16. Hayes FJ, Taylor AE, Martin KM, Hall JE. Use of gonadotropin-releasing hormone antagonist as a physiologic probe in polycystic ovary syndrome: assessment of neuroendocrine and androgen dynamics. J Clin Endocrinol Metab 1998; 83: 2343–2349.
17. Ilbanez L, Valls C, Potau A, Marcos MV, De Zheger F. Polycystic ovary syndrome after precious puberty – ontogeny of the low birth weight effect. Clin endocrinol 2001; 55:667–672.
18. Jonard S, Dewailly D. The follicular excess in polycystic ovaries, due to intraovarian hyperandrogenism, may be the main culprit for follicular arrest. Hum Reprod Upd 2004; 10:107–117.
19. Hillier SG. Hormonal control of folliculogenesis and luteinization. In Findlay, JK (eds) Molecular Biology of the Female Reproductive System. Academic Press Sand Diego, 1994; 1–37.
20. Jakimuik AJ, Weitsman SR, Navab A, Magoffin DA. Luteinizing hormone receptor, steroidogenesis acute regulatory protein, and steroidogenic enzyme messenger ribonucleic acids are overexpressed in thecal and granulosa cells from polycystic ovaries. J Clin Endocrinol Metab 2001; 86:1318–1323.
21. Pagan YL, Srouji SS, Jimenez Y, Emerson A, Gill S, Hall JE. Inverse relationship between luteinizing hormone and body mass index in polycystic ovary syndrome: investigation of hypothalamic and pituitary contributions. J Clin Endocrinol Metab 2006; 91:1309–1316.
22. Blank SK, McCartney CR, Marshall JC; The origins and sequelae of abnormal neuroendocrine function in polycystic ovary syndrome. Hum Reprod Update 2006; 12(4):351–316.
23. Adams JM, Taylor AE, Crowley Jr WF, Hall JE. Polycystic ovarian morphology with regular ovulatory cycles: insights into the pathophysiology of polycystic ovarian syndrome. J Clin Endocrinol Metab 2004; 89:4343–4350.
24. Gill S, Taylor A, Martin KA, Welt C, Adams J, Hall JE. Predictive factors of the responsive to pulsatile GnRH therapy in polycystic ovarian syndrome. J Clin Endocrinol Metab 2001; 86:2428–2436.

25. Imani B, Eijkemans MJC, Te Velde ER, Habbema JDF, Fauser BCJM. Predictores of patients remaining anovulatory during clomiphene citrate induction of ovulation in normogonadotropic oligoamenorrheic infertility. J Clin Endocrinol Metab 1998; 83:2361–2365.
26. Diamanti-Kandarakis E, Papailiou J, Palimeri S. Hyperandrogenemia: pathophysiology and its role in ovulatory dysfunction in PCOS. Pediatr Endocrinolog Rev 2006; 3(suppl 1):198–204.
27. Srouji SS, Pagan YL, D'Amato F, Dabela A, Jimenez Y, Supko JG, Hall JE. Pharmacokinetic factors contribute to the inverse relationship between luteinizing hormone and body mass index in polycystic ovary syndrome. J Clin Endocrinol Metab 2007; 92:1347–1352.
28. Sprizer PM, Poy M, Wiltgen D, Mylius LS, Capp E. Leptin concentrations in hirsute women with polycystic ovarian syndrome or idiopathic hirsutism: influence on LH and relationship with hormonal, metabolic and anthropometric measurements. Hum Reprod 2001; 16:1340–1346.
29. Welt CK, Taylor AE, Martin KA, Hall JE. Inhibin B in polycystic ovary syndrome: Regulation by insulin and luteinizing hormone. J Clin Endocrinol Metab 2002; 87:5559–5565.
30. Dunaif A. Insulin resistance and the polycystic ovarian syndrome: mechanism and implications for pathogeneiss. Endocr Rev 1997; 18:774–800.
31. Lord JM, Flight IH, Norman RJ. Insulin-sensitising drugs (metformin, troglitazone, rosiglitazone, pioglitazone, D-chiro-inositol) for polycystic ovary syndrome. Cochrane Database Syst Rev. 2003;(3):CD003053. Review
32. Barbieri RL, Makris A, Randall RW, Daniels G, Kistner RW and Ryan KJ. Insulin stimulates androgen accumulation in incubations of ovarian stroma obtained from women with hyperandrogenism. J Clin Endocrinol Metab 1986; 62:904–910.
33. Mitwally MF, Witchel SF, Casper RF. Trolgitazone: a possible modulator of ovarian steroidogenesis. J Soc Gynecol Investig 2002; 9:163–167.
34. Eagleson CA, Bellows AB, Hu K, Gingrich MB, Marshall JC. Obese patients with polycystic ovary syndrome: Evidence that metformin does not restore sensitivity of the gonadotropin-releasing hormone pulse generator to inhibition by ovarian steroids. J Clin Endocrinol Metab 2003; 88:5158–5162.
35. Lawson MA, Jain S, Sun S, Patel K, Malcolm PJ, Chang RJ; Evidence for insulin suppression of baseline luteinizing hormone in women with polycystic ovarian syndrome and normal women. J Clin Endocrinol Metab 2008 Jun;93(6):2089–2096.

Chapter 3
The Radiology of Polycystic Ovaries

Susan J. Barter

3.1 Introduction

The diagnostic conundrum of possible polycystic ovarian syndrome is one frequently encountered in both the primary care setting and in secondary care. As part of the diagnostic work-up, women are often referred for ultrasound. Transabdominal and, more recently, transvaginal ultrasound have become universally used for identification of polycystic ovaries, but for many years, there has been lack of agreement as to the ultrasound diagnostic features. All too often ovaries are described as looking polycystic in the imaging report without reference to the phase of the menstrual cycle, number or size of follicles, or volume of the ovaries. This has led to many women being incorrectly labelled as having polycystic ovaries in the past, without fulfilling any of the now accepted criteria.

The joint meeting of the ASRM and ESHRE in Rotterdam in 2003 [1] was key to the agreement of a refined definition of polycystic ovarian syndrome (PCOS) and for the first time included a specific description of the ultrasound morphology.

The definition required two out of three of the following criteria:

1. Oligo- and/or anovulation
2. Hyperandrogenism (clinical and/or biochemical)
3. Polycystic ovaries

and the exclusion of other aetiologies (congenital adrenal hyperplasias, androgen-secreting tumours, Cushing's syndrome).

This chapter will discuss the evidence for the international consensus definition of the ultrasound assessment of the polycystic ovary, and describe the imaging features.

3.2 Historical Perspective

The condition now known as polycystic ovarian syndrome (PCOS) was first described by Stein and Leventhal in 1935 [2] as amenorrhoea, severe hirsutism, obesity and characteristic ovarian morphology on histology of wedge resections of ovarian tissue taken at laparotomy. Further studies identified endocrine disturbances in such women, and the diagnosis of PCOS was based on a combination of clinical and endocrine features [3, 4]. However, it was noted that the clinical and biochemical features varied widely between women, and some women with histological confirmation of polycystic ovaries showed no other common symptoms of the disorder. Symptoms and signs for an individual may also change with time [5, 6].

S.J. Barter (✉)
Consultant Radiologist, Addenbrookes Hospital University Trust, Hills Road, Cambridge, CB2 2QQ, UK
e-mail: suebarter@btinternet.com

N.R. Farid, E. Diamanti-Kandarakis (eds.), *Diagnosis and Management of Polycystic Ovary Syndrome*,
DOI 10.1007/978-0-387-09718-3_3, © Springer Science+Business Media, LLC 2009

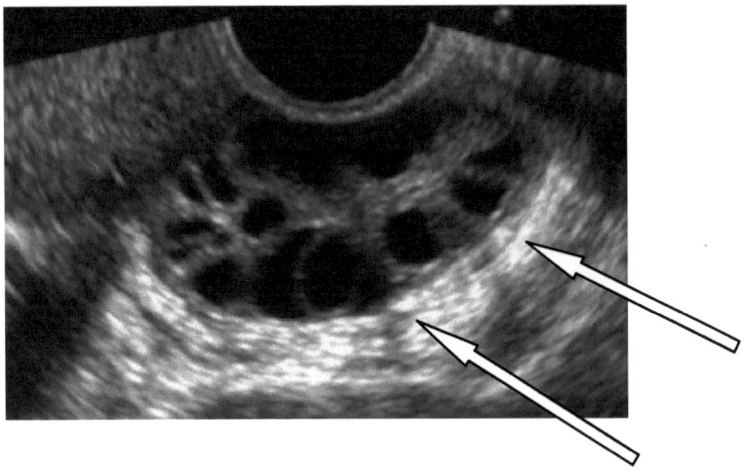

Fig. 3.1 A typical polycystic ovary as described by Adams [7] with more than 10 follicles of 2–8 mm in diameter in one plane, arranged peripherally around an echo dense stroma. (*arrows*)

For many years, wedge resection was the method of diagnosis, since it was the only treatment for PCO, but with the development of pelvic ultrasound in the 1980s, transabdominal (TA) ultrasound of the pelvis became the common method of non-invasive assessment of ovarian morphology.

In 1985, Adams et al. published a definition of a polycystic ovary, based on transabdominal (TA) ultrasound, which required 10 or more follicles of 2–8 mm in diameter in one plane, arranged peripherally around an echo dense stroma (Fig. 3.1) [7]. This definition has remained in widespread use even after the introduction of transvaginal (TV) ultrasound a decade later and was cited in many subsequent studies which used ultrasound to detect polycystic ovaries [8].

Transvaginal ultrasound has now largely replaced transabdominal ultrasound because of its greater resolution. The TV approach facilitates a more accurate view of ovarian morphology and is now considered the gold standard for investigation.

At the joint meeting of the ASRM and ESHRE in Rotterdam in 2003, it was recognized that an up-to-date definition of the sonographic appearances of the polycystic ovary was needed to reflect imaging advances. A Medline search of all reports of polycystic ovaries and PCOS since 1970 was performed. The literature was reviewed extensively and the definitions agreed (Table 3.1) [1, 8]. Despite this, many sonographers and radiologists remain unaware of the revised definitions and continue to make assessments of the ovaries without the mention of size, volume, number or size of follicles or reference to the phase of the cycle in the report.

3.3 Ultrasound

Polycystic ovaries (PCO) are often found incidentally in women undergoing ultrasound for any gynaecological symptom, e.g. pelvic pain or unscheduled bleeding. Previous ultrasound studies have reported that approximately 20% of young women have ovaries which appear polycystic and of these, about 25–70% have symptoms of infertility, menstrual irregularity or hirsutism, consistent with the diagnosis of PCOS [5, 9]. However, any woman with PCO in the absence of an ovulatory disorder or hyperandrogenism (‘asymptomatic’ PCO) should not be considered as having PCOS, until more is known regarding the clinical evolution of PCOS [1, 10].

Table 3.1 Ultrasound assessment of the polycystic ovary (PCO)

1. The polycystic ovary (PCO) should have at least one of the following: either 12 or more follicles measuring 2–9 mm in diameter or increased ovarian volume (>10 cm3). If there is evidence of a dominant follicle (>10 mm) or a corpus luteum, the scan should be repeated during the next cycle.
2. The subjective appearance of PCOs should not be substituted for this definition. The follicle distribution should be omitted as well as the increase in stromal echogenicity and/or volume. Although the latter is specific to polycystic ovary, it has been shown that the measurement of the ovarian volume is a good surrogate for the quantification of the stroma in clinical practice.
3. Only one ovary fitting this definition or a single occurrence of one of the above criteria is sufficient to define the PCO. If there is evidence of a dominant follicle (>10 mm) or corpus luteum, the scan should be repeated next cycle. The presence of an abnormal cyst or ovarian asymmetry, which may suggest a homogeneous cyst, necessitates further investigation.
4. This definition does not apply to women taking the oral contraceptive pill, as ovarian size is reduced, even though the 'polycystic' appearance may persist.
5. A woman having PCO in the absence of an ovulation disorder or hyperandrogenism ('asymptomatic PCO') should not be considered as having PCOS, until more is known about this situation.
6. In addition to its role in the definition of PCO, ultrasound is helpful to predict fertility outcome in patients with PCOS (response to clomiphene citrate, risk for ovarian hyperstimulation syndrome (OHSS), decision for in vitro maturation of oocytes). It is recognized that the appearance of PCOs may be seen in women undergoing ovarian stimulation for IVF in the absence of overt signs of PCOS. Ultrasound also provides the opportunity to screen for endometrial hyperplasia.

Source: International Consensus Definitions [1]

3.4 Some Practical Facts

3.4.1 Transabdominal and Transvaginal Ultrasound

The baseline ultrasound scan should be performed by both the transabdominal (TA) and transvaginal (TV) routes. A TA scan affords a wide field of view of the pelvis and is useful for detecting associated uterine or ovarian abnormalities, or if the ovaries are located high in the pelvic cavity. If not found between the uterus and the iliac vessels, the ovaries may lie caudally, in the iliac fossa close to the abdominal wall, or in the Pouch of Douglas.

Although a full bladder is required for visualization of the ovaries, theoretically an overfilled bladder can compress the ovaries, giving a falsely increased length. This emphasizes the need for assessing the ovarian size by measuring the volume (see below) or by repeating the measurement after partial micturition for those women who are unable to have a TV scan. The transvaginal route is of course omitted in girls and women who are virgo intacta or for a few patients who decline a transvaginal scan.

The TV scan using high-frequency probes (>6 MHz) has much better spatial resolution but less examination depth than TA scans and gives a high-definition view of the ovaries, enabling a much more specific assessment of the architecture. The ovaries, particularly in obese patients, can appear homogeneous on TA scans.

The Rotterdam ESHRE/ASRM-sponsored PCOS consensus workshop group recommends the TV route whenever possible, particularly in obese patients (Table 3.2). Several studies have reported that transvaginal ultrasound is a more sensitive method for the detection of polycystic ovaries. [8]

3.4.2 Timing of the Ultrasound Scan

It has been recommended that the baseline ultrasound scan of the pelvis is best performed in the early follicular phase of the menstrual cycle (days 3–5), when the ovaries are relatively quiescent [8]. However in clinical practice in a busy department, it is usually impractical if not logistically impossible to book the scan to coincide with this phase, and many women are uncomfortable with the idea of a TV scan when menstruating. Although this is the optimal approach in order to obtain consistency in the measurement of ovarian volume, this is probably only significant when performing scans for research studies, in which consistency is more relevant than the

Table 3.2 International consensus: Technical recommendations for ultrasound examination of polycystic ovaries

- State-of-the-art equipment is required and should be operated by appropriately trained personnel.
- Whenever possible, the transvaginal approach should be preferred, particularly in obese patients.
- Regularly menstruating women should be scanned in the early follicular phase (days 3–5). Oligo-/amenorrhoeic women should be scanned either at random or between days 3 and 5 after a progestogen-induced bleed.
- If there is evidence of a dominant follicle (>10 mm) or a corpus luteum, the scan should be repeated the next cycle.
- Calculation of ovarian volume is performed using the simplified formula for a prolate ellipsoid (0.5 3 length 3 width 3 thickness).
- Follicle number should be estimated both in longitudinal, transverse and antero-posterior cross-sections of the ovaries. Follicle size should be expressed as the mean of the diameters measured in the three sections.
- The usefulness of 3-D ultrasound, Doppler or MRI for the definition of PCO has not been sufficiently ascertained to date, and should be confined to research studies.

Source: Balen et al. [8]

pragmatic approach that is often taken in day-to-day practice. However, the presence of a follicle >10 mm diameter or a corpus luteum will result in an increased ovarian volume and therefore the scan should be repeated during the early days of the next cycle.

In oligo-amenorrhoeic women, the scan can be performed at random. It is recognized that women with PCOS are usually oligo-ovulatory rather than totally anovulatory, and so it is not uncommon to see a dominant follicle when assessing the ovaries.

3.5 Ultrasound Assessment of the Ovaries

As in Table 3.1, assessment of the size and number of follicles, and volume are key to making the sonographic diagnosis of PCO (Fig. 3.2).

The consensus definition is that a polycystic ovary should have 12 or more follicles of 2–9 mm in diameter. In the past, it was thought that the follicles in polycystic ovaries were arranged peripherally just beneath the surface of the ovary, but it is now accepted that the distribution of the follicles is unimportant [8, 11] (Fig. 3.3).

Increased stromal echogenicity of the ovary compared to the echogenicity of the myometrium is no longer considered to be an important diagnostic feature since this is a subjective assessment, depending on the operator, the settings of the ultrasound machine and the size of the patient. However, it has been shown that ovarian volume correlates well to the increase in stroma and therefore measurement of the ovarian volume remains crucial [1, 8].

The Rotterdam ESHRE/ASRM-sponsored PCOS consensus workshop group defines the increased volume as greater than 10 $cm^{3.}$ They specify that the ovarian volume should be calculated using the simplified formula for a prolate ellipsoid (0.5 3 length 3 width 3 thickness) (Table 3.2). In practice, modern ultrasound machines have this formula built in to the software programme for volume calculation. Studies have shown that normal ovaries never have a volume of greater than 8.0 cm^3. [8].

Wider use of TV US has also identified a small group of women with one polycystic ovary in whom the contralateral ovary can be clearly visualised and appears normal.

The consensus definition states that only one ovary fulfilling the criteria is sufficient to define PCO (Table 3.1) [1, 8].

The ultrasound findings fulfilling the criteria above have to be taken in the context of the clinical presentation, together with appropriate endocrine, biochemical and metabolic tests. For example, abnormalities of basal serum prolactin or FSH levels may indicate a coexistent hypothalamic-pituitary disorder or incipient ovarian failure.

There are also some instances where the above criteria do not fit, and this must be borne in mind until further studies clarify the position.

In women taking the combined oral contraceptive pill, the ovarian volume may be within the normal range, but the appearance may still be polycystic. Polycystic ovaries may also be found incidentally in post-menopausal women and whilst, not surprisingly, they are smaller than in pre-menopausal women with polycystic ovaries,

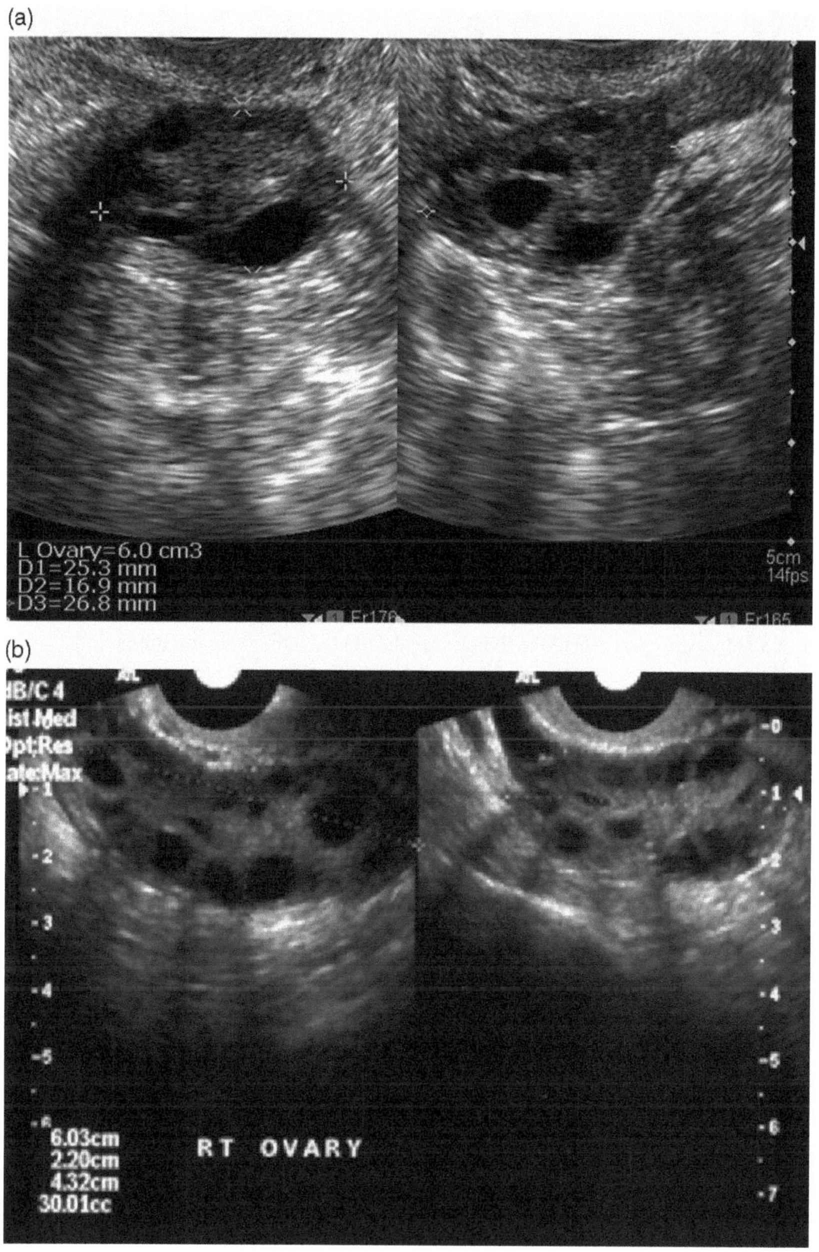

Fig. 3.2 Transvaginal scans of (**a**) normal ovary, (**b**) polycystic ovary. Note increased volume and multiple small follicles, mainly situated peripherally in the polycystic ovary

they are still larger (6.4 versus 3.7 cm^3) with more follicles (9.0 versus 1.7) than normal post-menopausal ovaries [8]. The significance of this is unknown.

3.5.1 Multifollicular Ovaries

Multifollicular ovaries were first described by Adams and colleagues [11] and are seen in mid to late normal puberty and in women recovering from hypothalamic amenorrhoea. In both situations, there is follicular growth

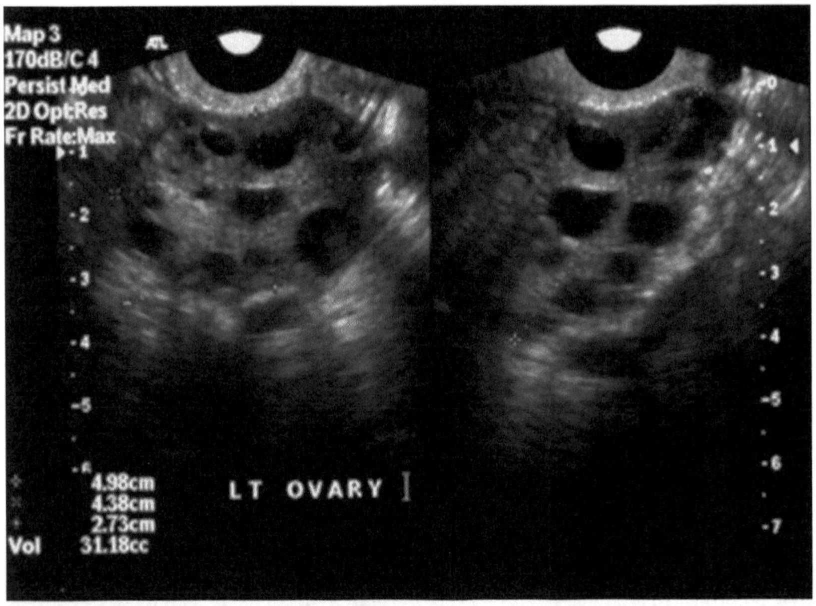

Fig. 3.3 An example of a polycystic ovary where the follicles are distributed throughout the stroma

without consistent formation of a dominant follicle. This condition can cause confusion among inexperienced ultrasonographers, radiologists and gynaecologists, resulting in some adolescent girls incorrectly acquiring the label of polycystic ovaries. Since it is thought that PCOS manifests for the first time during the adolescent years, it is very important these two conditions are not confused.

Multifollicular ovaries differ from PCO, having fewer cysts (>6 per ovary); and these tend to be larger (up to 10 mm in diameter), and there is no stromal hypertrophy [11].

3.5.2 Doppler Studies

Haemodynamic changes in blood flow to the ovaries in women with PCOs have been described, but the measurement of Doppler blood flow requires specific expertise and equipment, and is not considered necessary as part of the diagnostic criteria. [8]

3.5.3 Other Ultrasound Findings

It has been known for many years that severe oligo- and amenorrhoea in the presence of premenopausal levels of oestrogen can lead to endometrial hyperplasia and carcinoma. In women with PCOS, intervals between menstruations of more than three months may be associated with endometrial hyperplasia. Those with persistently thickened endometrium when measured by transvaginal ultrasound should be advised to have an endometrial biopsy and/or hysteroscopy to rule our endometrial hyperplasia. [12]

Ultrasound also has an important role to play in women with PCO undergoing fertility treatment. It is known that this group is more at risk of ovarian hyperstimulation.

PCO may also be seen in clinically normal women having a TV US before undergoing ovarian stimulation for IVF. These ovaries, when stimulated, behave like the ovaries of PCOS women and are also at increased risk for hyperstimulation. [1]

3.6 Technical Recommendations for Ultrasound Assessment of Ovaries in PCOS

Pelvic ultrasound scans should be performed and reported by appropriately trained personnel using modern high-resolution ultrasound machines with an appropriate selection of transducers (Table 3.2). Measurements should be obtained of the ovarian and uterine dimensions and total number and size of follicles recorded. Images should be recorded as either hard copy or electronically.

(a)

(b)

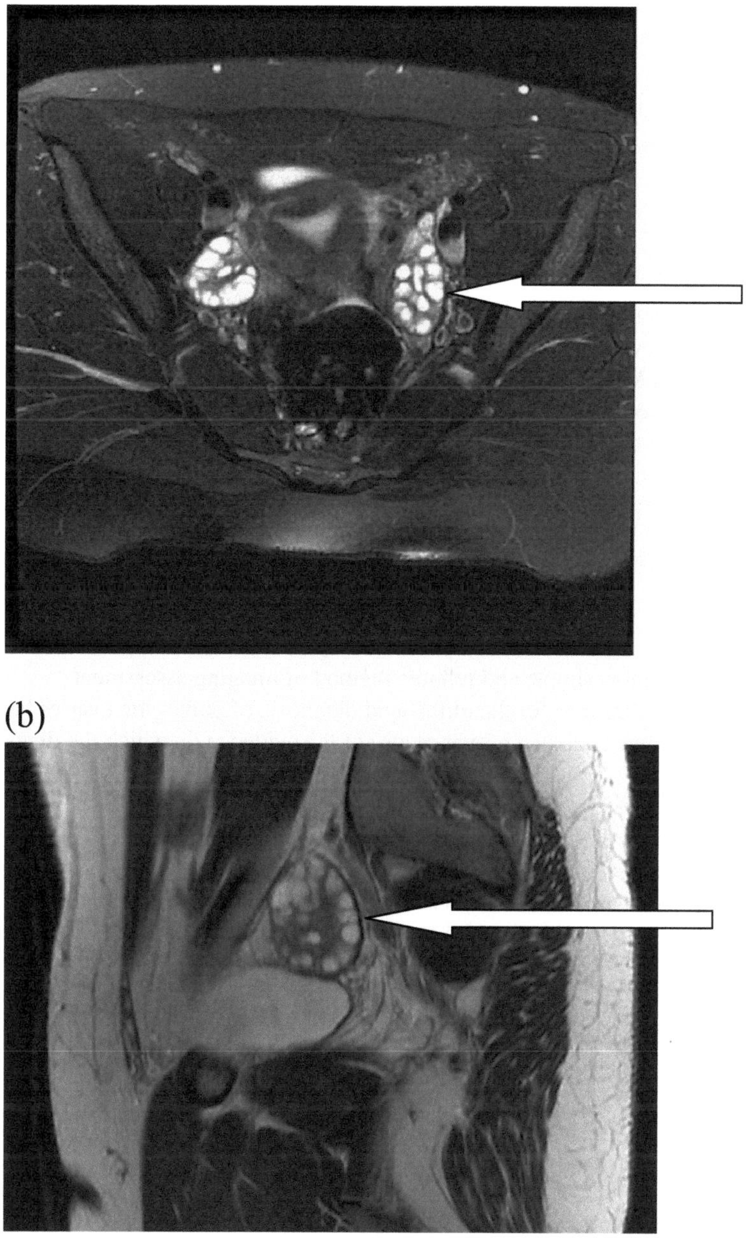

Fig. 3.4 MRI Scan of a patient with PCOS clearly showing large ovaries, with multiple small follicles. (*arrows*). (**a**) Axial T2-weighted image with fat suppression, (**b**) T2-weighted Sagittal image

The ultrasound scan report should include at least the following:

- Date of scan and relation to menstrual cycle
- Relevant treatment (COCP, GnRHa, etc.)
- Type of scan (transabdominal/transvaginal, etc.)
- The morphology and volume of each ovary
- No. and size/range of cysts
- Stromal echogenicity (if volume cannot be calculated)
- Uterine morphology, size measurements and endometrial thickness
- Other features
- Grade of person performing scan, and grade of person verifying scan and report (if relevant).

It is no longer professionally acceptable for a report to be issued on the impression of the sonographer without a proper record of the evidence on which the diagnosis has been made.

3.7 MRI

The use of MRI for the detection of PCO has been described and has been claimed to have even greater sensitivity than US [13, 14]. However, data on MRI for PCO are limited and some early papers were produced before TVS was in widespread use. MRI is expensive and rarely provides more information in PCOS than TVS. However, it may have a limited role where TVS is not practical or diagnostic (for example, in very obese patients or those who are virgo intacta). T2-weighted sequences in which fluid-containing structures are high signal elegantly demonstrate ovarian morphology (Fig. 3.4).

3.8 Key Points

Imaging has a key role to play in the diagnostic work-up of women with PCOS.
Ultrasound remains the most simple and reliable method of imaging assessment.
Internationally agreed definitions for the ultrasound diagnosis of polycystic ovaries have been published.
The ultrasound report must contain a proper record of the evidence on which the diagnosis has been made.

References

1. The Rotterdam ESHRE/ASRM-sponsored PCOS consensus workshop group. Revised 2003 consensus on diagnostic criteria and longterm health risks related to polycystic ovary syndrome (PCOS). Hum Reprod 2004; 19:41–47.
2. Stein IF, Leventhal ML. Amenorrhoea associated with bilateral polycystic ovaries. Am J Obstet Gynecol 1935; 29:181–191.
3. Franks S. Polycystic ovary syndrome: a changing perspective. Clin Endocrinol 1989; 31:87–120.
4. Conway GS, Honour JW, Jacobs HS. Heterogeneity of the polycystic ovary syndrome: clinical, endocrine and ultrasound features in 556 patients. Clin Endocrinol 1989; 30:459–470.
5. Polson DW, Adams J, Wadsworth J, Franks S. Polycystic ovaries—a common finding in normal women. Lancet 1988; 1:870–872.
6. Balen AH, Conway GS, Kaltsas G et al. Polycystic ovary syndrome: the spectrum of the disorder in 1741 patients. Hum Reprod 1995; 10:2107–2111.
7. Swanson M, Sauerbrei EE, Cooperberg PL. Medical implications of ultrasonically detected polycystic ovaries. J Clin Ultrasound 1981; 9:219–222.
8. Balen AH, Laven JS, Tan S et al. Ultrasound assessment of the polycystic ovary: international consensus definitions. Human Reproduction Update 2003; 9(6):505–514.
9. Clayton RN, Ogden V, Hodgkinson J, Worswick L, Rodin DA, Dyer S, et al. How common are polycystic ovaries in normal women and what is their significance for the fertility of the population? Clin Endocrinol 1992;37:127–134.

10. Dewailly D. Definition and significance of polycystic ovaries in hyperandrogenic states and hirsutism. Ball Clin Obstet Gynecol 1997;11:349–368.
11. Adams J, Polson DW, Abdulwahid N, Morris DV, Franks S, Mason HD, Tucker M, Price J, Jacobs HS. Multifollicular ovaries: clinical and endocrine features and response to pulsatile gonadotropin releasing hormone. Lancet 1985; 2:1375–1379.
12. The Royal College of Obstetricians and Gynaecologists. Long-term consequences of polycystic ovary syndrome. Guideline No 33; 2003
13. Kimura I, Togashi K, Kawakami S, et al. Polycystic ovaries: implications of diagnosis with MR imaging. Radiology 1996; 201:549–52.
14. Faure N, Bastide A, Lemay A Assessment of ovaries by magnetic resonance imaging in patients presenting with polycystic ovarian syndrome. Hum Reprod 1989; 4:468–472

Part II
Origins

Chapter 4
Insulin Resistance in PCOS

Evanthia Diamanti-Kandarakis and Charikleia D. Christakou

4.1 Introduction: Definition of Insulin Resistance

Insulin resistance refers to the state, wherein insulin action is insufficient to accomplish the metabolic demands of peripheral tissues, despite the increased amounts of insulin secreted in the circulation. However, this is only an approximate description of this disorder. Insulin resistance encompasses an elaborate clinical, pathophysiologic, and molecular spectrum, and therefore, a well-established definition remains elusive.

Insulin resistance (IR) is recognized to be an integral feature of PCOS. Both lean and obese women with PCOS appear to harbor a greater degree of insulin resistance, compared with their healthy counterparts [1].

The clinical and pathophysiologic implications of the inherent linkage of PCOS with insulin resistance have been the subject of intensive research. Although insulin resistance has been intuitively linked with the metabolic disarray in PCOS, there is growing understanding of its significant contribution to the endocrine and reproductive abnormalities of the syndrome [2].

Studies on cell cultures and insulin target tissue biopsies obtained from women with PCOS have been aimed to explore the etiology and the spectrum of insulin resistance. Molecular research continuously evolves to unveil postbinding defects of insulin signaling, which may account for a unique, PCOS-specific form of insulin resistance [1, 3].

4.2 Prevalence of Insulin Resistance in Women with PCOS

Two decades ago Dunaif et al. using the hyperinsulinemic-euglycemic clamp technique were the first to show that both lean and obese women with PCOS are more insulin resistant than their age- and BMI-matched controls [4]. A significant body of literature subsequently confirmed that insulin resistance is present in women with PCOS over a wide BMI range [5–16] (Table 4.1).

The hyperinsulinemic-euglycemic clamp [5–7] and the frequently sampled intravenous glucose tolerance test (FSIVGTT) [12] have revealed lower insulin sensitivity in women with PCOS compared to age/BMI-matched (Table 4.1).

Although PCOS appears to confer a specific burden of IR, some studies, particularly among European women with normal or modestly increased BMI, have shown normal insulin sensitivity [17], even when more sensitive methods were employed (Table 4.1) [18–21].

PCOS is characterized by clinical and pathophysiological heterogeneity, reflected by the presence or the absence of detectable IR, as well as the differences in the magnitude of IR among affected women [22]. This heterogeneity appears also to account for the variation between prevalence rates of IR reported by different investigators in the PCOS literature. In the majority of studies, prevalence falls between 44% and 70% [7, 8,

E. Diamanti-Kandarakis (✉)
Endocrine Section of the 1st Department of Medicine, University of Athens, Medical School, Athens, Greece
e-mail: akandara@otenet.gr

N.R. Farid, E. Diamanti-Kandarakis (eds.), *Diagnosis and Management of Polycystic Ovary Syndrome*,
DOI 10.1007/978-0-387-09718-3_4,

12, 15, 22–26], significantly higher than the corresponding rate of 10–25% among young, healthy subjects [27] (Table 4.2).

In an attempt to reappraise available literature, several points warrant consideration. Most studies addressing the presence (Table 4.1) or the prevalence (Table 4.2) of IR in the PCOS cohort have included small numbers of individuals, while study populations varied considerably in terms of anthropometric, demographic, clinical, and endocrine features. Some studies did not clarify the racial/ethnic composition of the study population [15, 20], whereas in others there was no control group or patients and controls were not well matched for all confounders [14, 15, 17, 22–25, 28] (Tables 4.1, 4.2). Our ability to draw clear conclusions is further constrained by the lack of a common definition and methodology for the assessment of insulin resistance. Even among the studies which used the same methodology, the reference limits for insulin resistance differed in the studied populations (Table 4.2).

Table 4.1 Studies comparing various insulin-sensitivity indexes between women with PCOS and controls

Study	Study population	Method	Comparison of Insulin sensitivity
AGE, BMI-MATCHED PATIENTS and CONTROLS			
NIH CRITERIA			
BMI≤ 25			
Ovesen 1993 [18]	7 PCOS age:27.1, BMI:22.2 7 controls NORTH EUROPEAN	Hyperinsul Euglycemic Clamp	PCOS = controls
Ducluzeau 2003 [7]	16 PCOS age:23.4, BMI:23.6 10 controls WHITE EUROPEAN	Hyperinsul Euglycemic Clamp	PCOS < Controls
Fulgeshu 2006 [8]	49 PCOS age:17.9, BMI:20.6 50 Controls WHITE EUROPEAN	HOMA-R AUC-I	PCOS < Controls
Palomba 2007 [9]	30 PCOS age: 24.3, BMI: 22.4 10 controls WHITE EUROPEAN	Hyperinsul Euglycemic Clamp	PCOS < Controls
Mixed (overweight/obese+lean)			
Dunaif 1996 [5]	13 LPCOS,age:26, BMI:22.1 15 OPCOS,age:30, BMI:36.2 29 Controls (14 O + 15 L) WHITE NON-HISPANIC & CARIBBEAN HISPANIC	FSIVGTT	PCOS < Controls
Diamanti-Kandarakis 1995 [6]	8 LPCOS,age:22, BMI:21.5 10 OPCOS, age:22, BMI:31.5 13 Controls (5 O,older + 8 L) EUROPEAN GREEK	Hyperinsul Euglycemic Clamp	PCOS < Controls
Heald 2005 [10]	25 PCOS age:29, BMI:32.9 25 Controls WHITE EUROPEAN	1/HOMA-R	PCOS < Controls
Micic 2007 [11]	8 L PCOS, BMI:20.52 8 OPCOS, BMI: 34.36 16 controls: 8 L+8 O WHITE EUROPEAN	hyperinsul euglycemic clamp	L PCOS < L controls O PCOS < O controls
Vrbikova 2004 [19]	53 LPCOS, age:24.2, BMI:21.5 30 OPCOS, age:22.2, BMI:29.6 15 controls, matched with LPCOS NORTH EUROPEAN	Hyperinsul Euglycemic Clamp	LPCOS = controls OPCOS < LPCOS & controls

Table 4.1 (continued)

Study	Study population	Method	Comparison of Insulin sensitivity
Ciampelli 1997 ¶ [20]	age:17-31 15 LPCOS, BMI:22.42/23.17 20 OPCOS, BMI:28.1/30.2 10 controls,matched with LPCOS ETHNICITY NOT DEFINED	Hyperinsul Euglycemic Clamp	LPCOS = controls OPCOS < controls
BMI>25			
Legro 1998 [12]	40 PCOS Age:26.9, BMI:39 15 age/BMI matched controls AMERICAN, WHITE NON-HISPANIC	FSIVGTT FGIR	PCOS < Controls
Jayagopal 2002 [13]	12 PCOS Age: 26.25, BMI: 33.18 11 controls WHITE EUROPEAN	HOMA-R	PCOS < Controls
ROTTERDAM CRITERIA BMI≤ 25			
Gennarelli 2005 [21] ⚔	20 PCOS age:26.5, BMI:20.8 20 controls WHITE EUROPEAN	FSIVGTT	PCOS = controls
PATIENTS and CONTROLS NOT MATCHED for AGE and/or BMI NIH CRITERIA Mixed(overweight/obese+lean)			
Park 2001 [14]	9 PCOS Age:25*, BMI:26 5 Controls older, ≈ BMI KOREAN	Hyperinsul Euglycemic Clamp	PCOS < controls
Vrbikova 2002 [17]	37 L PCOS age:23.5, BMI:21.8 27 O PCOS age:26.5, BMI:31 20 controls older,≈ BMI with L PCOS NORTH EUROPEAN	HOMA-R	OPCOS < controls & LPCOS LPCOS = controls
Diamanti-Kandarakis 2007 [32]	545 CPCOS age:24·36*, BMI 26·83 89 Non classic PCOS age 24.24*, BMI:26·03 108 controls older, BMI ≈ with patients EUROPEAN GREEK	QUICKI	CPCOS > Controls Non-classic PCOS ≈ Controls PHO > Controls HO > Controls No dif between PCOS groups
Barber 2007 [33]	191 PHO age 32·9, BMI:29·2* 76 PH age 34·8, BMI:23·7 42 PO age 32·1, BMI:23·9 76 controls older, BMI:24 (≈PO) WHITE EUROPEANS	HOMA-R	Adj. for BMI/age PHO > PH PHO > Controls PHO > PO PO = Controls
ROTTERDAM CRITERIA MIXED (OVERWEIGHT/OBESE+LEAN)			
dePaula Martins 2007 [15]	44 LPCOS BMI:20.81,age:21.34 61 OPCOS BMI:32.87,age:25.66 50 Controls (25 L, ≈BMI with LPCOS,older 26 O, ≈BMI with OPCOS, older)	1/HOMA-R QUICKI COMP	L PCOS < L Controls O PCOS < O Controls
Kowalska 2007 [16]	23 L PCOS age: 23.69, BMI: 21.39 47 O PCOS, age: 26.13, BMI :30.99 45 controls (25 L + 20 O) WHITE EUROPEAN	Hyperinsul Euglycemic Clamp	L PCOS < L Controls O PCOS < O Controls

Table 4.1 (continued)

Study	Study population	Method	Comparison of Insulin sensitivity
BMI>25			
Morin- Papunen 2000 [28] ☸	28 O PCOS age:30.1, BMI:34.5 15 L PCOS age:28.9, BMI:22.7 34 Controls (17 O ≈BMI with OPCOS,older,17 L Controls ≈BMI with LPCOS, older) NORTH EUROPEAN	Hyperinsul Euglycemic Clamp	trend LPCOS < L controls OPCOS < O controls

The provided values for age and BMI are means

Abbreviations
Adj.:adjusted
AUC-I:Area under the curve for insulin levels(OGTT 2 hours)
COMP:Composite insulin-sensitivity index (Matsuda)
CPCOS:Classic PCOS
HO: hyperandrogenemic and oligomenorrheic
IHA:Idiopathic hyperandrogenism (hyperandrogenism with ovulatory cycles and normal ovaries)
L:Lean
Non-classic PCOS: PCO morphology with hyperandrogenemia or oligomenorrhea
No dif: No difference
O:Overweight/obese
OV-PCOS:Ovulatory PCOS
PHO: hyperandrogenemic and oligomenorrheic with polycystic ovarian morphology
PH: hyperandrogenemic eumenorrheic with polycystic ovarian morphology
PO normoandrogenemic, oligomenorrheic with polycystic ovarian morphology
1/HOMA-R: 1/homeostasis model assessment-insulin resistance

Symbols-Clarifications
>: *Higher than*
≤: *Lower or equal to*
<: Lower insulin sensitivity
= Similar (BMI or insulin sensitivity)
≈ *similar*
⋆*Significantly higher BMI*
¶ *In the study by Ciampelli et al. (20) patients and controls were subgrouped as normo- or hyperinsulinemic .The authors provided two mean BMI values, one for the normoinsulinemic and one for the hyperinsulinemic subgroup of patients.*
⋉ *In the study by Gennarelli et al (21) the diagnosis of PCOS was based on the ultrasonographic evidence of polycystic ovaries, in association with a history of amenorrhea or menstrual irregularities, rather than hyperandrogenemia*
☸ *In the study by Morin–Papunen et al (28), the diagnosis of PCOS was based on the following criteria: polycystic ovaries on transvaginal ultrasonography (≥8 subcapsular follicles of 3–8 mm diam. in one plane in one ovary and increased stroma) and at least 1 of the following: oligo-/amenorrhea, clinical signs of hyperandrogenism &/or elevated serum testosterone levels.*

4.3 Determinants of Heterogeneity of IR in PCOS

4.3.1 Factors Specific to PCOS

4.3.1.1 Diagnostic Criteria – PCOS Phenotypes

The use of different diagnostic criteria [29, 30, 31] appears to significantly account for the variability in the reported prevalence rates of insulin resistance in PCOS. The different phenotypes introduced in the broadened spectrum of PCOS, as defined by the Rotterdam criteria [30] appear to harbor different degrees of insulin resistance.

Table 4.2 Studies addressing the prevalence of IR in women with PCOS with different BMIs and ethnic origins using different diagnostic criteria for PCOS and various methods of assessment

Study	Study population	Methods and Cut-offs	Prevalence of IR in PCOS
AGE, BMI-MATCHED PATIENTS & CONTROLS			
NIH CRITERIA			
BMI ≤25			
Ducluzeau 2003 [7]	16 PCOS age:23.4, BMI:23.6 10 controls WHITE EUROPEAN	Hyperinsul Euglycemic Clamp	50%
Fulgeshu 2006(8)	49 PCOS age:17.9, BMI:20.6 50 Controls EUROPEAN ITALIAN	AUC-I :11817μIU/ml	44%
BMI>25			
Legro 1998 [12]	40 PCOS Age:26.9, BMI:39 15 Controls AMERICAN NON-HISPANIC WHITE	FSIVGTT FGIR:4.5	53%
ROTTERDAM CRITERIA			
Mixed(Overweight/obese+Lean)			
Carmina 2005 [26]	Age-matched 204 CPCOS age:24.8, BMI:28.1⋆ 50 OV-PCOS BMI:23.8 33 IHA BMI≈:with OV-PCOS 85 L controls, BMI≈:with OV-PCOS,IHA 42 controls, BMI≈:with CPCOS EUROPEAN ITALIAN	QUICKI:0.333	CPCOS 68% OV-PCOS 36% IHA 26%
PATIENTS & CONTROLS NOT MATCHED for AGE and BMI &/or ETHNICITY OR NO CONTROLS			
NIH			
Mixed(Overweight/obese+Lean)			
Ciampelli 2005 [23]	93 PCOS Age: 25, BMI: 29.83 No controls EUROPEAN ITALIAN	Hyperinsul Euglycemic Clamp	66.1%
Carmina 2004 [24]	267 PCOS Age:22.1, BMI:27.6 [129 BMI>28, 138 BMI <27] 50 Controls EUROPEAN ITALIAN	ITT FGIR :6.4 1/HOMA-R:0.47 QUICKI: 0.33	Total PCOS FGIR: 65.4%, 1/HOMA-R:77%, QUICKI: 79.2%,ITT:78.3% PCOS BMI>28 ITT:92% PCOS BMI<27 FGIR: 56.5%, 1/HOMA-R: 60.9%, QUICKI: 63%, ITT:69%
DeUgarte 2005 [25]	271 PCOS age:27.4, BMI:36.4 260 Controls WHITE & BLACK AMERICANS	adjusted for race, age, BMI HOMA-R:3.9 FGIR:2.67	HOMA: 64.4% FGIR:19.7%
ROTTERDAM			
Mixed(Overweight/obese+Lean)			
dePaula Martins 2007 [15]	105 PCOS age:23.85, BMI:27.81 51 controls age:28.49, BMI:26.9 ETHNICITY NOT DEFINED	1/HOMA-R:0.47 QUICKI:0.333 COMP:4.75 AUC-I:7000μIU/ml New cutoffs 1/HOMA-R: 0.63 QUICKI: 0.356	Total PCOS 1/HOMA-R:51.4%, QUICKI: 44.8%, AUC-I: 70.5%, COMP:64.8% New cutoffs for 1/HOMA-R, QUICKI: 66.67%

Table 4.2 (continued)

Study	Study population	Methods: Cut-offs	Prevalence of IR in PCOS
Vigil 2007 [22]	69 PCOS, age:26.01, BMI:25.01 HISPANIC CHILEAN	octreotide modified insulin suppression test	52.17%

The provided values for age and BMI are means

Abbreviations
AUC-I:Area under the curve for insulin levels(OGTT 2 hours)
CPCOS:Classic PCOS
COMP:Composite-insulin sensitivity index (Matsuda)
Hyperinsul:hyperinsulinemic
IHA:Idiopathic Hyperandrogenism (hyperandrogenism with ovulatory cycles and normal ovaries)
ITT:Insulin tolerance test
L:Lean
O:Overweight/obese
OV-PCOS:Ovulatory PCOS
1/HOMA-R: 1/homeostasis model assessment-insulin resistance

Symbols-Clarifications
$>$: *Higher than*
$\leq$: *Lower or equal to*
$<$: *Lower than*
$\approx$ *Similar*
⋆ *Significantly higher than the BMIs in other groups*
☒ *In the study by Carmina et al (24),the ITT was performed in a subgroup of 60 women with PCOS and 20 controls*

Several investigators agree that the full-blown PCOS phenotype is more insulin resistant compared with the non-classic PCOS phenotypes, even after excluding the compounding effect of obesity, which is reportedly more common in women with classic PCOS [32–34] (Table 4.1).

In a large prospective study among women with PCOS, diagnosed by the Rotterdam Criteria, different subgroups of patients with comparable BMI were compared with each other and with BMI-matched controls. Patients with anovulation and hyperandrogenemia were the most insulin resistant in comparison with controls [32], a finding confirmed by Carmina et al. [26]. Sixty eight percent of women with classic PCOS were insulin-resistant, as compared with thirty six percent of ovulatory hyperandrogenemic women. However, the higher prevalence of obesity in the former group was a significant confounder. In addition, ovulatory, hyperandrogenemic women with PCOS were significantly more insulin resistant compared not only with BMI-matched controls, but also with BMI-matched women with idiopathic hyperandrogenism. The authors suggested that the polycystic ovary may be a significant determinant of the metabolic phenotype of PCOS [26]. Other investigators, however, showed that the combination of hyperandrogenemia and anovulation, independent of polycystic ovarian morphology, is a prerequisite for the emergence of metabolic aberrations [32].

Despite the controversy on the metabolic features of the non-classic hyperandrogenemic PCOS phenotype, normo-androgenemic women with PCOS do not appear to differ from BMI-matched controls in terms of insulin sensitivity [21, 32, 33] (Tables 4.1, 4.2).

More recently, the Androgen Excess Society (AES) has provided a contemporary version of the definition of PCOS [31]. Both the NIH and the AES definitions have declared hyperandrogenism as the core characteristic of PCOS [29, 31]. Considering the clinically evident association of hyperandrogenism with metabolic abnormalities, these two definitions fit better the metabolic phenotype of PCOS. Conversely, the Rotterdam criteria are less selective in metabolic terms, since they embrace a wider spectrum of women with less-pronounced endocrine and metabolic abnormalities [34]. On these grounds, the lack of significant difference in insulin sensitivity between PCOS women and controls, reported by some investigators, may be attributable to the inclusion of patients with milder phenotypes and particularly, those without [21, 28] hyperandrogenemia.

4.3.1.2 Obesity–Dietary Factors

Although insulin resistance is considered an inherent feature of PCOS, obesity is recognized as a significant aggravating factor [22]. The reported rates of obesity in the PCOS cohort vary widely from 30% to 75%, depending upon ethnicity, diagnostic criteria of PCOS, and recruitment criteria of the study population [35, 36]. Despite these variations, obesity prevails as a common phenotype among PCOS women [35, 36].

The coexistence between PCOS and obesity appears to have important clinical and pathological implications. In a sizeable cohort of women with PCOS, Vigil et al. showed that the steady-state plasma glucose (SSPG), an insulin resistance index derived from the modified insulin suppression test, is directly associated with BMI. Among patients with higher SSPG values 58% were obese, whereas the corresponding percentage was only 28% among women in the lowest SSPG range (lowest degree of insulin resistance) [22].

Reflecting the linkage between obesity and insulin resistance in PCOS, several studies among predominantly or exclusively lean patients have failed to confirm insulin resistance in the PCOS group [18, 19, 21]. It is recognized that insulin resistance is less frequent in lean patients as compared with their obese counterparts [22] (Table 4.1).

Additionally, there are data to suggest that obesity acts upon the hyperandrogenic phenotype to amplify the degree of insulin resistance and the occurrence of anovulation. Obesity has been suggested to be the environmental modulator of the deterioration from the phenotype of isolated hyperandrogenemia to PCOS [26].

Most important than obesity per se appears to be visceral adiposity, a common feature even in lean women with PCOS [37]. Interestingly, Lord et al. have reported that visceral adiposity is the most significant variable correlating with insulin resistance and metabolic dysfunction in women with PCOS [38]. In that regard, it would be intriguing to investigate insulin sensitivity in women with PCOS and controls matched not only for age and BMI, but also for visceral fat mass. In view of the influential role of total and central obesity, diet emerges as an important factor in the perpetuation of insulin resistance in PCOS. Chronic overnutrition is a widely acknowledged triggering factor of insulin resistance, particularly in susceptible individuals, like women with PCOS [39].

Currently, the quality of food [40] and specifically, diet enriched to Advanced Glycated end products (AGEs) are incriminated in metabolic abnormalities via the increase in circulating AGEs levels, which are known for their role in oxidative stress [41]. Young normoglycemic women with PCOS fed with a high-AGE diet demonstrated a further increase of serum AGEs levels [42], which were already increased at baseline [43]. Since serum AGEs levels are positively correlated with serum androgen levels and with indices of IR in PCOS women, dietary intake of AGEs may play a role in the pathophysiology of PCOS.

Nevertheless, obesity and dietary factors should not be considered as the sole cause of insulin resistance in PCOS. In a reanalysis of combined data from two prevalence studies of PCOS [44, 45], obesity was shown to have merely a modest exacerbating effect on the risk for PCOS [36].

It appears that the whole syndrome and its constituent parts originate from intrinsic pathogenic traits. Obesity and other potential environmental factors appear to be superimposed upon an abnormal inherent background to aggravate the insulin-resistant state in PCOS [46].

4.3.1.3 Family History PCOS – Family History of Type 2 Diabetes

The maternal history of PCOS appears to be a risk factor for insulin resistance in the female offspring, which can be detected in prepubertal period, before the onset of hyperandrogenism [47]. In a recent study, the 2 hour-insulin levels during the OGTT were higher in prepubertal and pubertal daughters of PCOS women compared with the respective levels in controls, whereas hyperandrogenemia was not detectable earlier than puberty [47]. These findings may be attributable partly to genetic traits [48, 49] and partly to intrauterine environmental influences that arouse fetal metabolic maladaptations [50].

The prevalence of PCOS among mothers and sisters of women with PCOS was 24% and 32%, respectively [51], that is four and five-fold higher compared with the one established in the general population [52]. However, in this PCOS population, the parameters of insulin sensitivity were not investigated [51].

A study among twin pairs (monozygotic and dizygotic), in which PCOS diagnosis was based on ultrasonographic and biochemical findings, suggested that fasting insulin levels were significantly influenced by genetic factors (reviewed in [49]). These data implicate a genetic component in the metabolic abnormalities associated with PCOS, but suggest a polygenic etiology leaving room for environmental factors to play an additional role.

The family history of metabolic abnormalities emerges as an additional determinant of insulin resistance in PCOS women. Clinical studies in individuals with PCOS have associated the family history of type 2 diabetes (T2D) with an increased risk for insulin resistance [53–55]. A recent study, using the hyperinsulinemic-euglycemic clamp in lean PCOS women, showed that only those patients with a family history of T2D had lower insulin sensitivity as compared to that of age and BMI-matched controls [56]. On that basis, the family history of T2D was proposed to be an independent risk factor for insulin resistance in PCOS.

These observations replicate what occurs in first-degree relatives of T2D patients without PCOS [57, 58]. More specifically, nondiabetic first-degree relatives of T2D families often carry inherited defects of peripheral insulin action which account for the common presence of insulin resistance in these subjects.

Thus, T2D and PCOS may share common genetic traits contributing to insulin resistance, an inborn or intrinsic feature in both disorders. Families of women with PCOS have a large number of individuals with disorders of glucose tolerance [54, 55, 59]. Almost 50% of parents of women with PCOS have IGT or frank T2D [55]. Insulin sensitivity was found to be significantly lower in first-degree relatives of PCOS women with normal glucose tolerance compared with controls, after adjustment for sex, age, and BMI [54, 55, 60, 61]. However, a specific insulin-signaling defect has been postulated to differentiate the molecular type of insulin resistance in PCOS women from the one in non-PCOS subjects with IGT or T2D [62]. To date, this speculation has not been supported by molecular data.

The familial predisposition to T2D appears to be attributable to the inherited defect of insulin sensitivity, but most importantly to a heritable trait of β-cell dysfunction [63, 64]. Women with PCOS display defective early phase insulin secretion, delayed hyperinsulinemia and reduced disposition index, a measure of β-cell secretory function adjusted for insulin sensitivity [5, 65]. Altuntas et al. [66]reported that even lean patients with a family history of T2D and reactive hypoglycemia in the fourth hour of the OGTT, reflective of late-phase insulin hypersecretion, carry an increased risk for the development of T2D. In one study, impaired insulin secretion was confined to those women with both PCOS and a family history of T2D [65]. Thus a family history of PCOS and/or of T2D should be considered as compounding factor, when studying insulin sensitivity and/or insulin secretion in women with PCOS.

4.3.2 Factors Independent of PCOS

4.3.2.1 Methodological Issues

Pitfalls in the laboratory evaluation of insulin resistance pose another difficulty in detecting and quantifying this disorder in the general population and specifically in PCOS [67]. Insulin resistance is commonly identified by its clinical corollaries, rather than being measurable in the laboratory setting [67].

In 1997, the Consensus Development Conference on Insulin Resistance of the American Diabetes Association [68] established that only the euglycemic hyperinsulinemic clamp and the minimal model method applied to a frequently sampled intravenous glucose tolerance test (FSIVGTT) can accurately estimate peripheral insulin resistance. Both methods are cumbersome and difficult to be carried out in clinical practice.

Several simplified mathematical models have been implemented for the assessment of insulin resistance in clinical practice. The most widely used are the fasting glucose to insulin ratio (FGIR), the homeostatic model of assessment (HOMA-R), and the quantitative insulin-sensitivity check index (QUICKI). They reflect spontaneous homeostatic characteristics based on insulin affecting hepatic glucose production in the fasting state, but unlike the euglycemic clamp, they cannot offer information for peripheral insulin action in the postprandial state.

Two studies have reported that FGIR is a reliable predictor of insulin resistance in obese [12] and nonobese [7] PCOS patients. Significant correlations between the clamp-derived insulin sensitivity index and surrogate markers, like the FGIR, the HOMA and the QUICKI were reported [69, 70, 71].

However, the correlation of the QUICKI or HOMA indices to the results obtained by the euglycemic-hyperinsulinemic clamp technique should not be considered equivalent a priori in every insulin-resistant population [72]. Metabolic or hormonal factors as well as ethnicity may influence this correlation, and the results may not correctly represent the degree of insulin resistance [72]. The considerable variance of the detection rates of IR by different surrogates further challenges their diagnostic utility in women with PCOS [15] (Table 4.2), as does the lack of standardized cut-off values. As a result, the applied cut-off points vary according to the population studied (Table 4.2).

Serum insulin measurements are vitiated by the poor performance of available immunoassays, highlighted by a working group of the American Diabetes Association [73]. Substantial inter-assay and inter-laboratory variations posit major concerns over the diagnostic value of serum insulin measurements [73]. Moreover, insulin resistance, assessed by HOMA, demonstrates greater inter-individual and intra-individual variability in women with PCOS, than the one in age/BMI-matched controls. The wider biological variation seen in PCOS may be inherent to the syndrome, rather than a methodological flaw of the HOMA method [13].

A recent study among PCOS women used the receiver-operating characteristic (ROC) curve to calculate new cut-off values for QUICKI and HOMA-R based on insulin sensitivity indices derived from the Oral Glucose Tolerance Test (OGTT). However, the reliability of these data is limited by the fact that the proposed cut-off points lack validation by the euglycemic clamp [15].

As a dynamic method, the OGTT may provide a relatively more precise estimate of insulin resistance [8, 15, 74]. Of the insulin sensitivity indexes based on the OGTT, the area under curve for insulin (AUC-I) and the composite insulin sensitivity index by Matsuda and DeFronzo (COMP) [75] were shown to have a high positive predictive value validated by the euglycemic clamp in PCOS patients [23]. This conclusion was challenged by another study showing no correlation of fasting or OGTT-derived measures with FSIVGTT in a heterogeneous population consisting of premenopausal women with or without PCOS and postmenopausal women [76].

In summary, surrogate indices, based on measurements either in the fasting state or during the OGTT cannot accurately mirror the presence and the degree of IR in women with PCOS and are not equivalent to the euglycemic clamp technique [72]. A false-negative estimate is particularly likely at the two extremities of the insulin-resistance spectrum. Caution should be exercised in individuals with subtle aberrations and in patients with impaired glucose tolerance (IGT) or frank diabetes [77, 78].

4.3.2.2 Race/Ethnicity

There are racial/ethnic variations in the prevalence of IR among individuals without PCOS [79, 80]. Different racial/ethnic groups differ in lifestyle and genetic factors, and therefore, the prevalence of IR is predictably modified by race/ethnicity. Studies in the general population have shown that racial differences in insulin sensitivity is determined by differences in fat distribution. South Asian adolescents tend to be more insulin resistant and display central fat accumulation, compared with white European adolescents [80]. Moreover, certain racial groups, like African-Americans may harbor an inherent type of insulin resistance, independent of adiposity [81].

The modifying role of ethnic and racial origin has been also confirmed within the PCOS cohort, with a greater prevalence of IR in Mexican and Carribean Hispanic as compared with non-Hispanic white women. In addition, South Asian and American women with PCOS are more insulin resistant than their white European counterparts [82–84] (Table 4.2). In particular, studies from North Europe did not detect significantly greater degrees of insulin resistance among lean women with PCOS [18, 19, 28]. Reports from other European regions also witnessed racial and ethnic variations of IR in PCOS, yet most of them agree that women with PCOS are more insulin-resistant than their healthy counterparts [6–11, 13, 16] (Table 4.1). The lower BMI, in addition to potential genetically determined factors should be considered as significant determinants of the more favorable metabolic status in European women with PCOS [40].

4.4 Target Tissues of Insulin Action in PCOS

Insulin acts on classic insulin-sensitive tissues, e.g., adipose tissue and skeletal muscle, as well as non-classic target tissues, like the ovary [85, 86] and the endothelium [87].

Insulin binding to its receptor causes phosphorylation of insulin receptor substrates (IRS), resulting in the activation of mitogen-activated kinase (MAPK) and phosphoinositide 3-kinase (PI3K) signaling pathways. This multiplicity of signaling pathways downstream of the insulin receptor may explain the pathway-specific defects of insulin action in insulin-resistant states [88].

A key feature of insulin resistance is that it is characterized by specific impairment in PI3K-dependent signaling pathways [89–93]. Compensatory hyperinsulinemia will overdrive unaffected pathways leading to an imbalance between insulin actions mediated by PI-3 K and those mediated by other signaling pathways. Moreover, insulin resistance is tissue selective in that a signaling pathway may be functional in one tissue, while impaired in another [94].

4.4.1 Insulin Action in Peripheral Tissues

4.4.1.1 Skeletal Muscle

Muscle biopsies, which were performed during a hyperinsulinemic euglycemic clamp study, revealed significantly lower insulin-mediated glucose uptake in women with PCOS [95] Moreover, insulin receptors partially purified from PCOS skeletal muscle had decreased insulin-induced tyrosine phosphorylation and increased insulin-independent serine phosphorylation, as that seen in PCOS skin fibroblasts cultured for many passages [62], a finding not confirmed in cultures of skeletal myotubes.

However, constitutively increased basal phosphorylation [96] was observed on Serine312 residues of insulin receptor substrate1 (IRS-1) [96]. Enhanced mitogenic signaling in cultured myotubes, as indicated by increased phosphorylation of extracellular signal-regulated kinase 1/2 (ERK ½), was incriminated in the increased serine312 phosphorylation of IRS-1 [97].

Skeletal muscle biopsies from women with PCOS showed several defects, including transiently decreased insulin stimulation of IRS-1-associated PI3-K activity and increased IRS-2 protein abundance [95, 97] with unaltered IRS-1 and IRS-2 mRNA expression [95].

Microarrays of skeletal muscle specimens from women with PCOS demonstrated that insulin resistance is associated with reduced expression of genes involved in mitochondrial oxidative metabolism and that reduced expression of peroxisome proliferator agonist receptor γ (PPARγ) coactivator 1α (PGC-1^{α}) could play an integral role in this defect [98]. These findings provided evidence for a causative association between insulin resistance and impaired mitochondrial oxidative metabolism (OXPHOS) in skeletal muscle of women with PCOS, independently of obesity and T2D. Transcriptional alterations in insulin-signaling pathways, fatty acid metabolism, and calcium homeostasis may also contribute to the potentially unique phenotype of insulin resistance in patients with PCOS [98].

In support of impaired mitochondrial oxidative metabolism in PCOS skeletal muscle, a clinical study has shown reduced maximal oxygen consumption (*V*o2max) in PCOS women [99], an abnormality which has been associated with the expression of OXPHOS genes in diabetic patients [100].

4.4.1.2 Adipose Tissue

Subcutaneous adipocytes from women with PCOS were found to have impaired insulin-stimulated glucose transport [101–103], likely related to decreased responsiveness rather than decreased sensitivity to insulin [104]. PCOS subcutaneous and omental adipocytes showed also decreased expression of glucose transporter GLUT-4 [107, 108], which mediates the rate-limiting step of insulin-stimulated glucose transport.

Diminished insulin-stimulated autophosphorylation of the insulin receptor initially demonstrated in cultured adipocytes from obese women with PCOS [101, 102] was recently extended to erythrocytes from insulin-resistant PCOS women, but not from insulin-sensitive patients [105].

Impaired insulin-stimulated phosphorylation of IRS-1 has emerged as an additional signaling defect in adipocytes from PCOS women [3] probably secondary to increased glycogen synthase kinase 3-beta (GSK-3-beta) resulting in increased IRS-1 serine phosphorylation [106].

Recent gene expression studies bolster the evidence of IR in omental adipose tissue from obese PCOS women [109]. Differential gene expression includes overexpression of ectonucleotide pyrophosphatase/phosphodiesterase 1 (ENPP1) (also termed PC-1), a negative regulator of insulin receptor tyrosine kinase activity, and overexpression of PI3KR1, encoding for the regulatory p85 α-subunit of PI3K, which could be involved in the pathogenesis of insulin resistance in these patients [109]. Several of the dysregulated genes were found to contain putative androgen response elements in their promoters [109] suggesting a role of androgen excess in IR in PCOS.

4.4.2 Insulin Action in the Ovarian Tissue: Clinical Aspects and Molecular Insights into the Paradox

Insulin has been implicated in endocrine and reproductive aberrations in PCOS in a dual fashion, through the modulation of both ovarian steroidogenesis and folliculogenesis. Studies in hyperandrogenic adolescents [110] and in adult women with PCOS [111] have shown positive associations of insulin resistance or hyperinsulinemia with biochemical hyperandrogenemia and anovulation [112]. The finding that inhibition of insulin secretion by diazoxide treatment caused a decline in androgen levels in PCOS women without detectable IR supports the notion that insulin action on theca cells contributes to increased androgen levels in PCOS [113]. In support of a detrimental role of hyperinsulinemia in reproductive function is also the fact that women with type 1 diabetes have a two-fold higher prevalence of PCOS than the one established in the general female population [114].

Conversely, treatment with insulin sensitizers or with an inhibitor of intestinal carbohydrate absorption as well as diet-induced weight loss improves hyperandrogenemia and anovulation [115–120]. All the aforementioned therapeutic interventions share a common mechanism of action, the reduction of insulin resistance/hyperinsulinemia. However, regarding metformin and thiazolinediones, a direct action upon the ovary should also be considered [121, 122].

Insulin receptors are present in theca and granulosa cells, where they mediate metabolic, steroidogenic, and mitogenic actions [123]. In porcine theca cells, insulin was shown to increase the LH-driven accumulation of cyclic AMP contributing to increased expression of genes encoding the steroidogenic acute regulatory (StAR) protein and the 17alpha-hydroxylase/17,20-lyase (CYP17A1) enzyme [124]. Most importantly, in human theca cells, insulin was shown to directly amplify the activity of 17-alpha hydroxylase (CYP17A1), acting through the PI3K pathway, independently of MAPK [125]. A positive crosstalk between insulin and LH was also confirmed at the level of the PI 3-K/Akt pathway in rat ovaries. This molecular interaction may have implications for insulin action in both theca and granulosa cells in the human ovary [126, 127].

In granulosa cells from normal ovaries, insulin enhances FSH-induced aromatase activity and interacts with LH to stimulate the expression of sterol-regulatory genes encoding the low-density lipoprotein (LDL) receptor, *stAR* protein, 3βhydroxysteroid-dehydrogenase (3β-HSD) and cytochrome P450 side-chain cleavage (*P450scc*) [128–131]. Wu et al. [132] has shown that IRS-1 is present in follicles from normal human ovaries, and the intensity of its expression increases with follicle growth. These findings suggest that insulin may regulate follicle growth, at least in part, by increasing the expression of its receptor substrates at the protein level [132]. Additionally, insulin enhances LH receptor expression in granulosa cells from growing human follicles [133].

Ovarian theca and granulosa cells from anovulatory women with PCOS appear to respond normally to insulin [123, 134, 135]. Cultured granulosa cells from anovulatory women with polycystic ovaries exhibited normal estradiol (E2) and progesterone secretion in response to physiological insulin concentrations, indicating that these cells remain insulin sensitive [94, 134].

Insulin excess characterizing PCOS is also incriminated in the premature LH receptor expression leading to premature luteinization of follicles smaller than 8 mm in diameter from these women [94, 134, 136, 137]. Insulin excess was also associated with premature follicle luteinization in prenatally androgenized female rhesus monkeys undergoing gonadotropin therapy for IVF [138].

The maintenance of insulin action on the ovary in the context of peripheral insulin resistance in PCOS has been a challenging area for research. Metabolic pathways appear to be intrinsically insulin resistant not only in peripheral tissues but also in granulosa cells from PCOS women [94, 139]. In particular, cultured granulosa cells from anovulatory patients were resistant to insulin action on glucose metabolism compared with those from normal women, despite maintaining normal steroidogenic output in response to physiological doses of insulin [94]. Thus, the dichotomy between insulin-dependent pathways is not merely a matter of tissue specificity, since it is also present within the same tissue.

Different subtypes of the insulin receptor [140], as well as divergent insulin-signaling pathways appear to contribute to the multiplicity of insulin's biologic roles in diverse tissues, as well as within the same tissue or cellular unit [123, 141]. Thereby, the signaling pathway responsible for glucose transport may be impaired, producing a state of insulin resistance, while the pathways mediating steroidogenic/mitogenic effects may continue to operate normally [91]. This molecular scenario may pathophysiologically couple ovarian and metabolic dysfunction in PCOS.

One study has demonstrated that insulin-stimulated androgen production in human theca cells from polycystic ovaries involves inositol-glycan mediators rather than the classic tyrosine kinase signaling system [123]. Likewise, insulin-stimulated progesterone production by human granulosa cells does not require the activation of PI3-K, which is the main substrate in metabolic insulin-signaling pathways, [141]. The steroidogenic activity of insulin has been also shown to be independent of extracellular signal receptor kinases (ERK)-1 and -2 in theca and granulosa cells from human ovaries [125, 142].

Another interesting finding was the abnormal pattern of expression of IRS-1 and -2 in follicles from polycystic ovaries [132]. Compared with follicles at a similar developmental stage in normal ovaries, the follicles in polycystic ovaries demonstrated increased intensity of IRS-2 staining in theca and granulosa cells, but reduced IRS-1 staining in granulosa cells. Strikingly, similar defects were detected in follicles from women with gestational diabetes compared with those from women who had uncomplicated pregnancy. These findings suggest that insulin resistance via decreased IRS-1 may selectively affect carbohydrate metabolism in granulosa cells inducing a compensatory increase of IRS-2 expression. Because IRS-2 is considered an antiapoptotic factor, the overexpression of IRS-2 in small antral follicles may suggest its involvement in the accumulation of cysts in the polycystic ovary. Additionally, increased IRS-2 in theca cells may contribute to increased androgen production [132].

Although in vitro findings indicate that insulin retains its ability to stimulate ovarian steroidogenesis in PCOS, an in vivo study in PCOS women has supported that insulin resistance affects not only metabolism, but also granulosa cell steroidogenesis [143]. This discrepancy could imply that hormonal or metabolic factors, which are active in vivo but absent in vitro, contribute to insulin resistance at the ovarian level. In this study, insulin had no effect on E2 responses to recombinant human (rh) FSH (75 IU) in PCOS women with baseline insulin resistance, whereas insulin-sensitizing treatment with pioglitazone restored the enhancing effect of insulin on rhFSH-induced E2 production. In addition to a greater magnitude of response, post-treatment peak levels of E2 were sustained for longer [143].

Overall, insulin may interact with gonadotropins in a dose-dependent manner, thus contributing to the regulation of ovarian function. The balance between insulin and FSH concentrations may be a critical "switch" in granulosa cell steroidogenesis [144]. A similar interaction appears to occur between LH and insulin, so that extremely elevated LH and/or insulin levels tend to distort normal steroidogenesis and follicular growth. However, insulin either through increased levels or through impaired action appears to be a "second hit," rather than the primary cause of anovulation in PCOS [145].

4.4.3 Insulin Action in the Cardiovascular System

Insulin resistance has been linked with cardiovascular aberrations in several insulin-resistant states, including PCOS [146–154]. Beyond metabolic aspects, insulin resistance has been directly associated with biochemical indicators of systemic and vascular inflammation [146–148], as well as dysfibrinolysis [152–154] in women with PCOS.

Most strikingly, insulin resistance has been shown to be an independent determinant of endothelial dysfunction and accelerated atherosclerosis, as determined by biochemical, functional, and morphological markers in women with PCOS [146–159]. Increased serum levels of endothelin-1, the most potent endothelial vasoconstrictor and a marker of endothelial dysfunction, were positively correlated with insulin resistance in women with PCOS across the entire BMI range [152, 154]. In PCOS similar associations have been reported between insulin resistance/hyperinsulinemia and decreased flow mediated dilatation in brachial arteries [146, 154, 157], as well as increased intima media thickness in carotid arteries [158]. These associations were found in obese patients and in lean PCOS women of early reproductive age [146, 154, 157, 158].

Other investigators have also provided pathophysiological insights into the endothelial impact of IR in PCOS. A functional defect in the ex vivo insulin action on resistance arteries from women with PCOS was described [155], which may be coupled with impaired insulin action on glucose metabolism, at least in obese women [156]. In another study, only the insulin-resistant subgroup stratified by HOMA index demonstrated blunted endothelial-dependent vasodilation, impaired endothelial release of tissue—plasminogen activator and sustained elevation of plasminogen activator inhibitor-1 (PAI-1) during insulin infusion, indicative of endothelial dysfunction and hypofibrinolysis [151]. Talbott et al. has provided data pointing to a temporal link of insulin resistance with subsequent subclinical coronary atherosclerosis observed at the 9-yr follow-up [159].

Moreover, insulin resistance/hyperinsulinemia appears to have an adverse impact on myocardiac function. Young women with PCOS were reported to have impaired left ventricular systolic outflow and a non-restrictive type of diastolic dysfunction, both associated with fasting hyperinsulinemia [160, 161]. Other investigators showed an obesity-independent increase in left ventricular mass, which was linearly correlated with insulin resistance in women with PCOS [162, 163]. Increased aldosterone levels reported in women with PCOS may mediate insulin resistance/hyperinsulinemia-related left ventricular hypertrophy and accelerated atheromatosis [164]. Contrariwise the beneficial effects of insulin sensitizers on structural and functional cardiovascular parameters in women with PCOS emphasize the role of IR in cardiovascular risk [157, 165–167].

These findings appear to be an indirect clinical expression of impaired insulin action upon the vasculature. Human endothelial cells possess insulin receptors and in physiological states, insulin binds with its receptor and activates both the PI3K and the MAPK-dependent signaling cascades in the endothelium [87]. Thus, in addition to direct PI3K-dependent metabolic actions of insulin to promote glucose uptake in peripheral tissues, the PI3K-dependent pathway serves to increase blood flow and capillary recruitment under healthy conditions [87]. In insulin-resistant states, like PCOS, the uncoupling between these two signaling pathways appears to govern the pathophysiology of vascular dysfunction. Specifically, in the setting of vascular insulin resistance, the impairment of the PI3K-dependent pathway leads to decreased activation of endothelial nitric oxide synthase and decreased production of nitric oxide (NO). By contrast, increased MAPK signaling, stimulated by hyperinsulinemia, promotes secretion of the vasoconstrictor endothelin-1 (ET-1), increases expression of cell adhesion molecules, including vascular cell adhesion molecule-1 (VCAM) and E-selectin, and activates cation pumps. Taken together, these MAPK-dependent functions contribute to endothelial dysfunction, increased peripheral vascular resistance, hypertension, and accelerated atherosclerosis [87].

Hyperinsulinemia has also sympatho-excitatory actions, and insulin resistance hyperactivates the renin–angiotensin system, promotes distal tubular sodium re-absorption, and inhibits compensatory natriuresis, thereby further contributing to mechanisms of cardiovascular dysfunction in insulin-resistant states [87].

4.5 Insulin Resistance in PCOS: The Aggravating Role of the Endocrine and Inflammatory Milieu

4.5.1 The Role of Androgens

Biochemical hyperandrogenemia is positively associated with measures of insulin resistance in women with PCOS [32]. These clinical findings are suggestive of an influential interrelationship between insulin resistance and hyperandrogenemia. Family studies have shown that in sisters of women with PCOS, insulin resistance is associated with hyperandrogenemia rather than with menstrual dysfunction [168], further suggesting that insulin resistance and hyperandrogenemia may share common pathogenic mechanisms.

Moreover, GnRH-induced suppression of ovarian androgens was accompanied with improved insulin sensitivity in women with PCOS [169]. Studies in PCOS women treated with antiandrogens [170] and in female-to-male transsexuals receiving cross-sex hormone therapy implicate androgens in the perpetuation of insulin resistance [171]. However, not all authors agree with the above outcomes [6, 172]

A potential linkage between IR and ovarian hyperandrogenism is also reflected by the beneficial metabolic effects of laparoscopic ovarian electrocautery (LOE) in women with PCOS. A relevant study showed improved insulin sensitivity in parallel with the reduction of androgen levels in patients who underwent LOE, possibly indicating an interrelationship between androgens and insulin resistance. Interestingly, the same investigators have provided molecular evidence of partial reversal of insulin-signaling defects in visceral adipocytes after LOE in this group of patients with PCOS [108]. Accordingly, insulin responsiveness in adipocytes from amenorrheic women with PCOS was found to be significantly enhanced in parallel with the reduction of testosterone levels after an ovulatory cycle [173].

Androgens may act directly upon the signaling cascade contributing to the impairment of insulin action. In an experimental study, chronic testosterone treatment induced metabolic insulin resistance acting via the androgen receptor in cultured human subcutaneous adipocytes. The signaling defect selectively affected the metabolic pathway of insulin, was independent of PI3K, and involved the impaired phosphorylation of protein kinase Cζ(PKCζ) [174]. Similarly, androgens were shown to induce insulin resistance in cultured rat skeletal myotubes via increased phosphorylation in Akt, mammalian target of rapamycin (mTOR), and ribosomal S6-kinase (S6K), leading to increased Serine 636/639 phosphorylation of IRS-1 [175].

Androgens may also contribute to insulin resistance through their triggering or aggravating role in visceral adiposity. Androgen excess during fetal life and infancy may precipitate the development of abdominal adiposity later in life [50]. In non-human primates, intrauterine exposure to androgen excess leads to phenotypic traits of PCOS accompanied by visceral fat accumulation, insulin resistance, and impaired insulin secretion [50]. Furthermore, the exposure of peripubertal rats to an androgenic milieu has been shown to induce central fat accumulation, deranged metabolic/endocrine function of the adipose tissue and impaired insulin sensitivity [176, 177]. Sex steroids have been also implicated in the modulation of cytokine secretion by adipose tissue in women with PCOS [16, 178–180].

Additionally, testosterone is a potent regulator of lipolysis in adipose tissue. However, this effect appears to rest upon the inhibition of catecholamine-induced lipolysis in subcutaneous adipocytes, independently of the antilipolytic insulin action [181]. In support of these in vitro observations are the findings by Diamanti-Kandarakis et al. [182], showing improvement of lipid profile in lean and obese PCOS women post antiandrogen treatment.

The role of adrenal androgens in PCOS-related insulin resistance is less studied. Few data imply an inverse association between adrenal androgens and disturbed glucose tolerance in PCOS [66]. Acute dehydroepiandrosterone (DHEA) treatment of adipocytes stimulates translocation of the glucose transporter GLUT 4 to the cell surface with resultant increases in glucose uptake [183, 184]. In bovine aortic endothelial cells, DHEA has been also shown to exert nongenomic, insulin-mimicking actions inducing a concomitant stimulation of PI3-K and MAPK-dependent pathways [185]. However, the biologic relevance of these findings to human physiology remains to be explored [185].

4.5.2 The Role of Inflammation, Adipokines, Oxidative Stress

Several studies in women with PCOS have unveiled the bidirectional relationship of insulin resistance with a wide array of inflammatory/oxidative markers, including C-reactive protein (CRP), reactive oxygen species (ROS), interleukin-18, protein cardonyls, soluble CD36, oxidized LDL and AGEs [42, 146, 186–190]. Beyond a simple association, there are data to support a causal, reciprocal relationship between inflammation/oxidative stress and insulin resistance in PCOS [191, 192].

Mononuclear (MNC)-derived macrophages, ubiquitously present in human tissues, appear to hold a driving role in this interplay. Specifically, MNC-derived macrophages from obese patients with PCOS were shown to overproduce ROS and TNF-a, in response to physiologic, postprandial hyperglycemia. [186, 192]. The in vivo setting may differ, since TNF-a serum levels are not consistently increased in PCOS women [193] and hyperinsulinemia during the OGTT suppressed TNFa levels in these women [194]. Nevertheless, dysfunctional macrophages appear to be key players in the cascades of inflammatory and metabolic stress in PCOS [191].

In macrophages from PCOS women, exposed to physiological hyperglycemia, increased nuclear translocation of nuclear factor (NF)κB and its catalytic subunit, p65, was shown to negatively correlate with insulin sensitivity. This response was positively associated with abdominal fat, but not total obesity suggesting that low-grade inflammation is perpetuated by central adiposity contributing to insulin resistance [192].

The migration of macrophages in adipose tissue is a major proinflammatory process that is accentuated in the presence of visceral adiposity [195], the latter being present even in lean patients with PCOS [37, 196, 197]. In the pathophysiologic context of PCOS, visceral adiposity, independently of obesity, has been incriminated as a major trigger of insulin resistance and low-grade chronic inflammation [38, 198, 199]. Nevertheless, the assessment of visceral fat mass with clinical measures, like waist circumference and waist-to-hip ratio may be insensitive to quantify the degree of visceral adiposity and unveil its correlations with other variables.

In states characterized by visceral fat accumulation, the interaction between macrophages and adipocytes appears to perpetuate inflammatory stress and insulin resistance in adipose tissue. Inflammatory cytokines, produced either by adipocytes or by macrophages in adipose tissue, collectively known as adipokines, are pivotal mediators in this process [200–202]. Specifically, macrophage-secreted cytokines were shown to inhibit insulin action in cultured adipocytes via downregulation of GLUT4 and IRS-1, decreased Akt phosphorylation, and impaired insulin-stimulated GLUT4 translocation [88, 201].

Beyond their effects on insulin action in metabolic tissues, mounting evidence suggests that adipokines contribute to vascular dysfunction either directly or through the induction of vascular insulin resistance [203]. In vitro studies unveil the molecular links between excessive/ectopic adiposity, insulin resistance, and endothelial dysfunction. Within this network, adipokines may modulate the balance between endothelium-derived vasodilators and vasoconstrictors, as well as antithrombotic and prothrombotic factors [203].

Adiponectin, the most abundant adipokine mainly secreted from visceral adipocytes cells, has been found to be decreased in lean [204, 205] and obese women with PCOS, as compared with BMI-matched controls [199, 204–210]. Insulin resistance/hyperinsulinemia has been directly associated with this aberration [7, 204, 206, 208, 210], although other investigators have published contradictory data [211]. Among overweight/obese young women with PCOS, adiponectin has been also correlated negatively with the progression of atherosclerotic disease, assessed by IMT [158], although no association was revealed between adiponectin and coronary arterial calcification [212].

Other adipokines, like resistin, retinol-binding protein (RBP)-4, visfatin, have been also studied in women with PCOS. Alterations in serum resistin levels appear to be mostly contingent on total obesity, independently of PCOS [205, 213]. Visfatin has been also reported to be at increased circulating levels in both obese and lean women with PCOS [16, 214]. Circulating visfatin levels were positively correlated with insulin resistance in PCOS women [16]. However, it remains unknown whether increased visfatin in PCOS is a compensatory response to tissue-specific insulin resistance or a marker of tissue-specific inflammation.

The role of RBP4 in PCOS is currently under investigation. RBP-4 may contribute to systemic insulin resistance in humans partly by decreasing insulin-induced IRS1 phosphorylation, as demonstrated by experiments in primary human adipocytes [215]. On the other hand, RBP4 mRNA was down regulated in subcutaneous adipose tissue in obese postmenopausal women, although these women were more insulin resistant than lean and overweight subjects [216]. Thus, the role of RBP-4 in insulin resistance in humans remains to be clarified. Available studies in PCOS patients have yielded inconsistent results, showing increased [217, 218], not significantly different [219, 220] or decreased levels [221] of RBP-4 as compared to the corresponding levels in controls. Furthermore, a substantial quantitative deviation of RBP4 serum levels between these studies was observed. Not all studies have confirmed a positive correlation of RBP-4 levels with insulin resistance assessed by the surrogate HOMA index [219–221]. However, Weiping et al. [217] have documented this correlation, using euglycemic clamp technique, a better method in assessing tissue sensitivity to insulin [72]. Differences in the mean BMI of study populations should be factored in the interpretation of discrepancies. However, three of the above studies restricting their measurements in lean PCOS patients have also reported discordant findings [218, 219, 221]. The methodology used for RBP4 measurements might have interfered in the estimation of serum RBP4 levels. Two of the aforementioned studies have used a competitive enzyme-linked immunoassay (EIAs) [218, 219], one has used a double-sandwich ELISA [221], while quantitative western blotting was used in another study [220]. Of the applied methods, quantitative western blotting is the most reliable one for assaying serum RBP4 elevations associated with insulin resistance [222], whereas the competitive EIAs underestimate serum RBP4 levels in insulin-resistant individuals [222]. Of the commercially available kits, double-sandwich ELISA is considered to be more accurate than the competitive EIAs; however, it may also underestimate the differences between insulin-sensitive and insulin-resistant people [222]. Another potential cause for assay inaccuracy is interference from serum transthyretin (TTR). TTR circulates in a three- to fivefold molar excess over RBP4. Circulating RBP4 is highly bound to TTR in a 1:1 stoichiometric ratio, and there is little or no "free RBP4" in circulation [222]. Using gel filtration chromatography to analyse the RBP4-TTR complex, the increased amount of serum RBP4 was shown to remain bound to TTR in insulin-resistant states. Nevertheless, because the affinity of RBP4-TTR binding is very strong, the relative stoichiometry and affinity of the two proteins in serum could conceivably influence kinetics of RBP4-antibody binding under the non-denaturing conditions employed by the commercial EIAs and ELISAs [222]. Therefore, the ratio RBP4/TTR may be a more accurate marker for RBP-4 circulating levels than absolute RBP-4 levels. To date, only one study has determined this marker in PCOS women showing that the RBP4 to TTR ratio is lower in lean patients as compared to that in lean controls [221].

Another group of molecules, advanced glycated end products (AGEs), known for their role in inflammatory and oxidative pathways [41], were found to be distinctly elevated in women with PCOS [42, 43]. Several data show that the interaction of AGEs with their receptor, RAGE impairs insulin signaling in a dual mode, through the direct stimulation of serine kinases [228] and through the NADPH oxidase-mediated generation of ROS [41]. Additionally, endogenous AGEs, partly deriving from dietary glycotoxins, act directly upon the endothelium to promote endothelial dysfunction [223]. On these grounds, increased serum AGEs levels in young normoglycemic women with PCOS prompts medical concern over the implications of this aberration for cardiometabolic and possibly for reproductive function [224, 225].

4.6 Genetics of Insulin Resistance in PCOS

Studies showing impaired insulin action in women with PCOS and the clustering of reminiscent abnormalities in PCOS families prompted research on the genetic basis of insulin resistance in PCOS and the role of genetics in the pathogenesis of the whole syndrome [61, 168]. Metabolic abnormalities of PCOS are tightly associated with hyperandrogenemia in female first-degree relatives, suggesting that these findings are causally related, reflect a common pathogenesis (e.g. same gene product), or are due to perturbations of genes within the same pathway [168].

Studies on the molecular aspects of PCOS and knowledge of the genetic origins of T2D have directed genetic research to specific areas of the genome [48, 49]. Candidate genes are those encoding proteins, which directly participate in the insulin-signaling pathway, as well as other proteins that co-modulate insulin action or secretion.

The insulin receptor gene has been a major target for research. An association of PCOS with a C/T single nucleotide polymorphism (SNP) in the tyrosine kinase domain of *the insulin receptor gene* was described [227]. A candidate susceptibility locus is the D19S884 allele A8, which maps to intron 55 of the fibrillin 3 gene, near the insulin receptor gene, on the chromosome 19p13.2. A8 of D19S884 was identified in association with the reproductive phenotype of PCOS and most recently, it was also associated with higher fasting insulin levels and HOMA-IR in women with PCOS, independently of obesity [228–230].

SNPs in genes encoding the IRS proteins have been also implicated in PCOS. An association of the Gly972Arg IRS1 variant with fasting insulin and HOMA values was described [231], whereas the Asp1057 IRS-2 variant was associated with increased insulin levels after an oral glucose load and an increased prevalence of IGT among women with PCOS [231]. However, a larger series showed the opposite effect of the Gly1057Asp IRS-2 polymorphism on glucose tolerance and no effect of the Gly972Arg IRS-1 polymorphism [232].

Other investigators have sought for polymorphisms in the *variable number tandem repeat* (VNTR) locus at the insulin gene (INS), known to regulate gene expression [233]. Waterworth *et al.* [234] found strong association between PCOS and the class III VNTR allele [157 repeats]. This allele was preferentially transmitted from heterozygous fathers, whereas maternal transmission was less frequent. However, other studies [235–237] failed to show any linkage between the INS VNTR alleles and hyperandrogenism or PCOS.

The 112/121 haplotype of the Calpain-10(CAPN10) gene, a cysteine protease modulating insulin secretion and action, has been associated with hyperinsulinemia in African–American women and an increased risk of PCOS in both African–American and White women [238]. Gonzalez *et al.* [239, 240] showed an association of the CAPN10 UCSNP-44 allele with PCOS in a Spanish population, whereas Haddad *et al.* [241] found no association between CAPN10 gene variation and PCOS. The common SNP Ala12 in the peroxisome proliferator-activated receptor-γ2 (PPAR-γ2) gene has been also studied in women with PCOS. Although its frequency was marginally significantly decreased in Finnish PCOS patients [242], no association was found in hyperandrogenic adolescents or PCOS women from other ethnic regions [243, 244].

Based on the role of oxidative stress in the perpetuation of insulin resistance, another study has explored potential polymorphisms in the gene encoding paraoxonase-1 (PON1), a serum high-density lipoprotein (HDL)-associated enzyme with antioxidant properties. Since the -108T alleles are associated with reduced PON1 expression, homozygosity for –108T alleles in PCOS women might be associated with an impairment of antioxidant mechanisms. This abnormality favoring oxidative stress may contribute to insulin resistance [244].

Available data add important information regarding the genetic background of insulin resistance in PCOS raising the possibility of multiple genetic components being involved. The elucidation of the genetics of insulin resistance and the identification of specific genes, related to PCOS are hampered by the heterogeneity in pathogenesis, the absence of pathognomonic clinical features, and the inadequate sample of studied populations. Although the current state of genetic studies seems rather discouraging, new tools investigating the genetic machinery and large well-defined pedigrees may facilitate and focus the analysis of this genetically complex disorder.

4.7 Conclusions

The prevailing concept is that PCOS is a polygenic trait that might result from the interaction of predisposing and protective genetic variants under the influence of environmental factors. PCOS is now recognized as a female subtype of the metabolic syndrome. The two major facets of metabolic syndrome, insulin resistance, and the compensatory hyperinsulinemia, are pathophysiologic denominators of cardiometabolic and reproductive abnormalities in PCOS. Metabolic disturbances, low-grade inflammation, and increased markers of oxidative stress have been all linked with insulin resistance in women with PCOS. It is well established that women diagnosed with PCOS, even at their twenties, demonstrate a cluster of metabolic and cardiovascular disturbances. There is also evidence that the impact of metabolic aberrations in PCOS may start earlier, in childhood or even in intrauterine life. It remains to be proved whether treatment or early management of insulin resistance will have a protective effect on the multifaceted spectrum of PCOS abnormalities.

References

1. Dunaif A. Insulin resistance and the polycystic ovary syndrome: mechanism and implications for pathogenesis. Endocr Rev 1997;18:774–800
2. Poretsky L, Cataldo N, Rosenwaks Z, Giudice L. The insulin-related ovarian regulatory system in health and disease. Endocr Rev 1999;20: 535–82
3. Diamanti-Kandarakis E. and Papavasiliou A. Molecular mechanisms of insulin resistance in polycystic ovary syndrome Trends Mol Med 2006;12:324–32
4. Dunaif A, Segal KR, Futterweit W, Dobrjansky A. Profound peripheral insulin resistance, independent of obesity, in polycystic ovary syndrome. Diabetes 1989; 38:1165–74
5. Dunaif A, Finegood DT. β-Cell dysfunction independent of obesity and glucose intolerance in the polycystic ovary syndrome. J Clin Endocrinol Metab 1996; 81:942–47
6. Diamanti-Kandarakis E, Mitrakou A, Hennes MM, Platanissiotis D, Kaklas N, Spina J, Georgiadou E, Hoffmann RG, Kissebah AH, Raptis S. Insulin sensitivity and antiandrogenic therapy in women with polycystic ovary syndrome. Metabolism 1995; 44(4):525–31
7. Ducluzeau P, Cousin P, Malvoisin E, Bornet H, Vidal H, Laville M, Pugeat M. Glucose-to-Insulin Ratio Rather than Sex Hormone-Binding Globulin and Adiponectin Levels Is the Best Predictor of Insulin Resistance in Nonobese Women with Polycystic Ovary Syndrome J Clin Endocrinol Metab 2003; 88(8):3626–31
8. Fulgeshu A, Angioni S, Portoghese E, Milano F, Batetta B, Paoletti A, Melis G. Failure of the homeostatic model assessment calculation score for detecting metabolic deterioration in young patients with polycystic ovary syndrome Fertil Steril 2006; 86:398–404.
9. Palomba S, Falbo A, Russo T, Manguso F, Tolino A, Zullo F, De Feo P, Orio F Jr. Insulin sensitivity after metformin suspension in normal-weight women with polycystic ovary syndrome. J Clin Endocrinol Metab 2007; 92(8):3128–35
10. Healds A, Whitehead S, Anderson S, Cruickshank K, Riste L, Laing I, Rudenski A, Buckler H. Screening for insulin resistance in women with polycystic ovarian Syndrome Gyn Endocrinol 2005; 20(2): 84–91
11. Micic D, Sumarac-Dumanovic M, Kendereski A, Cvijovic G, Zoric S, Pejkovic D, Micic J, Milic N, Dieguez C, Casanueva F. Total ghrelin levels during acute insulin infusion in patients with polycystic ovary syndrome J Endocrinol Invest 2007; 30: 820–27
12. Legro RS, Finegood D, Dunaif A. A fasting glucose to insulin ratio is a useful measure of insulin sensitivity in women with polycystic ovary syndrome J Clin Endocrinol Metab 1998; 83:2694–98
13. Jayagopal V, Kilpatrick ES, Holding PE, Jennings PE, Hepburn DA, Atkin SL. The biological variation of insulin resistance in polycystic ovarian syndrome J Clin Endocrinol Metab 2002; 87:1560–62
14. Park KH, Kim JY, Ahn CW, Song YD, Lim SK, Lee HC. Polycystic ovarian syndrome (PCOS) and insulin resistance Int J Gynecol Obstetr 2001; 74(3):261–67
15. de Paula Martins W, Santana LF, Nastri CO, Ferriani RA, de Sa MF, Dos Reis RM. Agreement among insulin sensitivity indexes on the diagnosis of insulin resistance in polycystic ovary syndrome and ovulatory women Eur J Obstet Gynecol Reprod Biol 2007; 133(2):203–7
16. Kowalska I, Straczkowski M, Nikolajuk A, Adamska A, Karczewska-Kupczewska M, Otziomek E, Wolczynski S and Gorska M Serum visfatin in relation to insulin resistance and markers of hyperandrogenism in lean and obese women with polycystic ovary syndrome Hum Reprod 2007; 22(7):1824–29
17. Vrbikova J, Bendlova B, Hill M, Vankova M, Vondra K, Starka L. Insulin sensitivity and beta-cell function in women with polycystic ovary syndrome. Diabetes Care 2002; 25:1217–22
18. Ovesen P, Moller J, Ingerslev HJ, Jorgensen JO, Mengel A, Schmitz O, Alberti KG, Moller N. Normal basal and insulin-stimulated fuel metabolism in lean women with the polycystic ovary syndrome. J Clin Endocrinol Metab 1993; 77(6): 1636–40
19. Vrbikova J, Cibula D, Dvorakova K, Stanicka S, Sindelka G, Hill M, Fanta M, Vondra K, Skrha J. Insulin sensitivity in women with polycystic ovary syndrome. J Clin Endocrinol Metab 2004; 89:2942–45
20. Ciampelli M, Fulghesu AM, Cucinelli F, Pavone V, Caruso A, Mancuso S, Lanzone A Heterogeneity in β-cell activity, hepatic insulin clearance and peripheral insulin sensitivity in women with polycystic ovary syndrome. Hum Reprod 1997; 12:1897–1901
21. Gennarelli G, Rovei V, Novi R, Holte J, Bongioanni F, Revelli A, Pacini G, Cavallo-Perin P, Massobrio M. Preserved insulin sensitivity and β-cell activity, but decreased glucose effectiveness in normal-weight women with the polycystic ovary syndrome. J Clin Endocrinol Metab 2005; 90:3381–86
22. Vigil P, Contreras P, Alvarado J, Godoy A, Salgado A, Cortes M. Evidence of subpopulations with different levels of insulin resistance in women with polycystic ovary syndrome Hum Reprod 2007; 22:2974–80
23. Ciampelli M, Leoni F, Cucinelli F, et al. Assessment of insulin sensitivity from measurements in the fasting state and during an oral glucose tolerance test in polycystic ovary syndrome and menopausal patients. J Clin Endocrinol Metab 2005; 90: 1398–406
24. Carmina E, Lobo R. Use of fasting blood to assess the prevalence of insulin resistance in women with polycystic ovary syndrome. Fertil Steril 2004; 82:661–65

25. DeUgarte CM, Bartolucci AA, Azziz R. Prevalence of insulin resistance in the polycystic ovary syndrome using the homeostasis model assessment. Fertil Steril 2005; 83(5):1454–60
26. Carmina E, Longo RA, Rini GB, Lobo RA. Phenotypic variation in hyperandrogenic women influences the finding of abnormal metabolic and cardiovascular risk parameters. J Clin Endocrinol Metabol 2005; 90:2545–49
27. McLaughlin T, Allison G, Abbasi F, Lamendola C, Reaven G. Prevalence of insulin resistance and associated cardiovascular disease risk factors among normal weight, overweight, and obese individuals. Metabolism 2004; 53(4):495–99
28. Morin-Papunen LC, Vauhkonen I, Koivunen RM, Ruokonen A, Tapanainen JS. Insulin sensitivity, insulin secretion, and metabolic and hormonal parameters in healthy women and women with polycystic ovarian syndrome. Hum Reprod 2000; 15(6):1266–74
29. Zawadski JK, Dunaif A. Diagnostic criteria for polycystic ovary syndrome: towards a rational approach. In: Polycystic Ovary Syndrome (Dunaif, A. et al., eds; Hershman, S.M., series ed.), Current Issues in Endocrinology and Metabolism, Blackwell Scientific Publications, Boston, 1992
30. The Rotterdam ESHRE ASRM-sponsored PCOS Consensus Workshop Group Revised 2003 consensus on diagnostic criteria and long-term health risks related to polycystic ovary syndrome. Fertil Steril 2004; 81:19–25
31. Azziz R, Carmina E, Dewailly D, Diamanti-Kandarakis E, Escobar-Morreale HF, Futterweit W, Janssen OE, Legro RS, Norman RJ, Taylor AE, Witchel SF, Androgen Excess Society Position statement: criteria for defining polycystic ovary syndrome as a predominantly hyperandrogenic syndrome: an Androgen Excess Society guideline. J Clin Endocrinol Metab 2006; 91:4237–45
32. Diamanti-Kandarakis E, Panidis D. Unravelling the phenotypic map of polycystic ovaries syndrome (PCOS): a prospective study of 634 women with PCOS. Clin Endocrinol 2007; 67:735–42
33. Barber TM, Wass JA, McCarthy MI, Franks S. Metabolic characteristics of women with polycystic ovaries and oligo-amenorrhoea but normal androgen levels: implications for the management of polycystic ovary syndrome. Clin Endocrinol (Oxf) 2007; 66(4):513–17
34. Amato MC, Galluzzo A, Finocchiaro S, Criscimanna A, Giordano C. The evaluation of metabolic parameters and insulin sensitivity for a more robust diagnosis of the polycystic ovary syndrome. Clin Endocrinol (Oxf) 2008; 69(1):52–60
35. Norman RJ, Davies MJ, Lord J, Moran LJ. The role of lifestyle modification in polycystic ovary syndrome. Trends Endocrinol Metab 2002; 13(6):251–57
36. Yildiz BO, Knochenhauer ES, Azziz R. Impact of obesity on the risk for polycystic ovary syndrome. J Clin Endocrinol Metab 2008; 93(1):162–8
37. Escobar-Morreale H, San Millan J. Abdominal adiposity and the polycystic ovary syndrome Trends in Endocrinol Metabol 2007; 18(7):266–72
38. Lord J, Thomas R, Fox B, Acharya U, Wilkin T The central issue? Visceral fat mass is a good marker of insulin resistance and metabolic disturbance in women with polycystic ovary syndrome. BJOG 2006; 113(10):1203–9
39. Kahn S, Hull R, Utzschneider K. Mechanisms linking obesity to insulin resistance and type 2 diabetes Nature 2006; 444(14):840–46
40. Carmina E, Legro RS, Stamets K, Lowell J, Lobo RA. Difference in body weight between American and Italian women with polycystic ovary syndrome. Human Reprod 2003; 11:2289–93
41. Vlassara H. Advanced glycation in health and disease: role of the modern environment Ann NY Acad Sci 2005; 1043: 452–60
42. Diamanti-Kandarakis E, Piperi C, Kalofoutis A and Creatsas G Increased levels of serum advanced glycation end-products in women with polycystic ovary syndrome Clin Endocrinol 2005; 62:37–43
43. Diamanti-Kandarakis E, Katsikis I, Piperi C, Kandaraki E, Piouka A, Papavassiliou AG, Panidis D. Increased serum Advanced Glycation End products is a distinct finding in lean women with PCOS. Clin Endocrinol (Oxf) 2008; 69(4): 634–41
44. Knochenhauer ES, Key TJ, Kahsar-Miller M, Waggoner W, Boots LR, Azziz R. Prevalence of the polycystic ovary syndrome in unselected black and white women of the southeastern United States: a prospective study. J Clin Endocrinol Metab 1998; 83(9):3078–82
45. Azziz R, Woods KS, Reyna R, Key TJ, Knochenhauer ES, Yildiz BO The prevalence and features of the polycystic ovary syndrome in an unselected population. J Clin Endocrinol Metab 2004; 89:2745–49
46. Diamanti Kandarakis E, Piperi C, Spina J, Argyrakopoulou G, Papanastasiou L, Bergiele A, Panidis D. Polycystic ovary syndrome: the influence of environmental and genetic factors. Hormones (Athens) 2006; 5:17–34
47. Sir Petermann T, Maliqueo M, Codner E, Echibur B, Crisosto N, Ptrez V, Ptrez-Bravo F, Cassorla F. Early metabolic derangements in daughters of women with PCOS J Clin Endocrin Metab 2007; 92(12):4637–42
48. Diamanti-Kandarakis E, Piperi C. Genetics of polycystic ovary syndrome: searching for the way out of the labyrinth. Hum Reprod Update 2005; 11: 631–43
49. Escobar-Morreale H, Luque-Ramirez M, San Millan J. The molecular-genetic basis of functional hyperandrogenism and the polycystic ovary syndrome. Endocr Rev 2005; 26F:251–82
50. Abbott DH, Barnett DK, Bruns CM, Dumesic DA. Androgen excess fetal programming of female reproduction: a developmental aetiology for polycystic ovary syndrome? Hum Reprod Update. 2005; 11(4):357–74
51. Kahsar-Miller MD, Nixon C, Boots LR, Go RC, Azziz R. Prevalence of polycystic ovary syndrome (PCOS) in first-degree relatives of patients with PCOS. Fertil Steril 2001; 75(1):53–8

52. Diamanti-Kandarakis E, Kouli CR, Bergiele AT, Filandra FA, Tsianateli TC, Spina GG, Zapanti ED, Bartzis MI. A survey of the polycystic ovary syndrome in the Greek island of Lesbos: hormonal and metabolic profile. J Clin Endocrinol Metab 1999; 84:4006–11
53. Ehrmann D, Kasza K, Azziz R, Legro R, Ghazzi M. Effects of Race and Family History of Type 2 Diabetes on Metabolic Status of Women with Polycystic Ovary Syndrome. J Clin Endocrinol Metab 2005; 90(1):66–71
54. Sir-Petermann T, Angel B, Maliqueo M, Carvajal F, Santos JL, Perez-Bravo F. Prevalence of type II diabetes mellitus and insulin resistance in parents of women with polycystic ovary syndrome. Diabetologia 2002; 45:959–64
55. Yildiz BO, Yarali H, Oguz H, Bayraktar M. Glucose intolerance, insulin resistance, and hyperandrogenemia in first degree relatives of women with polycystic ovary syndrome. J Clin Endocrinol Metab 2003; 88:2031–36
56. Vrbíková J, Grimmichová T, Dvoráková K, Hill M, Stanická S, Vondra K. Family history of diabetes mellitus determines insulin sensitivity and beta cell function in polycystic ovary syndrome. Physiol Res 2008; 57(4):547–53
57. Jackson S, Bagstaff S, Lynn S, Yeaman S, Turnbull D, Walker M. Decreased Insulin Responsiveness of Glucose Uptake in Cultured Human Skeletal Muscle Cells From Insulin-Resistant Nondiabetic Relatives of Type 2 Diabetic Families. Diabetes 2000; 49:1169–77
58. Axelsen M, Smith U, Eriksson JW, Taskinen M-R, Jansson P-A. Postprandial hypertriglyceridemia and insulin resistance in normoglycemic first-degree relatives of patients with type 2 diabetes. Ann Intern Med 1999; 131:27–31
59. Yilmaz M, Bukan N, Ersoy R, Karakoc A, Yetkin I, Ayvaz G, et al. Glucose intolerance, insulin resistance and cardiovascular risk factors in first degree relatives of women with polycystic ovary syndrome. Hum Reprod 2005; 20:2411–20.
60. Unlühızarcı K, Özocak M, Tanrıverdi F, Atmaca H and Kelestimur F. Investigation of hypothalamo-pituitary-gonadal axis and glucose intolerance among the first-degree female relatives of women with polycystic ovary syndrome Fertil Steril 2007; 87:1377–82
61. Diamanti-Kandarakis E, Alexandraki K, Bergiele A. Presence of metabolic risk factors in non-obese PCOS sisters: Evidence of heritability of insulin resistance. J Endocrinol Invest. 2004; 27:931–36
62. Dunaif A, Book CB, Schenker E, Tang Z. Excessive insulin receptor serine phosphorylation in cultured fibroblasts and in skeletal muscle. A potential mechanism for insulin resistance in the polycystic ovary syndrome. J Clin Invest 1995; 96:801–10
63. Colilla S, Cox NJ, Ehrmann DA. Heritability of insulin secretion and insulin action in women with polycystic ovary syndrome and their first degree relatives. J Clin Endocrinol Metab 2001; 86:2027–31
64. Salley K, Wickham E, Cheang K, Essah P, Karjane N, Nestler J. Position statement: Glucose Intolerance in Polycystic Ovary Syndrome—A Position Statement of the Androgen Excess Society J Clin Endocrinol Metab 2007; 92:4546–56
65. Ehrmann DA, Sturis J, Byrne MM, Karrison T, Rosenfield RL, Polonksy KS. Insulin secretory defects in polycystic ovary syndrome. Relationship to insulin sensitivity and family history of non-insulin-dependent diabetes mellitus. J Clin Invest 1995; 96:520–27
66. Altuntas Y, Bilir M, Ucak S, Gundogdu S. Reactive hypoglycemia in lean young women with PCOS and correlations with insulin sensitivity and with beta cell function. Eur J Obstet Gynecol Reprod Biol. 2005; 119:198–205
67. Samaras K, McElduff A, Twigg S, Proietto J, Prins J, Welborn T, Zimmet P, Chisholm D, Campbell L Insulin levels in insulin resistance: phantom of the metabolic opera? Med J Aust 2006; 185(3):159–61
68. American Diabetes Association Consensus Development Conference on Insulin Resistance; 5–6 November 1997. Diabetes Care 1998; 21:310–14
69. Cibula D, Skrha J, Hill M, Fanta M, Haaková L, Vrblková J, Zivný J. Prediction of insulin sensitivity in nonobese women with polycystic ovary syndrome. J Clin Endocrinol Metab 2002; 87(12):5821–25
70. Rabasa-Lhoret R, Bastard JP, Jan V, Ducluzeau PH, Andreelli F, Guebre F, Bruzeau J, Louche-Pellissier C, Maltrepierre C, Peyrat J, Chagné J, Vidal H, Laville M. Modified quantitative insulin sensitivity check index is better correlated to hyper-insulinemic glucose clamp than other fasting-based index of insulin sensitivity in different insulin-resistant states. J Clin Endocrinol Metab 2003; 88(10):4917–23
71. Skrha J, Haas T, Sindelka G, Prázný M, Widimský J, Cibula D, Svacina S. Comparison of the insulin action parameters from hyperinsulinemic clamps with homeostasis model assessment and QUICKI indexes in subjects with different endocrine disorders. J Clin Endocrinol Metab 2004; 89(1):135–41
72. Diamanti-Kandarakis E, Kouli C, Alexandraki K, Spina G. Failure of mathematical indices to accurately assess insulin resistance in lean, overweight, or obese women with polycystic ovary syndrome. J Clin Endocrinol Metab 2004; 89:1273–76
73. Marcovina S, Bowsher RR, Miller WG, Staten M, Myers G, Caudill SP, Campbell SE, Steffes MW. For the insulin standardization workgroup standardization of insulin immunoassays: report of the American Diabetes Association workgroup. Clinical Chemistry 2007; 53:711–716
74. Stumvoll M, Mitrakou A, Pimenta W, Jenssen T, Yki-Jarvinen H, Van Haeften T, Renn W, Gerich J. Use of the oral glucose tolerance test to assess insulin release and insulin sensitivity. Diabetes Care 2000; 23(3):295–301
75. Matsuda M, DeFronzo RA. Insulin sensitivity indices obtained from oral glucose tolerance testing: comparison with the euglycemic insulin clamp. Diabetes Care 1999; 22:1462–70
76. Cagnacci A, Arangino S, Renzi A, Cagnacci P, Volpe A. Insulin sensitivity in women: a comparison among values derived from intravenous glucose tolerance tests with different sampling frequency, oral glucose tolerance test or fasting Eur J Endocrinol 2001; 145:281–87
77. Quon MJ. Limitations of the fasting glucose to insulin ratio as an index of insulin sensitivity. J Clin Endocrinol Metab 2001; 86:4615–17

78. Abassi F, Reaven GM. Evaluation of the quantitative insulin sensitivity check index as an estimate of insulin sensitivity in humans. Metabolism 2002; 51:235–37
79. Bacha F, Saad R, Gungor N, Janosky J, Arslanian SA. Obesity, regional fat distribution, and syndrome X in obese black versus white adolescents: race differential in diabetogenic and atherogenic risk factors. J Clin Endocrinol Metab 2003; 88(6): 2534–40
80. Ehtisham S, Crabtree N, Clark P, Shaw N, Barrett T. Ethnic Differences in Insulin Resistance and Body Composition in United Kingdom Adolescents J Clin Endocrinol Metab 2005; 90(7):3963–69
81. Whincup PH, Gilg JA, Papacosta O, Seymour C, Miller GJ, Alberti KG, Cook DG. Early evidence of ethnic differences in cardiovascular risk: cross sectional comparison of British South Asian and white children. BMJ 2002; 324:635
82. Wijeyaratne CN, Balen AH, Barth JH, Belchetz PE. Clinical manifestations and insulin resistance (IR) in polycystic ovary syndrome (PCOS) among South Asians and Caucasians: is there a difference? Clin Endocrinol 2002; 57:343–50
83. Kauffman VM, Baker P, Dimarino T, Gimpel VD. Castracane, Polycystic ovarian syndrome and insulin resistance in white and Mexican American women: a comparison of two distinct populations, Am J Obstet Gynecol 2002; 187:1362–69
84. Dunaif A, Sorbara L, Delson R, Green G. Ethnicity and polycystic ovary syndrome are associated with independent and additive decreases in insulin action in Caribbean-Hispanic women. Diabetes 1993; 42:1462–68
85. Willis D, Franks S. Insulin action in human granulosa cells from normal and polycystic ovaries is mediated by the insulin receptor and not the type-I insulin-like growth factor receptor. J Clin Endocrinol Metab 1995; 80:3788–90
86. Samoto T, Maruo T, Ladines-Llave CA, Matsuo H, Deguchi J, Barnea ER, Mochizuki M. Insulin receptor expression in follicular and stromal compartments of the human ovary over the course of follicular growth, regression and atresia. Endocr J 1993; 40:715–26
87. Muniyappa R, Montagnani M, Koh KK, Quon MJ. Cardiovascular actions of insulin. Endocr Rev 2007; 28(5):463–91
88. Mlinar B, Marc J, Janež A, Pfeifer M. Molecular mechanisms of insulin resistance and associated diseases. Clin Chim Acta 2007; 375:20–35
89. Buchs A, Chagag P, Weiss M, Kish E, Levinson R, Aharoni D, Rapoport MJ. Normal p21Ras/MAP kinase pathway expression and function in PBMC from patients with polycystic ovary disease Int J Mol Med 2004; 13:595–99
90. Ciaraldi TP, Morales AJ, Hickman MG, Odom-Ford R, Yen SS, Olefsky JM. Lack of insulin resistance in fibroblasts from subjects with polycystic ovary syndrome. Metabolism 1998; 47:940–46
91. Poretsky L. Commentary: polycystic ovary syndrome – increased or preserved ovarian sensitivity to insulin? J Clin Endocrinol Metab 2006; 91:2859–60
92. Book CB, Dunaif A. Selective insulin resistance in the polycystic ovary syndrome. J Clin Endocrinol Metab 1999; 84: 3110–16
93. Venkatesan AM, Dunaif A, Corbould A. Insulin resistance in polycystic ovary syndrome: progress and paradoxes. Recent Prog Horm Res 2001; 56:295–308
94. Rice S, Christoforidis N, Gadd C, Nikolaou D, Seyani L, Donaldson A, Margara R, Hardy K, Franks S. Impaired insulin-dependent glucose metabolism in granulosa-lutein cells from anovulatory women with polycystic ovaries Hum. Reprod 2005; 20(2):373–81
95. Dunaif A, Wu X, Lee A, Diamanti-Kandarakis E. Defects in insulin receptor signaling in vivo in the polycystic ovary syndrome (PCOS). Am J Physiol Endocrinol Metab 2001; 281:E392–E399
96. Corbould A, Kim Y-B, Youngren JF, Pender C, Kahn BB, Lee A, Dunaif A. Insulin resistance in the skeletal muscle of women with PCOS involves intrinsic and acquired defects in insulin signaling. Am J Physiol Endocrinol Metab 2005; 288: E1047–E1054
97. Corbould A, Zhao H, Mirzoeva S, Aird F, Dunaif A. Enhanced mitogenic signaling in skeletal muscle of women with polycystic ovary syndrome. Diabetes 2006; 55:751–59
98. Skov V, Glintborg D, Knudsen S, Jensen T, Kruse T, Tan Q, Brusgaard K, Beck-Nielsen H, Højlund K. Reduced Expression of Nuclear-Encoded Genes Involved in Mitochondrial Oxidative Metabolism in Skeletal Muscle of Insulin-Resistant Women With Polycystic Ovary Syndrome. Diabetes 2007; 56:2349–55
99. Orio F Jr, Giallauria F, Palomba S, Cascella T, Manguso F, Vuolo L, Russo T, Tolino A, Lombardi G, Colao A, Vigorito C. Cardiopulmonary impairment in young women with polycystic ovary syndrome. J Clin Endocrinol Metab 2006; 91:2967–71
100. Mootha VK, Lindgren CM, Eriksson KF, et al. PGC-1alpha-responsive genes involved in oxidative phosphorylation are coordinately downregulated in human diabetes. Nat Genet 2003; 34:267–73
101. Ciaraldi TP, el-Roeiy A, Madar Z, Reichart D, Olefsky JM, Yen SS. Cellular mechanisms of insulin resistance in polycystic ovarian syndrome. J ClinEndocrinol Metab 1992; 75:577–583
102. Dunaif A, Segal KR, Shelley DR, Green G, Dobrjansky A, Licholai T. Evidence for distinctive and intrinsic defects in insulin action in polycystic ovary syndrome. Diabetes 1992; 41:1257–1266
103. Marsden PJ, Murdoch A, Taylor R Severe impairment of insulin action in adipocytes from amenorrheic subjects with polycystic ovary syndrome. Metabolism 1994; 43(12):1536–42
104. Lystedt E, Westergren H, Brynhildsen J, Lindh-Astrand L, Gustavsson J, Nystrom F, Hammar M, Stralfors P. Subcutaneous adipocytes from obese hyperinsulinemic women with polycystic ovary syndrome exhibit normal insulin sensitivity but reduced maximal insulin responsiveness. Eur J Endocrinol 2005; 153:831–35
105. Mor E, Zograbyan A, Saadat P, Bayrak A, Tourgeman D, Zhang C, Stanczyk F, Paulson R. The insulin resistant subphenotype of polycystic ovary syndrome: clinical parameters and pathogenesis Am J Obstet Gynecol 2004; 190:1654–60

106. Goodarzi MO, Antoine HJ, Pall M, Cui J, Guo X, Azziz R. Preliminary evidence of glycogen synthase kinase 3 beta as a genetic determinant of the polycystic ovary syndrome Fertil Steril 2007; 87:1473–76
107. Rosenbaum D, Haber RS, Dunaif A. Insulin resistance in PCOS:decreased expression of GLUT-4 glucose transporters in adipocytes. Am J Physiol 1993; 264(2 Pt 1):E197–202
108. Seow KM, Juan CC, Hsu YP, Hwang JL, Huang LW, Ho LT. Amelioration of insulin resistance in women with PCOS via reduced insulin receptor substrate-1 Ser312 phosphorylation following laparoscopic ovarian electrocautery Hum Reprod 2007; 22(4):1003–10
109. Corton M, Botella-Carretero JI, Benguría A, Villuendas G, Zaballos A, San Millán JL, Escobar-Morreale HF, Peral B. Differential gene expression profile in omental adipose tissue in women with polycystic ovary syndrome. J Clin Endocrinol Metab 2007; 92:328–337
110. Rosenfield R. Identifying Children at Risk for Polycystic Ovary Syndrome. J Clin Endocrinol Metab 2007; 92:787–96
111. Altuntas Y, Bilir M, Ozturk B. Comparison of various simple insulin sensitivity and β-cell function indices in lean hyperandrogenemic and normoandrogenemic young hirsute women. Fertil Steril 2003; 80:133–42
112. Pasquali R, Gambineri A, Pagotto U. The impact of obesity on reproduction in women with polycystic ovary syndrome. BJOG 2006; 113:1148–1159.
113. Baillargeon JP, Carpentier A. Role of insulin in the hyperandrogenemia of lean women with polycystic ovary syndrome and normal insulin sensitivity. Fertil Steril 2007; 88:886–93
114. Codner E, Escobar-Morreale HF. Hyperandrogenism and Polycystic Ovary Syndrome (PCOS) in Women with Type 1 Diabetes Mellitus. J Clin Endocrin Metab 2007; 92(4):1209–16
115. Huber-Buchholz MM, Carey DGP, Norman RJ. Restoration of reproductive potential by lifestyle modification in obese polycystic ovary syndrome: role of insulin sensitivity and luteinizing hormone. J Clin Endocrinol Metab 1999; 84:1470–74
116. Kiddy DS, Hamilton-Fairley D, Bush A, Short F, Anyaoku V, Reed MJ, Franks S. Improvement in endocrine and ovarian function during dietary treatment of obese women with polycystic ovary syndrome. Clin Endocrinol 1992; 36:105–11
117. Nestler JE, Jakubowicz DJ. Decreases in ovarian cytochrome p450c17a activity and serum free testosterone after reduction ofinsulin secretion in polycystic ovary syndrome. N Engl J Med 1996; 335:617–23
118. Diamanti-Kandarakis E, Kouli C, Tsianateli T, Bergiele A. Therapeutic effects of metformin on insulin resistance and hyperandrogenism in polycystic ovary syndrome. Eur J Endocrinol 1998; 138:269–74
119. Ryan CS, Nestler JE. Insulin-Sensitizing Drugs for the Treatment of Infertility in Polycystic Ovary Syndrome In Insulin resistance and polycystic ovarian syndrome: pathogenesis, evaluation and treatment. (Diamanti-Kandarakis, E. et al., eds), pp. 433–4747, Insulin Resistance and Polycystic Ovarian Syndrome:Edited by Evanthia Diamanti-Kandarakis, John Nestler, Dimitrios Panidis, Renato Pasquali Humana Press 2007
120. Ciotta L, Calogero AE, Farina M, De Leo V, la Marca A, Cianci A. Clinical, endocrine and metabolic effects of acarbose, an α-glucosidase inhibitor, in PCOS patients with increased insulin response and normal glucose tolerance. Hum Reprod 2001; 16:2066–72
121. Attia GR, Rainey WE, Carr BR. Metformin directly inhibits androgen production in human thecal cells. Fertil Steril 2001; 76:517–24
122. Seto-Young D, Paliou M, Schlosser J, Avtanski D, Park A, Patel P, Holcomb K, Chang P, Poretsky L. Direct thiazolidinedione action in the human ovary: insulin-independent and insulin-sensitizing effects on steroidogenesis and insulin-like growth factor binding protein-1 production. J Clin Endocrinol Metab 2005; 90:6099–105
123. Nestler JE, Jakubowicz DJ, de Vargas AF, Brik C, Quintero N, Medina F. Insulin stimulates testosterone biosynthesis by human thecal cells from women with polycystic ovary syndrome by activating its own receptor and using inositolglycan mediators as the signal transduction system. J Clin Endocrinol Metab 1998; 83:2001–5
124. Zhang G, Garmey JC, Veldhuis JD. Interactive stimulation by luteinizing hormone and insulin of the steroidogenic acute regulatory (StAR) protein and 17a-hydroxylase/17,20-lyase (CYP17) genes in porcine theca cells. Endocrinology 2000; 141:2735–42
125. Munir I, Yen HW, Geller DH, Torbati D, Bierden R, Weitsman S, Agarwal S, Magoffin D. Insulin augmentation of 17-α hydroxylase activity is mediated by phosphatidyl inositol 3-kinase but not extracellular signa lregulated kinase-1/2 in human ovarian theca cells. Endocrinology 2004; 145:175–83
126. Carvalho CRO, Carvalheira JB, Lima MH, Zimmerman SF, Caperuto LC, Amanso A, Gasparetti AL, Meneghetti V, Zimmerman LF, Velloso LA et al. Novel signal transduction pathway for luteinizing hormone and its interaction with insulin: activation of janus kinase/signal transducer and activator of transcription and phosphoinositol 3-kinase/Akt pathways. Endocrinology 2003; 144: 38–47
127. Lima M, Souza L, Caperuto L, Bevilacqua E, Gasparetti A, Zanuto R, Saad M, CarvalhoC. Up-regulation of the phosphatidylinositol 3-kinase/protein kinase B pathway in the ovary of rats by chronic treatment with hCG and insulin. J Endocrinol 2006; 190:451–59
128. Garzo VG, Dorrington JH. Aromatase activity in human granulosa cells during follicular development and the modulation by follicle stimulating hormone and insulin. Am J Obstet Gynecol 1984; 148:657–62
129. Greisen S, Ledet T, Ovesen P. Effects of androstenedione, insulin and LH on steroidogenesis in human granulosa luteal cells. Hum Reprod 2001; 16:2061–65
130. McGee E, Sawetawan C, Bird I, Rainey WE, Carr BR. The effects of insulin on 3 b-hydroxysteroid dehydrogenase expression in human luteinized granulosa cells. J Soc Gynecol Investig 1995; 2:535–41

131. Sekar N, Garmey JC, Veldhuis JD. Mechanisms underlying the steroidogenic synergy of insulin and luteinizing hormone in porcine granulosa cells: joint amplification of pivotal sterol-regulatory genes encoding the low-density lipoprotein (LDL) receptor, steroidogenic acute regulatory (stAR) protein and cytochrome P450 side-chain cleavage (P450scc) enzyme. Mol Cell Endocrinol 2000; 159:25–35
132. Wu XK, Sallinen K, Anttila L, Makinen M, Luo C, Pollanen P, and Erkkola, R Expression of insulin-receptor substrate-1and -2 in ovaries from women with insulin resistance and from controls. Fertil Steril 2000; 74:564–72
133. Franks S, Gilling-Smith C, Watson H, Willis D. Insulin action in the normal and polycystic ovary. Endocrinol Metab Clin North Am 1999; 28:361–78
134. Willis D, Mason H, Gilling-Smith C, Franks S. Modulation by insulin of follicle-stimulating hormone and luteinizing hormone actions in human granulosa cells of normal and polycystic ovaries. J Clin Endocrinol Metab 1996; 81:302–9
135. Baillargeon JP, Nestler JE. Polycystic ovary syndrome: a syndrome of ovarian hypersensitivity to insulin? J Clin Endocrinol Metab 2006; 91:22–4
136. Willis, D. Watson H, Mason H, Galea R, Brincat M, Franks S Premature response to LH of granulosa cells from anovulatory women with polycystic ovaries: relevance to mechanisms of anovulation. J Clin Endocrinol Metab 1998; 83: 3984–91
137. Jakimiuk AJ, Weitsman SR, Navab A, Magoffin DA. Luteinizing hormone receptor, steroidogenesis acute regulatory protein, and steroidogenic enzyme messenger ribonucleic acids are overexpressed in thecal and granulosa cells from polycystic ovaries. J Clin Endocrinol Metab 2001; 86:1318–23
138. Dumesic DA, Schramm RD, Peterson E, Paprocki AM, Zhou R, Abbott DH. Impaired developmental competence of oocytes in adult prenatally androgenized female rhesus monkeys undergoing gonadotropin stimulation for in vitro fertilization. J Clin Endocrinol Metab 2002; 87:1111–19
139. Wu XK, Zhou SY, Liu JX, Pollanen P, Sallinen K, Makinen M, Erkkola R. Selective ovary resistance to insulin signaling in women with polycystic ovary syndrome. Fertil Steril 2003; 80:954–65
140. Phy J, Conover C, Abbot D, Zschunke M, Walker D, Session D, Tummon I, Thornhill A, Lesnick T, Dumesic D. Insulin and Messenger Ribonucleic Acid Expression of Insulin Receptor Isoforms in Ovarian Follicles from Nonhirsute Ovulatory Women and Polycystic Ovary Syndrome Patients J Clin Endocrinol Metab 2004; 89:3561–66
141. Poretsky L, Seto-Young D, Shrestha A, S Dhillon, Mirjany M, Liu HC, Yih M, Rosenwaks Z Phosphatidyl-inositol-3 kinase-independent insulin action pathway(s) in the human ovary. J Clin Endocrinol Metab 2001; 86:3115–9
142. Seto-Young D, Zajac J, Liu HC, Rosenwaks Z, Poretsky L. The role of mitogen-activated protein kinase in insulin and insulin-like growth factor I (IGF-I) signaling cascades for progesterone and IGF-binding protein-1 production in human granulosa cells. J Clin Endocrinol Metab 2003; 88(7):3385–91
143. Coffler MS, Patel K, Dahan MH, Yoo RY, Malcom PJ, Chang RJ. Enhanced granulosa cell responsiveness to follicle-stimulating hormone during insulin infusion in women with polycystic ovary syndrome treated with pioglitazone. J Clin Endocrinol Metab 2003; 88:5624–31
144. Bhatia B, Price C. Insulin alters the effects of follicle stimulating hormone on aromatase in bovine granulosa cells in vitro. Steroids 2001; 66:511–9
145. Jonard S, Dewailly D. The follicular excess in polycystic ovaries, due to intraovarian hyperandrogenism, may be the main culprit for the follicular arrest Hum Reprod Update 2004; 10:107–17
146. Tarkun I, Arslan B, Canturk Z, Turemen E, Sahin T, Duman C. Endothelial dysfunction in young women with polycystic ovary syndrome: relationship with insulin resistance and low-grade chronic inflammation. J Clin Endocrinol Metab 2004; 89:5592–96
147. Diamanti-Kandarakis E, Paterakis T, Alexandraki K, Piperi C, Aessopos A, Katsikis I, Katsilambros N, Kreatsas G, Panidis D. Indices of low-grade chronic inflammation in polycystic ovary syndrome and the beneficial effect of metformin. Hum Reproduction 2006; 21(6):1426–31
148. Diamanti-Kandarakis E, Alexandraki K, Piperi C, Protogerou A, Katsikis I, Paterakis T, Lekakis J, Panidis D. Inflammatory and endothelial markers in women with polycystic ovary syndrome. Eur J Clin Invest 2006; 36(10):691–7
149. Atiomo WU, Fox R, Condon JE, Shaw S, Friend J, Prentice A et al. Raised plasminogen activator inhibitor–1 (PAI-1) is not an independent risk factor in the polycystic ovary syndrome (PCOS). Clin Endocrinol 2000; 52:487–92
150. Kelly CJ, Lyall H, Petrie JR, Gould GW, Connell JM, Rumley A, Lowe GD, Sattar N. A specific elevation in tissue plasminogen activator antigen in women with polycystic ovarian syndrome. J Clin Endocrinol Metab 2002; 87(7):3287–90
151. Carmassi F, De Negri F, Fioriti R, De Giorgi A, Giannarelli C, Fruzzetti F, Pedrinelli R, Dell'Omo G, Bersi C. Insulin resistance causes impaired vasodilation and hypofibrinolysis in young women with polycystic ovary syndrome. Thromb Res 2005; 116:207–14
152. Diamanti-Kandarakis E, Spina G, Kouli C, Migdalis I. Increased endothelin-1 levels in women with polycystic ovary syndrome and the beneficial effect of metformin therapy. J Clin Endocrinol Metab 2001; 86:4666–73
153. Charitidou C, Farmakiotis D, Zournatzi V, Pidonia I, Pegiou T, Karamanis N, Hatzistilianou M, Katsikis I, Panidis D. The administration of estrogens, combined with anti-androgens, has beneficial effects on the hormonal features and asymmetric dimethyl-arginine levels, in women with the polycystic ovary syndrome. Atherosclerosis 2008; 196(2):958–65
154. Orio Jr F, Palomba S, Cascella T, De Simone B, Di Biase S, Russo R, Labella D, Zullo F, Lombardi G, Colao A Early Impairment of Endothelial Structure and Function in Young Normal-Weight Women with Polycystic Ovary Syndrome J Clin Endocrinol Metab 2004; 89:4588–93

155. Kelly CJ, Speirs A, Gould GW, Petrie JR, Lyall H, Connell JM. Altered vascular function in young women with polycystic ovary syndrome. J Clin Endocrinol Metab 2002; 87:742–46
156. Paradisi G, Steinberg HO, Hempfling A, Cronin J, Hook G, Shepard MK, Baron AD. Polycystic ovary syndrome is associated with endothelial dysfunction. Circulation 2001; 103(10):1410–5
157. Diamanti-Kandarakis E, Alexandraki K, Protogerou A, Piperi C, Papamichael C, Aessopos A, Lekakis J and Mavrikakis M Metformin administration improves endothelial function in women with polycystic ovary syndrome. Eur J Endocrinol 2005; 152:749–756
158. Carmina E, Orio F, Palomba S, Longo RA, et al. Endothelial Dysfunction in PCOS: Role of Obesity and Adipose Hormones. Am J Med 2006; 119:356.e1–356.e6
159. Talbott E, Zborowski J, Rager J. Evidence for an association between metabolic cardiovascular syndrome and coronary and aortic calcification among women with polycystic ovary syndrome. J Clin Endocrinol Metab 2004; 89:5454–61
160. Prelevic GM, Beljic T, Balint-Peric L, Ginsburg J. Cardiac flow velocity in women with the polycystic ovary syndrome. Clin Endocrinol (Oxf) 1995; 43:677–81
161. Tiras MB, Yalcin R, Noyan V, Maral I, Yildirim M, Dortlemez O, Daya S. Alterations in cardiac flow parameters in patients with polycystic ovarian syndrome. Hum Reprod 1999; 14:1949–52
162. Orio F, Palomba S, Spinelli L, et al. The Cardiovascular risk of young women with polycystic ovary syndrome: an observational, analytical, prospective case-control study. J Clin Endocrinol Metab 2004; 89:3696–3701
163. Celik O, Sahin I, Celik N, Hascalik S, Keskin L, Ozcan H, Uckan A, Kosar F. Diagnostic potential of serum N-terminal pro-B-type brain natriuretic peptide level in detection of cardiac wall stress in women with polycystic ovary syndrome: a cross-sectional comparison study. Hum Reprod 2007; 22(11):2992–8
164. Cascella T, Palomba S, Tauchmanova L, Manguso F, Di Biase S, Labella D, Giallauria F, Vigorito C, Colao A, Lombardi G, Orio F Jr. Serum aldosterone concentration and cardiovascular risk in women with polycystic ovarian syndrome. J Clin Endocrinol Metab 2006; 91:4395–4400
165. Paradisi G, Steinberg HO, Shepard MK, Hook G, Baron AD. Troglitazone therapy improves endothelial function to near normal levels in women with polycystic ovary syndrome. J Clin Endocrinol Metab 2003; 88(2):576–80
166. Orio F, Palomba S, Cascella T, De Simone B, Manguso F, et al. Improvement in Endothelial Structure and Function after Metformin Treatment in Young Normal-Weight Women with Polycystic Ovary Syndrome: Results of a 6-Month Study. J Clin Endocrinol Metab 2005; 90(11):6072–76
167. Diamanti-Kandarakis E. Pharmaceutical Intervention in Metabolic and Cardiovascular Risk Factors in Polycystic Ovary Syndrome. In Insulin resistance and polycystic ovarian syndrome: pathogenesis, evaluation and treatment (Diamanti-Kandarakis, E. et al., eds), pp. 367–387, Insulin Resistance and Polycystic Ovarian Syndrome:Edited by Evanthia Diamanti-Kandarakis, John Nestler, Dimitrios Panidis, Renato Pasquali: Humana Press 2007
168. Legro RS, Bentley-Lewis R, Driscoll D, Wang SC, Dunaif A. Insulin resistance in the sisters of women with polycystic ovary syndrome: association with hyperandrogenemia rather than menstrual irregularity. J Clin Endocrinol Metab 2002; 87:2128–33
169. Cagnacci A, Paoletti AM, Arangino S, Melis GB, Volpe A. Effect of ovarian suppression on glucose metabolism of young lean women with and without ovarian hyperandrogenism. Hum Reprod 1999; 14: 893–7
170. Moghetti P, Tosi F, Castello R, et al. The insulin resistance in women with hyperandrogenism is partially reversed by antiandrogen treatment: evidence that androgens impair insulin action in women. J Clin Endocrinol Metab 1996; 81:952–60
171. Polderman K, Gorren L, Asscheman H, Bakker A, Heine R. Induction of insulin resistance by androgens and estrogens. J Clin Endocrinol Metab 1994; 79:265–27
172. Elbers J, Giltay E, Teerlink T, Scheffer P, Asscheman H, Seidell J. Gooren LEffects of sex steroids on components of the insulin resistance syndrome in transsexual subjects. Clin Endocrinol 2003; 58:562–571
173. Marsden PJ, Murdoch AP, Taylor R. Adipocyte insulin action following ovulation in polycystic ovarian syndrome. Hum Reprod 1999; 14(9):2216–22
174. Corbould A. Chronic testosterone treatment induces selective insulin resistance in subcutaneous adipocytes of women. J Endocrinol 2007; 192(3):585–94
175. Allemand MC, Asmann Y, Klaus K, Nair K. S An in vitro model for PCOS related insulin resistance: the effects of testosterone on phosphorylation of intracellular insulin signalling proteins in rat skeletal muscle primary culture. Fertil Steril Abstracts 2005; 84(Suppl 1):S30–31
176. Mannerås L, Cajander S, Holmäng A, Seleskovic Z, Lystig T, Lönn M, Stener Victorin E. A new rat model exhibiting both ovarian and metabolic characteristics of polycystic ovary syndrome. Endocrinology 2007; 148(8):3781–91
177. Perello M, Castrogiovanni D, Giovambattista A, Gaillard RC, Spinedi E. Impairment in insulin sensitivity after early androgenization in the post-pubertal female rat. Life Sci 2007; 80(19):1792–8
178. Nishizawa H, Shimomura I, Kishida K, Maeda N, Kuriyama H, Nagaretani H, Matsuda M, Kondo H, Furuyama N, Kihara S, Nakamura T, Tochino Y, Funahashi T, Matsuzawa Y. Androgens decrease plasma adiponectin, an insulin-sensitizing adipocyte-derived protein. Diabetes. 2002; 51(9):2734–41
179. Panidis D, Kourtis A, Farmakiotis D, Mouslech T, Rousso D, Koliakos G. Serum adiponectin levels in women with polycystic ovary syndrome. Hum Reprod 2003; 18(9):1790–96
180. Xu A, Chan KW, Hoo RL, Wang Y, Tan KC, Zhang J, Chen B, Lam MC, Tse C, Cooper GJ, Lam KS. Testosterone Selectively Reduces the High Molecular Weight Form of Adiponectin by Inhibiting Its Secretion from Adipocytes J Biol Chem 2005; 280(18):18073–80

181. Arner P. Effects of testosterone on fat cell lipolysis. Species differences and possible role in polycystic ovarian syndrome. Biochimie 2005; 87(1):39–43
182. Diamanti-Kandarakis E, Mitrakou A, Raptis S, Tolis G, Duleba AJ. The effect of a pure antiandrogen receptor blocker, flutamide, on the lipid profile in the polycystic ovary syndrome. J Clin Endocrinol Metab 1998; 83:2699–2705
183. Perrini S, Natalicchio A, Laviola L, Belsanti G, Montrone C, Cignarelli A, Minielli V, Grano M, De Pergola G, Giorgino R, Giorgino F. Dehydroepiandrosterone stimulates glucose uptake in human and murine adipocytes by inducing GLUT1 and GLUT4 translocation to the plasma membrane. Diabetes 2004; 53:41–52
184. Ishizuka T, Kajita K, Miura A, Ishikawa M, Kanoh Y, Itaya S, Kimura M, Muto N, Mune T, Morita H, Yasuda K. DHEA improves glucose uptake via activations of protein kinase C and phosphatidylinositol 3-kinase. Am J Physiol 1999; 276: E196–E204
185. Formoso G, Chen H, Kim J, Montagnani M, Consoli A, Quon M. Dehydroepiandrosterone mimics acute actions of insulin to stimulate production of both nitric oxide and endothelin 1 via distinct phosphatidylinositol 3-kinase and mitogen-activated protein kinase- dependent pathways in vascular endothelium. Mol Endocrinol 2006; 20:1153–63
186. González F, Rote NS, Minium J, Kirwan JP. Reactive oxygen species induced oxidative stress in the development of insulin resistance and hyperandrogenism in polycystic ovary syndrome. J Clin Endocrinol Metab 2006a; 91:336–340
187. Escobar-Morreale HF, Botella-Carretero JI, Villuendas G, Botella-Carretero J, Villuendas G., Sancho J, San Millan JL. Serum interleukin-18 concentrations are increased in the polycystic ovary syndrome: relationship to insulin resistance and to obesity. J Clin Endocrinol Metab 2004; 89:806–11
188. Zhang YF, Yang YS, Hong J, Gu WQ, Shen CF, Xu M, Du PF, Li XY, Ning G. Elevated serum levels of interleukin-18 are associated with insulin resistance in women with polycystic ovary syndrome. Endocrine 2006; 29(3):419–23
189. Fencki V, Fenkci S, Yilmazer M, Serteser M. Decreased total antioxidant status and increased oxidative stress in women with polycystic ovary syndrome may contribute to the risk of cardiovascular disease Fertil Steril 2003; 80:123–27
190. Glintborg D, Højlund K, Andersen M, Henriksen JE, Beck-Nielsen H, Handberg A. Soluble CD36 and risk markers of insulin resistance and atherosclerosis are elevated in polycystic ovary syndrome and significantly reduced during pioglitazone treatment. Diab Care 2008; 31(2):328–34
191. González F, Rote N, Minium J, Kirwan J. In vitro evidence that hyperglycemia stimulates TNF- α release in obese women with polycystic ovary syndrome. J Endocrinol 2006b; 188:521–29
192. Gonzalez F, Rote N, Minium J, Kirwan J. Increased activation of nuclear factor B triggers inflammation and insulin resistance in polycystic ovary syndrome. J Clin Endocrinol Metab 2006c; 91:1508–12
193. Naz RK, Thurston D, Santoro N. Circulating tumor necrosis factor (TNF)-a in normally cycling women and patients with premature ovarian failure and polycystic ovaries. Am J Reprod Immunol 1995; 34:170–75
194. Puder JJ, Varga S, Nusbaumer CPG,. Zulewski H, Bilz S, Müller B, Keller U. Women with polycystic ovary syndrome are sensitive to the TNF-a lowering effect of glucose-induced hyperinsulinaemia. Eur J Clin Inves 2006; 36:883–89
195. Wellen K, Hotamisligil G. Inflammation, stress, and diabetes. J Clin Invest 2005; 115(5):1111–19
196. Carmina E, Bucchieri S, Esposito A, Del Puente A, Mansueto P, Orio F, Di Fede G, Rini GB. Abdominal fat quantity and distribution in women with polycystic ovary syndrome and extent of its relation to insulin resistance. J Clin Endocrinol Metab 2007; 92:2500–5
197. Yildirim B, Sabir N, Kaleli B. Relation of intra-abdominal fat distribution to metabolic disorders in nonobese patients with polycystic ovary syndrome Fertil Steril 2003; 79:1358–64
198. Puder JJ, Varga S, Kraenzlin M, De Geyter C, Keller U, Muller B. Central fat excess in polycystic ovary syndrome: relation to low-grade inflammation and insulin resistance. J Clin Endocrinol Metab 2005; 90(11):6014–21
199. Glintborg D, Andersen M, Hagen C, Frystyk J, Hulstrom V, Flyvbjerg A, Hermann AP. Evaluation of metabolic risk markers in polycystic ovary syndrome (PCOS). Adiponectin, ghrelin, leptin and body composition in hirsute PCOS patients and controls. Eur J Endocrinol 2006; 155:337–45
200. Curat CA, Wegner V, Sengenes C, et al. Macrophages in human visceral adipose tissue: increased accumulation in obesity and a source of resistin and visfatin. Diabetologia 2006; 49:744–47
201. Lumeng C, Deyoung S, Saltiel A. Macrophages block insulin action in adipocytes by altering expression of signaling and glucose transport proteins. Am J Physiol Endocrinol Metab 2007; 292:E166–E174
202. Weisberg SP, McCann D, Desai M, Rosenbaum M, Leibel RL, Ferrante JrAW. Obesity is associated with macrophage accumulation in adipose tissue. J Clin Invest 2003; 112:1796–1808
203. Lau DC, Dhillon B, Yan H, Szmitko PE, Verma S. Adipokines: molecular links between obesity and atherosclerosis. Am J Physiol Heart Circ Physiol. 2005; 288:H2031–H2041
204. Ardawi MS, Rouzi AA. Plasma adiponectin and insulin resistance in women with polycystic ovary syndrome. Fertil Steril 2005; 83:1708–16
205. Escobar-Morreale HF, Villuendas G, Botella-Carretero JI. Adiponectin and resistin in PCOS: a clinical, biochemical and molecular genetic study. Human Reprod 2006; 21(9):2257–65
206. Glintborg D, Frystyk J, Højlund K, Andersen KK, Henriksen JE, Hermann AP, Hagen C, Flyvbjerg A, Andersen M. Total and high molecular weight (HMW) adiponectin levels and measures of glucose and lipid metabolism following pioglitazone treatment in a randomized placebo-controlled study in polycystic ovary syndrome. Clin Endocrinol 2008; 68(2):165–74
207. Sepilian V, Nagamani M. Adiponectin levels in women with polycystic ovary syndrome and severe insulin resistance. J Soc Gynecol Invest 2005; 12:129–34

208. Aroda V, Ciaraldi T, Chang S, Dahan MH, Chang RJ, Henry RR. Circulating and cellular adiponectin in polycystic ovary syndrome: relationship to glucose tolerance and insulin action. Fertil Steril 2008; 89(5):1200–8
209. Sieminska L, Marek B, Kos-Kudla B, Niedziolka D, Kajdaniuk D, Nowak M, Glogowska-Szelag J. Serum adiponectin in women with polycystic ovarian syndrome and its relation to clinical, metabolic and endocrine parameters. J Endocrinol Invest 2004; 27:528–34
210. Spranger J, Möhlig M, Wegewitz U, Ristow M, Pfeiffer A, Schill T, Schlösser H, Brabant G, Schöfl C. Adiponectin is independently associated with insulin sensitivity in women with polycystic ovary syndrome. Clin Endocrinol 2004; 61:738–46
211. Orio Jr F, Palomba S, Cascella T, Milan G, Mioni R, Pagano C, Zullo F, Colao A, Lombardi G, Vettor R. Adiponectin levels in women with polycystic ovary syndrome. J Clin Endocrinol Metab 2003; 88:2619–23
212. Shroff R, Kirschner A, Michelle M, Van Beek E, Jagasia D, Dokras A. Young Obese Women with Polycystic Ovary Syndrome have Evidence of Early Coronary Atherosclerosis. J Clin Endocrin Metab 2007; 92(12):4609–14
213. Panidis D, Koliakos G, Kourtis A. Serum resistin levels in women with polycystic ovary syndrome. Fertil Steril 2004; 81: 361–66
214. Chan TF, Chen YL, Chen HH, Lee CH, Jong SB, Tsai EM. Increased plasma visfatin concentrations in women with polycystic ovary syndrome. Fertil Steril 2007; 88(2):401–5
215. Ost A, Danielsson A, Liden M, Eriksson U, Nystrom FH, Stralfors P. Retinol-binding protein-4 attenuates insulin-induced phosphorylation of IRS1 and ERK1/2 in primary human adipocytes. FASEB J 2007; 21(13):3696–704
216. Janke J, Engeli S, Boschmann M, Adams F, Böhnke J, Luft FC, Sharma AM, Jordan J. Retinol-binding protein 4 in human obesity. Diabetes 2006; 55:2805–10
217. Weiping L, Qingfeng C, Shikun M, Xiurong L, Hua Q, Xiaoshu B, Suhua Z, Qifu L. Elevated serum RBP4 is associated with insulin resistance in women with polycystic ovary syndrome. Endocrine 2006; 30:283–88
218. Lee JW, Im JA, Lee DC. Retinol binding protein in non-obese women with polycystic ovary syndrome. Clin Endocrinol 2008; 68:786–790
219. Hahn S, Backhaus M, Broecker-Preuss M, Tan S, Dietz T, Kimmig R, Schmidt M, Mann K, Janssen OE. Retinol-binding protein 4 levels are elevated in polycystic ovary syndrome women with obesity and impaired glucose metabolism. Eur J Endocrin 2007; 157:201–207
220. Hutchison SK, Harrison C, Stepto N, Meyer C, Teede HJ. Retinol-binding protein 4 and insulin resistance in polycystic ovary syndrome. Diabetes Care 2008; 31(7):1427–32
221. Diamanti-Kandarakis E, Livadas S, Kandarakis S, Papassotiriou I and Margeli A. Low free plasma levels of Retinol-binding Protein 4 (RBP4) in insulin resistant subjects with Polycystic Ovary Syndrome. J Endocrinol Invest 2008, in Press.
222. Graham TE, Wason CJ, Blüher M, Kahn BB. Shortcomings in methodology complicate measurements of serum retinol binding protein (RBP4) in insulin-resistant human subjects. Diabetologia 2007; 50(4):814–23
223. Miele C, Riboulet A, Maitan MA, Oriente F, Romano C, Formisano P, Giudicelli J, Beguinot F, Van Obberghen E. Human glycated albumin affects glucose metabolism in L6 skeletal muscle cells by impairing insulin-induced insulin eceptor substrate (IRS) signalling through a protein kinase C-α mediated mechanism. J Biol Chem 2003; 278:47376–87
224. Uribarri J, Stirban A, Sander D, Cai W, Negrean M, Buenting CE, Koschinsky T, Vlassara H. Single oral challenge by advanced glycation end products acutely impairs endothelial function in diabetic and nondiabetic subjects. Diabetes Care 2007; 30(10):2579–82
225. Diamanti-Kandarakis E, Piperi C, Patsouris E, Korkolopoulou P, Panidis D, Pawelczyk L, Papavassiliou AG, Duleba AJ. Immunohistochemical localization of advanced glycation end-products (AGEs) and their receptor (RAGE) in polycystic and normal ovaries. Histochem Cell Biol 2007; 127:581–89
226. Diamanti-Kandarakis E, Piperi C, Korkolopoulou P, Kandaraki E, Levidou G, Papalois A, Patsouris E, Papavassiliou AG. Accumulation of dietary glycotoxins in the reproductive system of normal female rats. J Mol Med 2007; 85(12):1413–20
227. Siegel S, Futterweit W, Davies TF, Concepcion ES, Greenberg DA, Villanueva R, Tomer Y. A C/T single nucleotide polymorphism at the tyrosine kinase domain of the insulin receptor gene is associated with polycystic ovary syndrome. Fertil Steril 2002; 78:1240–43
228. Urbanek M, Sam S, Legro RS, Dunaif A. Identification of a polycystic ovary syndrome susceptibility variant in fibrillin-3 and association with a metabolic phenotype. J Clin Endocrinol Metab 2007; 92(11):4191–98
229. Tucci S, Futterweit W, Concepcion ES, Greenberg DA, Villanueva R, Davies TF, Tomer Y. Evidence for association of polycystic ovary syndrome in caucasian women with a marker at the insulin receptor gene locus. J Clin Endocrinol Metab 2001; 86:446–49
230. Ukkola O, Rankinen T, Gagnon J, Leon AS, Skinner JS, Wilmore JH, Rao DC, Bouchard C. A genome-wide linkage scan for steroids and SHBG levels in black and white families: the HERITAGE Family Study. J Clin Endocrinol Metab 2002; 87:3708–20
231. El Mkadem SA, Lautier C, Macari F, Molinari N, Lefebvre P, Renard E, Gris JC, Cros G, Daures JP, Bringer J, White MF, Grigorescu F. Role of allelic variants Gly972Arg of IRS-1 and Gly1057Asp of IRS-2 in moderate-to-severe insulin resistance of women with polycystic ovary syndrome. Diabetes 2001; 50:2164–68
232. Ehrmann DA, Tang X, Yoshiuchi I, Cox NJ, Bell GI Relationship of insulin receptor substrate-1 and -2 genotypes to phenotypic features of polycystic ovary syndrome. J Clin Endocrinol Metab 2002a; 87:4297–4300
233. Bennett ST, Lucassen AM, Gough SC, Powell EE, Undlien DE, Pritchard LE, Merriman ME, Kawaguchi Y, Dronsfield MJ, Pociot F et al. Susceptibility to human type 1 diabetes at IDDM2 is determined by tandem repeat variation at the insulin gene minisatellite locus. Nat Genet 1995; 9:284–92

234. Waterworth DM, Bennett ST, Gharani N, McCarthy MI, Hague S, Batty S, Conway GS, White D, Todd JA, Franks S et al. Linkage and association of insulin gene VNTR regulatory polymorphism with polycystic ovary syndrome. Lancet 1997; 349:986–90
235. Urbanek M, Legro RS, Driscoll DA, Azziz R, Ehrmann DA, Norman RJ, Strauss JF 3rd, Spielman RS, Dunaif A. Thirty-seven candidate genes for polycystic ovary syndrome: strongest evidence for linkage is with follistatin. Proc Nat Acad Sci USA 1999; 96:8573–78
236. Calvo RM, Telleria D, Sancho J, San Millan JL, Escobar-Morreale HF. Insulin gene variable number of tandem repeats regulatory polymorphism is not associated with hyperandrogenism in Spanish women. Fertil Steril 2002; 77:666–68.
237. Vankova M, Vrbikova J, Hill M, Cinek O, Bendlova B. Association of insulin gene VNTR polymorphism with polycystic ovary syndrome. Ann N Y Acad Sci 2002; 967:558–65
238. Ehrmann DA, Schwarz PE, Hara M, Tang X, Horikawa Y, Imperial J, Bell GI, Cox NJ. Relationship of calpain-10 genotype to phenotypic features of polycystic ovary syndrome. J Clin Endocrinol Metab 2002b; 87:1669–73
239. Gonzalez A, Abril E, Roca A, Aragon MJ, Figueroa MJ, Velarde P, Royo JL, Real LM, Ruiz A. Comment: CAPN10 alleles are associated with polycystic ovary syndrome. J Clin Endocrinol Metab 2002; 87:3971–76
240. Gonzalez A, Abril E, Roca A, Aragon MJ, Figueroa MJ, Velarde P, Ruiz R, Fayez O, Galan JJ, Herreros JA et al. Specific CAPN10 gene haplotypes influence the clinical profile of polycystic ovary patients. J Clin Endocrinol Metab 2003; 88: 5529–36
241. Haddad L, Evans JC, Gharani N, Robertson C, Rush K, Wiltshire S, Frayling TM, Wilkin TJ, Demaine A, Millward A et al. Variation within the type 2 diabetes susceptibility gene calpain-10 and polycystic ovary syndrome. J Clin Endocrinol Metab 2002; 87:2606–10
242. Hara M, Alcoser SY, Qaadir A, Beiswenger KK, Cox NJ, Ehrmann DA. Insulin resistance is attenuated in women with polycystic ovary syndrome with the Pro (12) Ala polymorphism in the PPARgamma gene. J Clin Endocrinol Metab 2002; 87:772–75
243. Witchel SF, White C, Siegel ME, Aston CE. Inconsistent effects of the proline12→alanine variant of the peroxisome proliferator-activated receptor-gamma2 gene on body mass index in children and adolescent girls. Fertil Steril 2001; 76: 741–47
244. San Millan JL, Corton M, Villuendas G, Sancho J, Peral B, Escobar-Morreale HF. Association of the polycystic ovary syndrome with genomic variants related to insulin resistance, type 2 diabetes mellitus, and obesity. J Clin Endocrinol Metab 2004; 89:2640–46

Chapter 5
Genetics of Metabolic Syndrome and Genetic Lipodystrophies

Tisha R. Joy and Robert A. Hegele

5.1 Introduction

Polycystic ovary syndrome (PCOS) affects ~7% of reproductive-aged women and is associated with several metabolic abnormalities including insulin resistance, type 2 diabetes (DM2), and dyslipidemia [1–3]. Although the presence of interfamilial and intrafamilial variation in the phenotype of PCOS-affected individuals points to an important role for environmental influences, studies demonstrating familial aggregation of PCOS and its associated metabolic disturbances also signify a critical genetic component to this syndrome [4–6]. Since the two key long-term sequelae of PCOS are type 2 diabetes and cardiovascular disease (CVD), PCOS can be seen as a common variant of the metabolic syndrome (MetS) with insulin resistance, dyslipidemia, and obesity as salient shared features. Thus, understanding the genetics of MetS may shed light on the genetic aspects of PCOS. Similarly, a discussion of the genetic basis of certain rare monogenic disorders of lipid distribution (genetic lipodystrophies) characterized by insulin resistance, dyslipidemia, increased cardiovascular risk, and polycystic ovaries may also aid in our understanding of common PCOS. We will focus on describing selected genetic aspects of MetS as well as of specific monogenic lipodystrophies (congenital generalized lipodystrophy [CGL] or familial partial lipodystrophy [FPLD]), where polycystic ovaries are a predominant feature. Furthermore, the similarities in candidate genes examined for MetS, genetic lipodystrophies, and PCOS will be briefly discussed.

5.2 Complex VS. Monogenic Traits

Both PCOS and MetS represent complex genetic traits since the clinical phenotypes usually arise from the intricate interaction of a number of genetic and environmental influences. For complex traits, large effects from the environment are superimposed on cumulative small effects arising from common genetic alterations. Conversely, monogenic disorders such as FPLD and CGL result from the large effect of a single genetic alteration with relatively little additional effect from the environment.

Complex traits can be influenced by genetic, environmental, and time-dependent factors. For example, complex traits may result through polygenic or "threshold" inheritance of mutations at different loci or through differential effects on physiological systems that share a final common phenotypic expression. In addition, with locus heterogeneity, a number of genetic loci may independently lead to disease susceptibility. Some complex traits are influenced by epistasis or gene interactions, where mutations in several genes confer disease susceptibility depending on the concomitant contribution of other genetic variations.

The genetic variant may confer susceptibility to the phenotype only under certain environmental conditions (e.g., obesity in the face of an imbalance between dietary intake and physical activity). Even time is influential

R.A. Hegele (✉)
Director, Blackburn Cardiovascular Genetics Laboratory, Scientist, Vascular Biology Research Group, Robarts Research Institute, 406 – 100 Perth Drive, N6A 5K8 London, Ontario, Canada, N6A 5K8
e-mail: hegele@robarts.ca

N.R. Farid, E. Diamanti-Kandarakis (eds.), *Diagnosis and Management of Polycystic Ovary Syndrome*,
DOI 10.1007/978-0-387-09718-3_5, © Springer Science+Business Media, LLC 2009

to the development of complex traits since certain genes can have their most pronounced effect at a certain age or developmental stage (e.g., in autism). Aging may lead to increased phenotypic expression of certain complex traits, as evidenced by the increased prevalence of MetS with increasing age. The age-related expression of complex traits may occur through varied genetic mechanisms, including increased mutational rate, poor DNA repair, programmed senescence, or integration of the cumulative environmental exposures required for phenotypic expression [7]. Thus, determining the genetic basis of complex traits such as PCOS or MetS is a complex feat. But, genetic strides in MetS may be helpful to PCOS. Similarly, genetic determination of monogenic syndromes such as CGL or FPLD which share similar traits to PCOS may also provide possible candidate genes for PCOS.

5.3 Metabolic Syndrome

5.3.1 Clinical Features and Epidemiology

MetS is characterized by the clustering of four main risk factors for CVD, including abdominal obesity, hypertension, dysglycemia, and dyslipidemia (increased triglyceride and decreased high-density lipoprotein [HDL]-cholesterol levels). There are at least six different published definitions for this syndrome, based on varying combinations of the above-listed risk factors [8–13] (Table 5.1). Despite the controversy regarding the lack of a unified definition, MetS is the focus of much research, especially given its high prevalence. Data from the Third National Health and Nutrition Examination Survey (NHANES III) revealed that the overall age-adjusted prevalence of MetS (using the National Cholesterol Education Program Adult Treatment Panel [NCEP/ATP] III definition [9]) in the United States was ~ 24% [14]. Further analysis revealed several risk factors associated with an increased odds of the MetS including older age, postmenopausal status, Mexican-American ethnicity, physical inactivity, current smoking, lack of alcohol intake, low household income, high carbohydrate dietary intake, and higher body-mass index [15]. Although the growing obesity epidemic has certainly contributed to its high prevalence, MetS is also diagnosed among ~5% of normal-weight individuals in NHANES III [15]. The prevalence of each component of the MetS seems to be dependent on age, gender, and ethnicity [15]. In NHANES III, the overall prevalence of each component was 38.6% for increased waist circumference, 30.0% for hypertriglyceridemia, 37.1% for low HDL-cholesterol levels, 34.0% for hypertension, and 12.6% for dysglycemia [14].

PCOS and MetS share many overlapping features, including abdominal obesity, insulin resistance, and future-increased risk for DM2. The reported prevalence of MetS among women with PCOS has been quite variable, anywhere from 2 to 47%, depending on the type of study (case-control, retrospective, or prospective) and the particular criteria chosen [16–23]. A prospective trial using the NCEP/ATP III criteria for MetS revealed a prevalence of 46% among 138 women with PCOS with the prevalence for each individual component of MetS being 33% for hypertriglyceridemia, 65% for low HDL-cholesterol levels, 45% for hypertension, 86% for increased waist circumference, and 5% for dysglycemia [20]. Thus, the true prevalence for MetS among those with PCOS probably lies somewhere between 33% and 50%. However, the reverse statistic – i.e., the prevalence of polycystic ovaries among women with MetS – remains to be determined and may be an under-recognized problem.

5.3.2 Pathophysiology of Mets

The exact mechanism responsible for the development of common MetS remains to be determined. Dysregulation of adipose tissue together with inflammation are thought to be important instigators leading to the development of MetS. Obesity has been associated with increased macrophage accumulation and elevated circulating free fatty acids (FFA), the latter inducing skeletal muscle resistance by inhibiting insulin-mediated glucose uptake [24–26]. FFA can also directly induce apoptosis of pancreatic beta cells, leading to impaired

Table 5.1 Definitions of MetS

Criteria	AACE [12]	AHA/NHLBI [13]	EGIR [11]	IDF [10]	NCEP/ATP III [9]	WHO [8]
Adiposity	BMI ≥ 25 kg/m^2	WC ≥ 102 cm (M) or ≥ 88 cm (F)	WC ≥ 94 cm (M) or ≥ 80 cm (F)	Ethnicity-specific WC: • Europid* ≥94 cm (M) or ≥80 cm (F) • South Asian** or Chinese ≥90 cm (M) or ≥80 cm (F) • Japanese ≥85 cm (M) or ≥90 cm (F)	WC > 102 cm (M) or >88 cm (F)	WHR > 0.9 (M) or > 0.85 (F) and/or BMI > 30 kg/m^2
Dysglycemia	Glucose intolerance defined as: - IFG (FBG 6.1–6.9 mmol/L) Or - IGT (2 h PPG ≥7.8 mmol/L)	IFG (FBG ≥5.6 mmol/L) Or Drug treatment for diabetes	IR defined as hyperinsulinemia (non-diabetic fasting insulin in top 25%) IFG (FBG ≥6.1 mmol/L)	IFG (FBG ≥5.6 mmol/L) Or Pre-existing DM2	IFG (FBG ≥6.1 mmol/L)	Any one of the following: - DM2 - IFG (FBG ≥6.1 mmol/L) - IGT (2 h PPG ≥ 7.8 mmol/L) - Lowest 25% for hyperinsulinemic euglycemic clamp glucose uptake
Dyslipidemia • Tg • HDL-C	 ≥ 1.69 mmol/L < 1.04 mmol/L (M) Or < 1.29 mmol/L (F)	 ≥ 1.7 mmol/L < 1.03 mmol/L(M) Or < 1.3 mmol/L (F)	 > 2.0 mmol/L < 1.0 mmol/L	 ≥ 1.69 mmol/L < 1.0 mmol/L(M)¶ Or < 1.3 mmol/L (F)¶	 ≥ 1.69 mmol/L¶ < 1.04 mmol/L (M)¶ Or < 1.29 mmol/L (F)¶	 ≥ 1.7 mmol/L < 0.9 mmol/L (M) Or < 1.0 mmol/L (F)
Hypertension	BP ≥ 130/85 mmHg	BP ≥ 130/85 mmHg And/or Use of antihypertensive medication	BP ≥ 140/90 mmHg And/or Use of antihypertensive medication	BP ≥ 130/85 mmHg And/or Use of antihypertensive medication	BP ≥ 130/85 mmHg And/or Use of antihypertensive medication	BP ≥ 140/90 mmHg And/or Use of antihypertensive medication

Table 5.1 (continued)

Criteria	AACE [12]	AHA/NHLBI [13]	EGIR [11]	IDF [10]	NCEP/ATP III [9]	WHO [8]
Other	- Family history of DM2, CVD, or hypertension - High risk ethnic group for DM2 or CVD - PCOS -sedentary lifestyle - advancing age	None	None	None	None	Microalbuminuria (≥20 μg/min albumin excretion rate Or Albumin:creatinine ratio ≥ 30 mg/g)
Minimum criteria for diagnosis	Clinical judgment based on all features		IR + 2 other features	Adiposity + 2 other features	Any 3 features	Dysglycemia + 2 other features

Abbreviations: WHO, World Health Organization; EGIR, European Group for the Study of Insulin Resistance; NCEP/ATP III, National Cholesterol Education Program Adult Treatment Panel III; AACE, American Association of Clinical Endocrinology; AHA/NHLBI, American heart Association/National Heart, Lung, and Blood Institute; IDF, International Diabetes Federation; WHR, waist-to-hip ratio; M, male; F, female; BMI, body mass index; WC, waist circumference; IFG, impaired fasting glucose; FBG, fasting blood glucose; IGT, impaired glucose tolerance; 2 h PPG, 2-hour post-prandial glucose (after oral glucose tolerance test); IR, insulin resistance; BP, blood pressure; DM2, type 2 diabetes, CVD, cardiovascular disease; PCOS, polycystic ovary syndrome; Tg, triglycerides; HDL-C, high density lipoprotein cholesterol

* Europid criteria for individuals of European, Sub-Saharan African, or Middle Eastern descent.

**South Asian criteria for individuals of South Asian, South, or Central American descent.

¶ Or specific treatment with anti-cholesterol medication for either of these problems insulin secretion, likely through oxidative stress [27, 28]. Visceral obesity leads to altered secretion of several adipokines, including hyposecretion of adiponectin and hypersecretion of leptin, tumor necrosis factor α (TNF- α), and interleukin-6 (IL-6). Adiponectin is inversely associated with insulin resistance through effects on insulin signaling, endogenous glucose production, and fatty acid oxidation [29–31]. Both TNF- α and IL-6 impair insulin signaling at several steps, leading to insulin resistance and increased lipolysis (since insulin has a major anti-lipolytic role) [32, 33]. These two cytokines also decrease the secretion of adiponectin by adipose cells [34, 35]. The resultant insulin-resistant state together with excessive FFA flux to the liver is believed to drive hepatic triglyceride (TG) synthesis. As more TG is produced, HDL-cholesterol levels decrease partly due to the transfer of TG to HDL in exchange for cholesterol from HDL through the cholesteryl ester transfer protein (CETP). Despite the tendency for normal plasma levels of LDL-cholesterol among patients with MetS, the LDL particles are often smaller and denser, a pattern that is often associated with increased CVD risk [36, 37].

Meanwhile, the increased presence of angiotensinogen and angiotensinogen-converting enzyme (ACE) from the visceral adipose compartment as observed in obesity leads to increased angiotensin II levels [38]. Although the increased production of angiotensin II (a potent vasoconstrictor) plays a role in the development of hypertension, excessive FFA and TNF-α have been proposed to inhibit the vasodilator effects of insulin, resulting in insulin-mediated vasoconstriction and microvascular dysfunction [39]. Thus, many different players are postulated in the pathogenesis of the MetS phenotype.

5.3.3 Genetic Features

Obesity, physical inactivity, and high carbohydrate intake (particularly fructose) have been nominated as important environmental factors contributing to the high prevalence of MetS [15]. However, the importance of a genetic contribution to this syndrome has been implied by the high clustering of MetS factors in family and twin studies. A seminal study of 2508 male twin pairs revealed concordance for the clustering of three MetS components (hypertension, diabetes, and obesity) among monozygotic pairs (31.6%) vs. dizygotic pairs (6.3%) [40]. Similarly, in a study of 236 female twin pairs, heritability estimates for obesity, insulin/glucose, and dyslipidemia were found to be 0.61, 0.87, and 0.25, respectively, indicating an important genetic contribution to the development of each of these components [41]. These findings support other studies also demonstrating heritability of the MetS components among Japanese Americans and Chinese individuals [42, 43]. The Northern Manhattan Family Study, evaluating 803 individuals from 89 Caribbean-Hispanic families, demonstrated that the heritability of MetS itself was found to be 24% while heritability analysis revealed significant genetic effects for lipids/glucose/obesity (44%) and hypertension (20%) [44]. Although the variability in heritability among the different studies is most likely attributable to ethnic/racial influences, the above studies point toward the importance of genetic contributions to MetS development. Consequently, several investigators have studied genetic contributions for MetS using either linkage analysis or genetic association studies.

5.3.4 Linkage Analysis

Linkage scanning uses genotypic and phenotypic data from large pedigrees to find a chromosomal region that is preferentially inherited among family members with MetS. As causative genes for MetS are passed down through generations, nearby markers that are in close linkage to these genes are also passed down. As a result, co-segregation of markers with MetS or its components helps identify chromosomal regions harboring genes possibly causative for MetS. These are termed "positional candidate" genes. However, linkage analysis in MetS is associated with two significant problems. First, the lack of a standard definition for MetS and the multiple possible combinations of phenotypes may result in the discovery of multiple different linked loci that might be specific only for one sub-phenotype. Secondly, the detection of a discrete and unique linkage signal may be obscured by the possibility that MetS results from the interplay among multiple genes on different chromosomes.

A wide range of loci have thus far been linked to MetS, including 3q27, 17p12, chromosome 6 (D6S403, D6S264), chromosome 7 (D7S479-D7S471), and 1q23-31 [45–47], although consistent evidence for linkage to MetS has been demonstrated for chromosomes 1q, 2p, 2q, 3p, 6q, 7q, 9q, and 15q [46–55]. Even within a single study examining North American families, several chromosomal regions – 1p34.1, 1q41, 2p22.3, 7q31.3, 9p13.1, 9q21.1, 10p11.2, 19q13.4 – were linked with MetS [50]. Meanwhile, evaluation of 234 Chinese families from the Hong Kong Family Diabetes Study demonstrated several major regions of suggestive linkage on chromosomes 1, 2, and 16 for MetS and related metabolic traits [52]. Significant linkage of MetS with chromosome 1q21-q25, an area previously linked to type 2 diabetes across different ethnicities, has also been found [56–60]. In addition, 1p36.13 as a possible locus for MetS was suggested after examination of 250 German families [61]. Thus, these studies demonstrate that no single locus is reproducibly linked with MetS across all populations, which may be due to differences in ethnicity, the variable definition of MetS itself, or perhaps false-positive results arising from numerous studies of this type. Therefore, linkage studies regarding MetS must be interpreted with caution.

5.3.5 Genetic Association Studies

Genetic association studies use cohort, case-control, or family-based studies to determine relationships between genetic factors and the desired phenotype (i.e., MetS). These studies often use single nucleotide polymorphism (SNP) markers for genomic interrogation of a large number of individuals. A SNP is a locus where 2 or more base pair alternatives occur in the population with frequency $\geq 1\%$, and SNPs are common ($\sim$1 per 300–400 base pairs). This type of analysis using SNP markers can indirectly mark the location of an actual causative mutation. SNP variants are typically chosen from candidate genes, based on their functional role in the pathophysiology of the desired phenotype.

Adipokines, inflammation, adipose distribution, and insulin signaling are thought to play crucial roles in the pathogenesis of MetS and also PCOS. Thus, examining candidate genes from these areas for MetS may be relevant as potential candidate genes for PCOS (Table 5.2).

5.3.5.1 Adipokine Candidate Genes

SNPs of the human adiponectin (*ADIPOQ*) and resistin (*RSTN*) genes have been studied for association with MetS due to their potential relationships with insulin resistance [62–66]. Among elderly Taiwanese individuals, the G allele of *ADIPOQ* SNP276 in intron 2 was associated with decreased risk of obesity, MetS, and type 2 diabetes [67]. Meanwhile, examination of the -420C→G SNP in *RSTN* revealed that G/G homozygotes had an increased prevalence of MetS. A follow-up study revealed that the *RSTN* -420C→G SNP was associated with an increased prevalence of MetS, but did not influence MetS prevalence amongst individuals at high cardiovascular risk [68]. Unfortunately, the exact role of genetic variants of resistin in insulin resistance or obesity remains unsettled, but warrants further investigation.

5.3.5.2 Candidate Genes in Inflammation

Pro-inflammatory cytokines, such as IL-6 and TNF-α, have been implicated in the pathogenesis of MetS, and thus are potential candidate genes for MetS. In a study of Caucasian Danes, the AGC/AGC composite genotypes were more frequent amongst controls without the MetS, while the AGC/GGG composite genotype of three common *IL6* promoter polymorphisms, -597G→A, -572G→C, and -174G→C, were more frequent amongst those with MetS [69]. Similarly, among 571 Caucasian individuals, individuals with the CC genotype for the *IL6* -174G→C promoter polymorphism had a higher prevalence of MetS than those who did not [70]. Meta-analysis of 31 studies revealed that the *TNFA* -308G→A polymorphism was not significantly associated with the composite phenotype of MetS despite having conferred a risk of 1.23 for obesity as well as an increase in

Table 5.2 Association studies of similar candidate genes examined for metabolic syndrome and polycystic ovary syndrome

Gene	Polymorphism	Association with MetS Population studied P Value (definition)	Association with PCOS Population studied P value (definition)
ADIPOQ	SNP276 (GT vs. GG genotype)	1433 Taiwanese, >65 years old [67] OR 1.33; p = 0.011(NCEP/ATP III*) OR 1.47; p = 0.001 (IDF)	114 Spanish; NSA (NIH) [135] 116 Spanish; NSA (NIH) [136] 240 Greeks; NSA (NIH) [137]
	45T→G	NR	114 Spanish; NSA (NIH) [135] 116 Spanish; NSA (NIH) [136] 240 Greeks; NSA (NIH) [137]
RSTN	–420C→G (GG vs. CG genotype)	1542 Italians [68] p = 0.042 (NCEP/ATP III) †	116 Spanish; NSA (NIH) [136]
IL6	–597G→A, –572G→C, and –174G→C	2828 Danes [69] OR 1.25 for composite genotype AGC/GGG; p<0.01 (WHO)	156 Austrian; NSA found for –174G→C (Rotterdam**) [151]
	–174G→C (CC vs. GG genotype)	571 Caucasians with DM2 [70] p = 0.007 (WHO)†	See above
TNFA	–308G→A	1195 French [156] NSA (NCEP/ATP III)	258 Australian; NSA (Rotterdam**) [149]
	C-850T	NR	202 Finnish; NSA [150]
HSD11B1	g.4478T→G, g.10733G→C, g.4437–4438insA	36 French-Canadian men NSA (NCEP/ATP III) [72]	NR
	83557insA	NR	192 Italian; NSA (Rotterdam) [146]
	rs12086634	NR	1018 Caucasian; NSA (Rotterdam) [147]
GRB		322 Europid and 262 South Asian; NSA (WHO or NCEP/ATP III) [76]	NR
GR	N363S	NR	206 Caucasian; NSA (NIH) [148]
LMNA	13 SNPs	1572 Caucasians; NSA (WHO) [79]	NR
PPARG	Pro12Ala	Conflicting results: • 1155 French; NSA for Pro12Ala, but significant association between GTGC haplotype and MetS as well as between the Ala12 allele on a background of 1431CC and MetS [OR 2.48, p = 0.002] (NCEP/ATP III) [83] • 2245 Danes; the Ala/Ala phenotype was associated with a lower propensity for MetS [OR 0.24; p = 0.02] (EGIR) [157]	Conflicting results: • 250 Finnish women; Ala substitution allele associated with decreased risk for PCOS [OR 0.61; p=0.045] (Rotterdam**) [158] • 200 Italians; NSA (NIH) [159]
INS	VNTR I/I haplotype	320 Italian obese children and adolescents [86] CR 2.5; P = 0.006 (definition ‡)	3047 Caucasian; NSA (Rotterdam) [140]

Table 5.2 (continued)

Gene	Polymorphism	Association with MetS Population studied P Value (definition)	Association with PCOS Population studied P value (definition)
INSR	Eight restriction fragment length polymorphisms 1085 C/T SNP	163 Mexicans; NSA [87]	NR Conflicting results: • 267 Koreans; NSA (Rotterdam) [160] • 235 Caucasians; p = 0.03 (NIH + polycystic ovaries on ultrasound) [161]
IRS1	Eight restriction fragment length polymorphisms Gly972Arg	163 Mexicans; NSA [87] NR	NR Conflicting results: • 152 Chileans; higher frequency among those with PCOS p<0.02) [141] • 227 Caucasians and African Americans; NSA (NIH) [142]
CAPN10	haplotypes (based on SNPS-43, −19, −63)	382 Koreans with DM2 111/121 haplotype 111/121 haplotype associated with OR = 1.9 (p = 0.042)(WHO and NCEP/ATP III) [89]	Conflicting studies: • 212 women different ethnicities; 112/121 haplotype associated with OR for PCOS 2.18 for African Americans and Caucasians (NIH) [143] • 856 Caucasians; NSA between any haplotypes and PCOS (Rotterdam) [144]
ESR1		548 African Americans [96]	NR
	rs6902771	p = 0.012	
	rs9340799	OR 1.53; p = 0.029	
	rs2431260	OR 2.51; p = 0.005	
	rs1033182	p = 0.02	
	rs2175898	OR 2.51; p = 0.006 (NCEP/ATP III)	
CYP19	–	NR	25 Mexican women; NSA (Rotterdam) [152] 150 nuclear families; NSA (NIH) [153]

DM2, type 2 diabetes; EGIR, European Group for the Study of Insulin Resistance; MetS, metabolic syndrome; NCEP ATP III – US National Cholesterol Education Program Adult Treatment Panel III; NIH, National Institutes of Health Consensus (PCOS guidelines) [162]; NR, not reported; NSA, not statistically significant association; OR, odds ratio; PCOS, polycystic ovary syndrome; Rotterdam criteria for PCOS [163]; VNTR-variable number of tandem repeats, WHO – World Health Organization

*NCEP ATP III – variation in waist circumference criteria ± use of body mass index (BMI) criteria ± lower fasting blood glucose cut-off value

** Rotterdam criteria modified to have all 3 criteria (menstrual irregularities, polycystic ovaries on ultrasound, and clinical or biochemical hyperandrogenism)

† No OR available

‡ MetS defined as three of the following criteria: BMI exceeding the 97th percentile, systolic blood pressure and/or diastolic blood pressure exceeding the 95th percentile, triglyceride levels higher than 110 mg/dl, high-density lipoprotein cholesterol lower than 40 mg/dl for males and 50 mg/dl for females, and impaired glucose tolerance (glucose level greater than 140 mg/dl but less than 200 mg/dl after 2 h from the beginning of the oral glucose tolerance test

systolic blood pressure by 3.5 mmHg [71]. Further studies are needed to replicate the role of genetic alterations in these two cytokine genes in relation to MetS.

5.3.5.3 Candidate Genes in Adipose Distribution

The adipose distribution of MetS shares many clinical features with rarer disorders such as Cushing's syndrome. Thus, candidate genes involved in glucocorticoid metabolism such as 11-β-hydroxysteroid dehydrogenase type 1 (*HSD11B1*) and the glucocorticoid receptor (*GR*) have been examined. Although overexpression of *HSD11B1* leads to MetS phenotype in mice, *HSD11B1* SNPs have not been associated with MetS [72, 73]. The effects of glucocorticoids through the GR occur through the functional isomer GRα, whose activity is inhibited by GRβ [74]. The *GRB* 3669A→G SNP, which leads to increased GRβ protein expression, has been reported to not be associated with the composite MetS. Instead, an association with reduced central obesity among European women and a more favorable lipid profile (increased HDL and decreased total cholesterol) among European men was made with this SNP [75, 76].

Moreover, since the adipose distribution between MetS-affected and FPLD-affected patients is similar, a few studies have examined the relation of the known molecular causes of FPLD (peroxisome proliferator-activated receptor-γ [*PPARG*] and lamin A [*LMNA*] – see below) in relation to MetS. Lamins belong to the intermediate filament family of proteins and have functions related to the structural integrity of the nuclear envelope, transcriptional regulation, nuclear pore functioning, and heterochromatin organization [77, 78]. Polymorphisms in LMNA have not been associated with MetS [79], although a more recent study revealed novel LMNA non-codon 482 mutations among individuals with severe MetS phenotypes [80].

PPARG is a nuclear transcription factor involved in adipose differentiation, adipokine release, and insulin sensitivity. Unfortunately, conflicting results for the *PPARG* Pro12Ala polymorphism have been reported [81, 82]. In a French sample, the *PPARG* GTGC haplotype was associated with a higher risk for MetS (odds ratio [OR] 2.37) [83]. Yet, a recent meta-analysis of 57 studies in non-diabetic individuals demonstrated no significant association of *PPARG* Pro12Ala polymorphism with diabetes-related traits. Only amongst Caucasians and obese individuals was there an association of the Pro12Ala allele with greater body mass index (BMI) and greater insulin sensitivity [84]. Thus, whether *PPARG* or *LMNA* play any role in common MetS still remains to be conclusively proven.

5.3.5.4 Candidate Genes in Insulin and Glucose Metabolism

Since insulin resistance is a prominent feature for individuals with MetS, a few studies have examined the influence of molecules involved in insulin action and secretion. Among children with obesity, the insulin gene variable number of tandem repeats (*INS VNTR*) genotype was examined in relation to the presence of MetS. The VNTR polymorphism regulates the transcriptional rate of the *INS* gene [85]. Children who demonstrated the I/I genotype were at a significantly higher risk for developing MetS (OR = 2.5) [86]. Studies have yet to determine the relation between the *INS VNTR* genotype and MetS among adults.

Binding of insulin to the insulin receptor leads to phosphorylation and activation of insulin receptor substrates 1 and 2 (IRS-1 and IRS-2) necessary for insulin signaling. Thus, other candidate genes examined for MetS include the insulin receptor (*INSR*) gene and the IRS-1 (*IRS1*) gene. Among 163 Mexican individuals, the *Pst*I polymorphism of *INS* was associated with hypertriglyceridemia and the presence of at least one MetS abnormality while the *Mae*III polymorphism of *INS* was associated with fasting hyperinsulinemia. However, none of the *INSR* or *IRS1* polymorphisms examined were associated with MetS [87]. These data imply a possible role for the *INS* gene in MetS phenotype that may be more apparent in larger studies.

Calpain-10 (*CAPN10*) represents a cysteine protease that is important in insulin secretion and action [88]. Since haplotype combinations created by alleles of three *CAPN10* SNPs (SNP-43, -19, and -63) have been associated with the risk of type 2 diabetes, examination of *CAPN10* haplotypes in relation to MetS has been recently reported [89–91]. Among 382 Korean patients with type 2 diabetes, those who possessed the 111/121 haplotype combination had a significantly greater risk of MetS (OR = 1.927) compared to other haplotype combinations examined [89]. As with other candidate gene studies, these results need to be replicated in larger and more diverse ethnic populations before a definitive link can be established.

5.3.5.5 Candidate Genes from Sex Hormone Metabolism

Estrogen is a possible candidate gene for MetS based on the presence of MetS components (dyslipidemia, dysglycemia, obesity) in reported cases of estrogen-deficient men bearing mutations in either the estrogen receptor-α (*ESR1*) or aromatase (*CYP19*) genes and supported by data among *ESR1*-knockout mice [92–95]. Thus, these 2 genes (*ESR1* and *CYP19*) have been proposed as MetS candidate genes. Among 548 African Americans, 5 SNPs (rs6902771, rs9340799, rs2431260, rs1033182, and rs2175898) from introns 1 and 2 of *ESR1* were associated with an increased risk of MetS (OR 1.53–2.51) [96]. No association studies have yet been reported for *CYP19* and MetS. More recently, low sex hormone binding globulin (SHBG) levels in both genders have correlated with an increased risk for MetS, thereby signifying *SHBG* as another potential candidate gene for MetS although genetic association studies have yet to be reported [97, 98].

5.4 Genetic Lipodystrophies

5.4.1 Definition

Lipodystrophy represents a clinically heterogeneous group of disorders characterized by adipose tissue loss in either localized or generalized regions of the body [99, 100]. Similar to MetS and PCOS, it is often accompanied by metabolic abnormalities such as insulin resistance, glucose intolerance, lipid disorders (hypertriglyceridemia and low HDL-cholesterol levels), hypertension, polycystic ovaries, and hepatic steatosis. An increased risk of premature CVD occurs in some affected individuals, particularly females [101]. As a result of these clinical features, lipodystrophies share features with MetS and PCOS.

Lipodystrophies have been traditionally classified into two broad categories: acquired and genetic. They may also be a component of rare inherited syndromes such as SHORT syndrome and the progeroid syndromes [99]. (Table 5.3) Unlike the complex traits such as common MetS and PCOS, genetic lipodystrophies are monogenic disorders. Two genetic lipodystrophies where polycystic ovaries have been often observed are CGL and FPLD.

Table 5.3 Classification of lipodystrophies

A. Congenital:
1. Congenital generalized lipodystrophy (CGL, Berardinelli–Seip)
   a) CGL1 (due to mutations in *AGPAT2*)
   b) CGL2 (due to mutations in *BSCL2*)
2. Familial partial lipodystrophy (FPLD)
   a) FPLD1 (Kobberling)
   b) FPLD2 (Dunnigan, due to mutations in *LMNA*)
   c) FPLD3 (due to mutations in *PPARG*)

B. Acquired:
1. HIV-related lipodystrophy
2. Acquired generalized lipodystrophy (AGL)
3. Acquired partial lipodystrophy (APL, Barraquer–Simons; some cases are associated with mutations in *LMNB2*)

C. Lipodystrophy as part of another syndrome
1. Mandibuloacral dysplasia
2. SHORT syndrome
3. Neonatal progeroid syndrome
4. Hutchinson–Gilford progeria syndrome
5. Werner syndrome

5.4.2 Congenital Generalized Lipodystrophy (Berardinelli–Seip Syndrome)

5.4.2.1 Clinical Features

CGL is an autosomal-recessive disorder characterized by the generalized near-absence of adipose tissue usually recognized in affected individuals soon after their birth [99, 102, 103]. During childhood, affected individuals are distinguished by the presence of muscular phenotype, voracious appetite, acceleration in linear growth, advanced bone age, acromegaloid features, and typically, marked acanthosis nigricans [104, 105]. Cardiomyopathy and mental retardation may occur, but is strongly dependent on genotype [106]. More importantly, endocrine complications include hypertriglyceridemia (sometimes resulting in pancreatitis), fasting hyperglycemia, diabetes (often with significant insulin resistance), and markedly low levels of adiponectin and leptin [107]. Hepatic steatosis with consequent hepatomegaly can also occur. As well, among women, hirsutism, polycystic ovaries (PCOS), and menstrual irregularities can occur, whereas among men, reproductive function has been reported to be normal [108].

5.4.2.2 Pathophysiology and Molecular Genetics

The two main molecular forms of CGL are (1) type 1 caused by mutations in the *AGPAT2* gene (MIM 608594) and (2) type 2 caused by mutations in the *BSCL2* gene (MIM 606158). Since not all patients affected with CGL have mutations in one of these two genes, additional loci or pathways may exist.

AGPAT2, located on chromosome 9q34, encodes 1-acylglycerol-3-phosphate O-acyltransferase 2, also called LPA acyltransferase (LPAAT)-β or 1-acyl-sn-glycerol-3-phosphate acetyltransferase (EC 2.3.1.51) [109, 110]. This enzyme plays a critical role in catalyzing reactions in TG synthesis and is also linked to increased transcription and synthesis of cytokines including IL-6 and TNF-α [111]. CGL1 caused by *AGPAT2* often results from nonsense or aberrant splicing mutations. Thus far, no obvious correlation between mutation severity and phenotypic severity has been shown.

BSCL2 gene in the CGL2 locus located on chromosome 11q13 encodes the protein "seipin" [112]. Seipin, expressed mainly in the brain and testes, is a 398-amino acid integral membrane protein that localizes to the endoplasmic reticulum of eukaryotic cells [112, 113]. The function of this protein is yet to be determined. Yet, compared to patients with *AGPAT2*-caused CGL, patients with *BSCL2*-caused CGL tend to have a more severe phenotype characterized by earlier onset of diabetes and higher prevalence of cardiomyopathy and mild mental delay [106]. To date, >12 mutations in *BSCL2* have been identified, and these are typically of the nonsense or aberrant splicing variety. Similar to *AGPAT2*-caused CGL, *BSCL2*-caused CGL does not demonstrate any obvious correlation between mutation severity and phenotype severity.

5.4.3 Familial Partial Lipodystrophy

5.4.3.1 Clinical Features

FPLD is an autosomal dominant syndrome, subdivided into 3 varieties – FPLD1 (or Kobberling-type MIM; 608600), FPLD2 (or Dunnigan-type; MIM 151660) caused by *LMNA* mutations, and FPLD3 (MIM 604367) caused by *PPARG* mutations [114–116]. FPLD is characterized by gradual but progressive subcutaneous adipose tissue loss from the extremities typically commencing at puberty. The onset of FPLD3, however, may be later in adulthood. Unlike individuals affected with CGL, FPLD-affected individuals cannot be easily distinguished from unaffected individuals during childhood. There is also variable degree of adipose tissue loss in the face and trunk depending on sub-type. In FPLD1, there is normal or increased fat deposition in the face, neck, and trunk, whereas in FPLD2, there is decreased fat deposition in the trunk and increased deposition in the neck and labia. Affected individuals with FPLD3 demonstrate decreased to absent facial fat. Yet, all three sub-types tend to have increased fat deposition within the muscles and within the liver [117–120].

Endocrine manifestations of FPLD include low HDL-cholesterol levels, hypertriglyceridemia, diabetes, acanthosis nigricans, and among women, hirsutism, polycystic ovaries, and menstrual irregularities [121]. Importantly, premature CVD is more prevalent among individuals who have FPLD2 and diabetes [122, 123].

5.4.3.2 Pathophysiology and Molecular Genetics

The genetic basis for FPLD1 remains unknown. Meanwhile, heterozygous mutations in the *LMNA* gene encoding nuclear lamin A/C (MIM 150330) are responsible for the majority of FPLD2 cases [124]. The majority of causative *LMNA* mutations for FPLD2 are missense, with only one splicing mutation described thus far. The exact mechanisms by which *LMNA* mutations cause lipodystrophy remain unknown. *LMNA* mutations typically occur downstream of the nuclear localization sequence (NLS), which divides lamin A into the structural rod domain on the amino-terminal side and the DNA-binding domain on the carboxy-terminal side. Thus, a possible mechanism for the FPLD2 phenotype through *LMNA* mutations may involve altered interactions of transcription factors or other DNA-binding molecules [77]. However, two FPLD2 mutations – *LMNA* D230N and R399C – have been recently found upstream of the lamin A NLS [125], signifying possible pathophysiologic importance of the secondary and/or tertiary structure of lamin A [77]. Deletions or duplications of *LMNA* for FPLD2 have not yet been found (Hegele, unpublished observations). LMNA exhibits a great deal of transcriptional variability, which may lead to the identification of novel mutation-bearing regions for FPLD2 as well as other laminopathies.

Heterozygous mutations in the *PPARG* gene (PPARγ; MIM 601487) are causative for FPLD3 (MIM 604367) [126–132]. There are 2 main proposed mechanisms for mutated *PPARG* in the pathogenesis of FPLD3: (a) "dominant-negative", in which the mutant receptor competes with the wild type for DNA binding and (b) "haploinsufficiency", in which the function of the PPARγ receptor is adversely affected by a 50% reduction in gene expression. Careful cellular assays indicate that seven PPARγ mutations (C114R, C131Y, C162W, FS315X, R357X, P467L, and V290M) act via a dominant negative mechanism [127, 132], and six (-14A>G, F388L, E138fsΔAATG, Y355X, R194W, and R425C) via haploinsufficiency [128–131, 133, 134].

Despite our knowledge thus far regarding the molecular basis of FPLD, ~50% of FPLD patients do not possess mutations in either *LMNA* or *PPARG* genes (Hegele, unpublished observations), possibly due to (1) presence of alternate mutation types not detected by DNA sequence analysis, such as copy number variations; (2) genetic heterogeneity from new causative genes yet to be identified; and/or (3) presence of mutations in unrecognized regions of *LMNA* or *PPARG*. Yet, despite these caveats, the search for determining other players in the molecular basis of FPLD continues since this may have relevance to other traits such as MetS or PCOS.

5.5 Genetics of Mets and Genetic Lipodystrophies: Relation to PCOS

Since PCOS shares many clinical features with both the genetic lipodystrophies and MetS, candidate genes from the latter two have been examined among patients with PCOS (Table 5.2). For a thorough discussion of all genetic influences on PCOS and its component traits, the reader is referred to another book chapter. Here, we focus solely on candidate genes in PCOS derived from genetic lipodystrophies or MetS.

Focusing on insulin resistance, candidate genes of *ADIPOQ*, *RSTN*, *INS*, *INSR*, and *IRS1* have been examined in PCOS. Several studies have not found a significant association between *ADIPOQ* polymorphisms (T45G and G276T) and PCOS, despite the fact that adiponectin is inversely correlated with insulin sensitivity [135–137]. Furthermore, the allelic and genotypic frequencies for the -420C→G *RSTN* polymorphism were not different between PCOS-affected patients and controls [136]. Although there have been several studies examining the relation between the *INS VNTR* genotype and PCOS, a recent examination of different datasets including a total of more than 3000 individuals revealed no significant relation [138–140]. Meanwhile, conflicting results have been demonstrated for the Gly972Arg polymorphism of *IRS1* [141, 142] or the *CAPN10* genotypes in relation to PCOS [143, 144].

Although conclusive evidence regarding the relationship between *PPARG* and MetS remains to be demonstrated [81–83], mutations in *PPARG* are causative for FPLD [126–128]. Similar to MetS, conflicting results have been obtained for the relation of Pro12Ala *PPARG* polymorphism to metabolic parameters of PCOS [135, 145]. To date, no studies have evaluated the influence of *LMNA*, *AGPAT2*, or *BSCL2* in relation to PCOS. Meanwhile, the influence of *HSD11β1* variants on susceptibility for PCOS has not been demonstrated [146, 147], and the N363S variant of the *GR* (glucocorticoid receptor gene) has not yet been correlated either with the PCOS phenotype or with hyperandrogenemia among PCOS patients [148].

The cytokine genes *TNF-α* and *IL6* have also been examined in PCOS. Several polymorphisms for *TNF-α* [149, 150] have not been linked to PCOS while one study demonstrated no link between the -174G→C *IL6* promoter polymorphisms to PCOS itself, but rather an association to the clinical characteristics of increased body mass index, elevated serum testosterone levels, and dysglycemia [151]. Conversely, studies of sex hormone-related candidate genes have provided more conclusive results. No relation has been demonstrated between the aromatase gene (*CYP19*) and the PCOS phenotype [152, 153]. Studies on the relation between *ESR1* and PCOS are awaited. Thus far, only one study among Greek women has demonstrated a significant association between the $(TAAAA)_n$ *SHBG* polymorphism and PCOS, although two studies have demonstrated that longer $(TAAAA)_n$ alleles are associated with lower SHBG levels, implying a possible genetic influence of *SHBG* [154, 155]. Therefore, determining the genetic basis of PCOS using candidate genes derived from an understanding of MetS, CGL, or FPLD requires further study.

5.6 Conclusions

Since PCOS shares many clinical features with both genetic lipodystrophies and MetS, understanding the genetic basis for the latter two clinical entities may shed light on the genetic basis of PCOS. Moreover, unlike genetic lipodystrophies, both MetS and PCOS represent common complex genetic traits, and thus genetic discernment remains difficult. Importantly, due to the lack of consensus definitions, both clinical entities (MetS and PCOS) are characterized by difficulties in accurate phenotype assignment. PCOS is further plagued by the uncertainty regarding definition of a male phenotype. Consequently, phenotypic variability negatively influences reproducibility of genetic associations. As well, differences in ethnicity or small sample sizes have contributed to the conflicting results demonstrated in genetic association and linkage studies, thereby limiting the validity and reproducibility of the genetic results obtained for both PCOS and MetS. Interestingly, examining PCOS by linkage studies poses an additional problem of possible selection bias for families with milder variants of PCOS since infertility (a key feature for PCOS) can limit the size of pedigrees that can be analyzed. Thus, linkage studies for PCOS need to be interpreted with caution. Hopefully, newer information from HapMap and genome-wide sets of markers as well as the use of more novel genetic interrogation strategies in MetS and genetic lipodystrophies will eventually help clarify the genetic basis of PCOS.

Acknowledgments This work was supported by operating grants from the Canadian Institutes of Health Research (MOP-13430 and MOP-79533), the Heart and Stroke Foundation of Ontario (T6018; NA6059 and PRG5657), and Genome Canada through the Ontario Genomics Institute. Dr. Hegele is a Career Investigator of the Heart and Stroke Foundation of Ontario and holds the Edith Schulich Vinet Canada Research Chair (Tier I) in Human Genetics and the Jacob J. Wolfe Distinguished Medical Research Chair.

References

1. Azziz R, Woods KS, Reyna R, et al. The prevalence and features of the polycystic ovary syndrome in an unselected population. The Journal of clinical endocrinology and metabolism 2004; 89(6):2745–9.
2. Ovalle F, Azziz R. Insulin resistance, polycystic ovary syndrome, and type 2 diabetes mellitus. Fertility and sterility 2002; 77(6):1095–105.
3. Diamanti-Kandarakis E, Papavassiliou AG, Kandarakis SA, et al. Pathophysiology and types of dyslipidemia in PCOS. Trends in endocrinology and metabolism 2007; 18(7):280–5.
4. Yildiz BO, Yarali H, Oguz H, et al. Glucose intolerance, insulin resistance, and hyperandrogenemia in first degree relatives of women with polycystic ovary syndrome. The Journal of clinical endocrinology and metabolism 2003; 88(5):2031–6.
5. Sam S, Legro RS, Bentley-Lewis R, et al. Dyslipidemia and metabolic syndrome in the sisters of women with polycystic ovary syndrome. The Journal of clinical endocrinology and metabolism 2005; 90(8):4797–802.

6. Diamanti-Kandarakis E, Alexandraki K, Bergiele A, et al. Presence of metabolic risk factors in non-obese PCOS sisters: evidence of heritability of insulin resistance. Journal of endocrinological investigation 2004; 27(10):931–6.
7. Schork NJ. Genetics of complex disease: approaches, problems, and solutions. American journal of respiratory and critical care medicine 1997; 156(4 Pt 2):S103–9.
8. WHO. Definition, diagnosis, and classification of diabetes mellitus and its complications. Report of a WHO Consultation. Available at: http://www.staff.newcastle.ac.uk/philip.home/who˙dmc.htm 1999.
9. Executive Summary of the Third Report of The National Cholesterol Education Program (NCEP) Expert Panel on Detection, Evaluation, and Treatment of High Blood Cholesterol In Adults (Adult Treatment Panel III). The journal of the American medical association 2001; 285(19):2486–97.
10. Alberti KG, Zimmet P, Shaw J. The metabolic syndrome–a new worldwide definition. Lancet 2005; 366(9491):1059–62.
11. Balkau B, Charles MA. Comment on the provisional report from the WHO consultation. European Group for the Study of Insulin Resistance (EGIR). Diabetic medicine 1999; 16(5):442–3.
12. Einhorn D, Reaven GM, Cobin RH, et al. American College of Endocrinology position statement on the insulin resistance syndrome. Endocrine practice 2003; 9(3):237–52.
13. Grundy SM, Cleeman JI, Daniels SR, et al. Diagnosis and management of the metabolic syndrome: an American Heart Association/National Heart, Lung, and Blood Institute Scientific Statement. Circulation 2005; 112(17):2735–52.
14. Ford ES, Giles WH, Dietz WH. Prevalence of the metabolic syndrome among US adults: findings from the third National Health and Nutrition Examination Survey. The journal of the American medical association 2002; 287(3):356–9.
15. Park YW, Zhu S, Palaniappan L, et al. The metabolic syndrome: prevalence and associated risk factor findings in the US population from the Third National Health and Nutrition Examination Survey, 1988–1994. Archives of internal medicine 2003; 163(4):427–36.
16. Margolin E, Zhornitzki T, Kopernik G, et al. Polycystic ovary syndrome in post-menopausal women–marker of the metabolic syndrome. Maturitas 2005; 50(4):331–6.
17. Taponen S, Martikainen H, Jarvelin MR, et al. Metabolic cardiovascular disease risk factors in women with self-reported symptoms of oligomenorrhea and/or hirsutism: Northern Finland Birth Cohort 1966 Study. The Journal of clinical endocrinology and metabolism 2004; 89(5):2114–8.
18. Apridonidze T, Essah PA, Iuorno MJ, et al. Prevalence and characteristics of the metabolic syndrome in women with polycystic ovary syndrome. The Journal of clinical endocrinology and metabolism 2005; 90(4):1929–35.
19. Legro RS. Detection of insulin resistance and its treatment in adolescents with polycystic ovary syndrome. Journal of Pediatric Endocrinology & Metabolism 2002; 15(Suppl 5):1367–78.
20. Glueck CJ, Papanna R, Wang P, et al. Incidence and treatment of metabolic syndrome in newly referred women with confirmed polycystic ovarian syndrome. Metabolism: clinical and experimental 2003; 52(7):908–15.
21. Dokras A, Bochner M, Hollinrake E, et al. Screening women with polycystic ovary syndrome for metabolic syndrome. Obstetrics and gynecology 2005; 106(1):131–7.
22. Vural B, Caliskan E, Turkoz E, et al. Evaluation of metabolic syndrome frequency and premature carotid atherosclerosis in young women with polycystic ovary syndrome. Human reproduction (Oxford, England) 2005; 20(9):2409–13.
23. Ehrmann DA, Liljenquist DR, Kasza K, et al. Prevalence and predictors of the metabolic syndrome in women with polycystic ovary syndrome. The Journal of clinical endocrinology and metabolism 2006; 91(1):48–53.
24. Weisberg SP, McCann D, Desai M, et al. Obesity is associated with macrophage accumulation in adipose tissue. The Journal of clinical investigation 2003; 112(12):1796–808.
25. Dresner A, Laurent D, Marcucci M, et al. Effects of free fatty acids on glucose transport and IRS-1-associated phosphatidylinositol 3-kinase activity. The Journal of clinical investigation 1999; 103(2):253–9.
26. Belfort R, Mandarino L, Kashyap S, et al. Dose-response effect of elevated plasma free fatty acid on insulin signaling. Diabetes 2005; 54(6):1640–8.
27. Lupi R, Dotta F, Marselli L, et al. Prolonged exposure to free fatty acids has cytostatic and pro-apoptotic effects on human pancreatic islets: evidence that beta-cell death is caspase mediated, partially dependent on ceramide pathway, and Bcl-2 regulated. Diabetes 2002; 51(5):1437–42.
28. Oprescu AI, Bikopoulos G, Naassan A, et al. Free fatty acid-induced reduction in glucose stimulated insulin secretion evidence for a role of oxidative stress in vitro and in vivo. Diabetes 2007; 56(12):2927–2937.
29. Combs TP, Berg AH, Obici S, et al. Endogenous glucose production is inhibited by the adipose-derived protein Acrp30. The Journal of clinical investigation 2001; 108(12):1875–81.
30. Tomas E, Tsao TS, Saha AK, et al. Enhanced muscle fat oxidation and glucose transport by ACRP30 globular domain: acetyl-CoA carboxylase inhibition and AMP-activated protein kinase activation. Proceedings of the National Academy of Sciences of the United States of America 2002; 99(25):16309–13.
31. Yamauchi T, Kamon J, Minokoshi Y, et al. Adiponectin stimulates glucose utilization and fatty-acid oxidation by activating AMP-activated protein kinase. Nature medicine 2002; 8(11):1288–95.
32. Rotter V, Nagaev I, Smith U. Interleukin-6 (IL-6) induces insulin resistance in 3T3-L1 adipocytes and is, like IL-8 and tumor necrosis factor-alpha, overexpressed in human fat cells from insulin-resistant subjects. The Journal of biological chemistry 2003; 278(46):45777–84.
33. Aguirre V, Werner ED, Giraud J, et al. Phosphorylation of Ser307 in insulin receptor substrate-1 blocks interactions with the insulin receptor and inhibits insulin action. The Journal of biological chemistry 2002; 277(2):1531–7.

34. Sopasakis VR, Sandqvist M, Gustafson B, et al. High local concentrations and effects on differentiation implicate interleukin-6 as a paracrine regulator. Obesity research 2004; 12(3):454–60.
35. Ruan H, Lodish HF. Insulin resistance in adipose tissue: direct and indirect effects of tumor necrosis factor-alpha. Cytokine & growth factor reviews 2003; 14(5):447–55.
36. Brunzell JD, Hokanson JE. Dyslipidemia of central obesity and insulin resistance. Diabetes care 1999; 22(Suppl 3):C10–3.
37. Ginsberg HN, Huang LS. The insulin resistance syndrome: impact on lipoprotein metabolism and atherothrombosis. Journal of cardiovascular risk 2000; 7(5):325–31.
38. Cooper R, McFarlane-Anderson N, Bennett FI, et al. ACE, angiotensinogen and obesity: a potential pathway leading to hypertension. Journal of human hypertension 1997; 11(2):107–11.
39. Serne EH, de Jongh RT, Eringa EC, et al. Microvascular dysfunction: a potential pathophysiological role in the metabolic syndrome. Hypertension 2007; 50(1):204–11.
40. Carmelli D, Cardon LR, Fabsitz R. Clustering of hypertension, diabetes, and obesity in adult male twins: same genes or same environments? American journal of human genetics 1994; 55(3):566–73.
41. Edwards KL, Newman B, Mayer E, et al. Heritability of factors of the insulin resistance syndrome in women twins. Genetic epidemiology 1997; 14(3):241–53.
42. Austin MA, Edwards KL, McNeely MJ, et al. Heritability of multivariate factors of the metabolic syndrome in nondiabetic Japanese Americans. Diabetes 2004; 53(4):1166–9.
43. Li JK, Ng MC, So WY, et al. Phenotypic and genetic clustering of diabetes and metabolic syndrome in Chinese families with type 2 diabetes mellitus. Diabetes/metabolism research and reviews 2006; 22(1):46–52.
44. Lin HF, Boden-Albala B, Juo SH, et al. Heritabilities of the metabolic syndrome and its components in the Northern Manhattan Family Study. Diabetologia 2005; 48(10):2006–12.
45. Kissebah AH, Sonnenberg GE, Myklebust J, et al. Quantitative trait loci on chromosomes 3 and 17 influence phenotypes of the metabolic syndrome. Proceedings of the National Academy of Sciences of the United States of America 2000; 97(26):14478–83.
46. Arya R, Blangero J, Williams K, et al. Factors of insulin resistance syndrome–related phenotypes are linked to genetic locations on chromosomes 6 and 7 in nondiabetic Mexican-Americans. Diabetes 2002; 51(3):841–7.
47. Langefeld CD, Wagenknecht LE, Rotter JI, et al. Linkage of the metabolic syndrome to 1q23-q31 in Hispanic families: the Insulin Resistance Atherosclerosis Study Family Study. Diabetes 2004; 53(4):1170–4.
48. McQueen MB, Bertram L, Rimm EB, et al. A QTL genome scan of the metabolic syndrome and its component traits. BMC genetics 2003; 4(Suppl 1):S96.
49. Hamet P, Merlo E, Seda O, et al. Quantitative founder-effect analysis of French Canadian families identifies specific loci contributing to metabolic phenotypes of hypertension. American journal of human genetics 2005; 76(5):815–32.
50. Loos RJ, Katzmarzyk PT, Rao DC, et al. Genome-wide linkage scan for the metabolic syndrome in the HERITAGE Family Study. The Journal of clinical endocrinology and metabolism 2003; 88(12):5935–43.
51. Olswold C, de Andrade M. Localization of genes involved in the metabolic syndrome using multivariate linkage analysis. BMC genetics 2003; 4(Suppl 1):S57.
52. Ng MC, So WY, Lam VK, et al. Genome-wide scan for metabolic syndrome and related quantitative traits in Hong Kong Chinese and confirmation of a susceptibility locus on chromosome 1q21-q25. Diabetes 2004; 53(10):2676–83.
53. Stein CM, Song Y, Elston RC, et al. Structural equation model-based genome scan for the metabolic syndrome. BMC genetics 2003; 4(Suppl 1):S99.
54. Tang W, Miller MB, Rich SS, et al. Linkage analysis of a composite factor for the multiple metabolic syndrome: the National Heart, Lung, and Blood Institute Family Heart Study. Diabetes 2003; 52(11):2840–7.
55. Bosse Y, Despres JP, Chagnon YC, et al. Quantitative trait locus on 15q for a metabolic syndrome variable derived from factor analysis. Obesity Silver Spring, Md 2007; 15(3):544–50.
56. Hsueh WC, St Jean PL, Mitchell BD, et al. Genome-wide and fine-mapping linkage studies of type 2 diabetes and glucose traits in the Old Order Amish: evidence for a new diabetes locus on chromosome 14q11 and confirmation of a locus on chromosome 1q21-q24. Diabetes 2003; 52(2):550–7.
57. Ng MC, So WY, Cox NJ, et al. Genome-wide scan for type 2 diabetes loci in Hong Kong Chinese and confirmation of a susceptibility locus on chromosome 1q21-q25. Diabetes 2004; 53(6):1609–13.
58. Das SK, Hasstedt SJ, Zhang Z, et al. Linkage and association mapping of a chromosome 1q21-q24 type 2 diabetes susceptibility locus in northern European Caucasians. Diabetes 2004; 53(2):492–9.
59. Vionnet N, Hani EH, Dupont S, et al. Genomewide search for type 2 diabetes-susceptibility genes in French whites: evidence for a novel susceptibility locus for early-onset diabetes on chromosome 3q27-qter and independent replication of a type 2-diabetes locus on chromosome 1q21-q24. American journal of human genetics 2000; 67(6):1470–80.
60. Thameem F, Farook VS, Bogardus C, et al. Association of amino acid variants in the activating transcription factor 6 gene (ATF6) on 1q21-q23 with type 2 diabetes in Pima Indians. Diabetes 2006; 55(3):839–42.
61. Hoffmann K, Mattheisen M, Dahm S, et al. A German genome-wide linkage scan for type 2 diabetes supports the existence of a metabolic syndrome locus on chromosome 1p36.13 and a type 2 diabetes locus on chromosome 16p12.2. Diabetologia 2007; 50(7):1418–22.
62. Stumvoll M, Tschritter O, Fritsche A, et al. Association of the T-G polymorphism in adiponectin (exon 2) with obesity and insulin sensitivity: interaction with family history of type 2 diabetes. Diabetes 2002; 51(1):37–41.

63. Yang WS, Tsou PL, Lee WJ, et al. Allele-specific differential expression of a common adiponectin gene polymorphism related to obesity. Journal of molecular medicine (Berlin, Germany) 2003; 81(7):428–34.
64. Kondo H, Shimomura I, Matsukawa Y, et al. Association of adiponectin mutation with type 2 diabetes: a candidate gene for the insulin resistance syndrome. Diabetes 2002; 51(7):2325–8.
65. Hara K, Boutin P, Mori Y, et al. Genetic variation in the gene encoding adiponectin is associated with an increased risk of type 2 diabetes in the Japanese population. Diabetes 2002; 51(2):536–40.
66. Yang WS, Hsiung CA, Ho LT, et al. Genetic epistasis of adiponectin and PPARgamma2 genotypes in modulation of insulin sensitivity: a family-based association study. Diabetologia 2003; 46(7):977–83.
67. Yang WS, Yang YC, Chen CL, et al. Adiponectin SNP276 is associated with obesity, the metabolic syndrome, and diabetes in the elderly. The American journal of clinical nutrition 2007; 86(2):509–13.
68. Norata GD, Ongari M, Garlaschelli K, et al. Effect of the -420C/G variant of the resistin gene promoter on metabolic syndrome, obesity, myocardial infarction and kidney dysfunction. Journal of internal medicine 2007; 262(1):104–12.
69. Hamid YH, Rose CS, Urhammer SA, et al. Variations of the interleukin-6 promoter are associated with features of the metabolic syndrome in Caucasian Danes. Diabetologia 2005; 48(2):251–60.
70. Stephens JW, Hurel SJ, Lowe GD, et al. Association between plasma IL-6, the IL6 -174G>C gene variant and the metabolic syndrome in type 2 diabetes mellitus. Molecular genetics and metabolism 2007; 90(4):422–8.
71. Sookoian SC, Gonzalez C, Pirola CJ. Meta-analysis on the G-308A tumor necrosis factor alpha gene variant and phenotypes associated with the metabolic syndrome. Obesity research 2005; 13(12):2122–31.
72. Robitaille J, Brouillette C, Houde A, et al. Molecular screening of the 11beta-HSD1 gene in men characterized by the metabolic syndrome. Obesity research 2004; 12(10):1570–5.
73. Seckl JR, Morton NM, Chapman KE, et al. Glucocorticoids and 11beta-hydroxysteroid dehydrogenase in adipose tissue. Recent progress in hormone research 2004; 59:359–93.
74. Oakley RH, Jewell CM, Yudt MR, et al. The dominant negative activity of the human glucocorticoid receptor beta isoform. Specificity and mechanisms of action. The Journal of biological chemistry 1999; 274(39):27857–66.
75. Derijk RH, Schaaf MJ, Turner G, et al. A human glucocorticoid receptor gene variant that increases the stability of the glucocorticoid receptor beta-isoform mRNA is associated with rheumatoid arthritis. The Journal of rheumatology 2001; 28(11):2383–8.
76. Syed AA, Irving JA, Redfern CP, et al. Association of glucocorticoid receptor polymorphism A3669G in exon 9beta with reduced central adiposity in women. Obesity Silver Spring, Md 2006; 14(5):759–64.
77. Hegele R. LMNA mutation position predicts organ system involvement in laminopathies. Clinical Genetics 2005; 68(1):31–4.
78. Capell BC, Collins FS. Human laminopathies: nuclei gone genetically awry. Nature Reviews Genetics 2006; 7(12):940–52.
79. Mesa JL, Loos RJ, Franks PW, et al. Lamin A/C polymorphisms, type 2 diabetes, and the metabolic syndrome: case-control and quantitative trait studies. Diabetes 2007; 56(3):884–9.
80. Decaudain A, Vantyghem MC, Guerci B, et al. New metabolic phenotypes in laminopathies: LMNA mutations in patients with severe metabolic syndrome. The Journal of clinical endocrinology and metabolism 2007; 92(12):4835–44.
81. Mousavinasab F, Tahtinen T, Jokelainen J, et al. The Pro12Ala polymorphism of the PPAR gamma 2 gene influences sex hormone-binding globulin level and its relationship to the development of the metabolic syndrome in young Finnish men. Endocrine 2006; 30(2):185–90.
82. Rhee EJ, Oh KW, Lee WY, et al. Effects of two common polymorphisms of peroxisome proliferator-activated receptor-gamma gene on metabolic syndrome. Archives of medical research 2006; 37(1):86–94.
83. Meirhaeghe A, Cottel D, Amouyel P, et al. Association between peroxisome proliferator-activated receptor gamma haplotypes and the metabolic syndrome in French men and women. Diabetes 2005; 54(10):3043–8.
84. Tonjes A, Scholz M, Loeffler M, et al. Association of Pro12Ala polymorphism in peroxisome proliferator-activated receptor gamma with Pre-diabetic phenotypes: meta-analysis of 57 studies on nondiabetic individuals. Diabetes care 2006; 29(11):2489–97.
85. Kennedy GC, German MS, Rutter WJ. The minisatellite in the diabetes susceptibility locus IDDM2 regulates insulin transcription. Nature genetics 1995; 9(3):293–8.
86. Santoro N, Cirillo G, Amato A, et al. Insulin gene variable number of tandem repeats (INS VNTR) genotype and metabolic syndrome in childhood obesity. The Journal of clinical endocrinology and metabolism 2006; 91(11):4641–4.
87. Sanchez-Corona J, Flores-Martinez SE, Machorro-Lazo MV, et al. Polymorphisms in candidate genes for type 2 diabetes mellitus in a Mexican population with metabolic syndrome findings. Diabetes research and clinical practice 2004; 63(1): 47–55.
88. Sreenan SK, Zhou YP, Otani K, et al. Calpains play a role in insulin secretion and action. Diabetes 2001; 50(9):2013–20.
89. Kang ES, Nam M, Kim HJ, et al. Haplotype combination of Calpain-10 gene polymorphism is associated with metabolic syndrome in type 2 diabetes. Diabetes research and clinical practice 2006; 73(3):268–75.
90. Lynn S, Evans JC, White C, et al. Variation in the calpain-10 gene affects blood glucose levels in the British population. Diabetes 2002; 51(1):247–50.
91. Cassell PG, Jackson AE, North BV, et al. Haplotype combinations of calpain 10 gene polymorphisms associate with increased risk of impaired glucose tolerance and type 2 diabetes in South Indians. Diabetes 2002; 51(5):1622–8.
92. Rochira V, Balestrieri A, Madeo B, et al. Congenital estrogen deficiency in men: a new syndrome with different phenotypes; clinical and therapeutic implications in men. Molecular and cellular endocrinology 2002; 193(1–2):19–28.

93. Smith EP, Boyd J, Frank GR, et al. Estrogen resistance caused by a mutation in the estrogen-receptor gene in a man. The New England journal of medicine 1994; 331(16):1056–61.
94. Ohlsson C, Hellberg N, Parini P, et al. Obesity and disturbed lipoprotein profile in estrogen receptor-alpha-deficient male mice. Biochemical and biophysical research communications 2000; 278(3):640–5.
95. Maffei L, Rochira V, Zirilli L, et al. A novel compound heterozygous mutation of the aromatase gene in an adult man: reinforced evidence on the relationship between congenital oestrogen deficiency, adiposity and the metabolic syndrome. Clinical endocrinology 2007; 67(2):218–24.
96. Gallagher CJ, Langefeld CD, Gordon CJ, et al. Association of the estrogen receptor-alpha gene with the metabolic syndrome and its component traits in African-American families: the Insulin Resistance Atherosclerosis Family Study. Diabetes 2007; 56(8):2135–41.
97. Kupelian V, Page ST, Araujo AB, et al. Low sex hormone-binding globulin, total testosterone, and symptomatic androgen deficiency are associated with development of the metabolic syndrome in nonobese men. The Journal of clinical endocrinology and metabolism 2006; 91(3):843–50.
98. Weinberg ME, Manson JE, Buring JE, et al. Low sex hormone-binding globulin is associated with the metabolic syndrome in postmenopausal women. Metabolism: clinical and experimental 2006; 55(11):1473–80.
99. Garg A. Acquired and inherited lipodystrophies. The New England journal of medicine 2004; 350(12):1220–34.
100. Garg A, Misra A. Lipodystrophies: rare disorders causing metabolic syndrome. Endocrinology and metabolism clinics of North America 2004; 33(2):305–31.
101. Hegele RA. Monogenic forms of insulin resistance: apertures that expose the common metabolic syndrome. Trends in endocrinology and metabolism 2003; 14(8):371–7.
102. Berardinelli W. An undiagnosed endocrinometabolic syndrome: report of 2 cases. The Journal of clinical endocrinology and metabolism 1954; 14(2):193–204.
103. Seip M. Lipodystrophy and gigantism with associated endocrine manifestations. A new diencephalic syndrome? Acta paediatrica 1959; 48:555–74.
104. Westvik J. Radiological features in generalized lipodystrophy. Acta Paediatrica Supplement 1996; 413:44–51.
105. Seip M, Trygstad O. Generalized lipodystrophy, congenital and acquired (lipoatrophy). Acta Paediatrica Supplement 1996; 413:2–28.
106. Agarwal AK, Simha V, Oral EA, et al. Phenotypic and genetic heterogeneity in congenital generalized lipodystrophy. The Journal of clinical endocrinology and metabolism 2003; 88(10):4840–7.
107. Haque WA, Shimomura I, Matsuzawa Y, et al. Serum adiponectin and leptin levels in patients with lipodystrophies. The Journal of clinical endocrinology and metabolism 2002; 87(5):2395.
108. Agarwal AK, Garg A. Genetic basis of lipodystrophies and management of metabolic complications. Annual review of medicine 2006; 57:297–311.
109. Garg A, Wilson R, Barnes R, et al. A gene for congenital generalized lipodystrophy maps to human chromosome 9q34. The Journal of clinical endocrinology and metabolism 1999; 84(9):3390–4.
110. Agarwal AK, Arioglu E, De Almeida S, et al. AGPAT2 is mutated in congenital generalized lipodystrophy linked to chromosome 9q34. Nature genetics 2002; 31(1):21–3.
111. Agarwal AK, Garg A. Congenital generalized lipodystrophy: significance of triglyceride biosynthetic pathways. Trends in endocrinology and metabolism 2003; 14(5):214–21.
112. Magre J, Delepine M, Khallouf E, et al. Identification of the gene altered in Berardinelli–Seip congenital lipodystrophy on chromosome 11q13. Nature genetics 2001; 28(4):365–70.
113. Lundin C, Nordstrom R, Wagner K, et al. Membrane topology of the human seipin protein. FEBS letters 2006; 580(9): 2281–4.
114. Kobberling J, Willms B, Kattermann R, et al. Lipodystrophy of the extremities. A dominantly inherited syndrome associated with lipatrophic diabetes. Humangenetik 1975; 29(2):111–20.
115. Kobberling J, Dunnigan MG. Familial partial lipodystrophy: two types of an X linked dominant syndrome, lethal in the hemizygous state. Journal of medical genetics 1986; 23(2):120–7.
116. Dunnigan MG, Cochrane MA, Kelly A, et al. Familial lipoatrophic diabetes with dominant transmission. A new syndrome. The Quarterly journal of medicine 1974; 43(169):33–48.
117. Garg A, Peshock RM, Fleckenstein JL. Adipose tissue distribution pattern in patients with familial partial lipodystrophy (Dunnigan variety). The Journal of clinical endocrinology and metabolism 1999; 84(1):170–4.
118. Garg A, Vinaitheerthan M, Weatherall PT, et al. Phenotypic heterogeneity in patients with familial partial lipodystrophy (dunnigan variety) related to the site of missense mutations in lamin a/c gene. The Journal of clinical endocrinology and metabolism 2001; 86(1):59–65.
119. Hegele RA. Lessons from human mutations in PPARgamma. International journal of obesity 2005; 29(Suppl 1):S31–5.
120. Ludtke A, Genschel J, Brabant G, et al. Hepatic steatosis in Dunnigan-type familial partial lipodystrophy. The American journal of gastroenterology 2005; 100(10):2218–24.
121. Garg A. Gender differences in the prevalence of metabolic complications in familial partial lipodystrophy (Dunnigan variety). The Journal of clinical endocrinology and metabolism 2000; 85(5):1776–82.
122. Hegele RA. Premature atherosclerosis associated with monogenic insulin resistance. Circulation 2001; 103(18): 2225–9.

123. Vantyghem MC, Pigny P, Maurage CA, et al. Patients with familial partial lipodystrophy of the Dunnigan type due to a LMNA R482W mutation show muscular and cardiac abnormalities. The Journal of clinical endocrinology and metabolism 2004; 89(11):5337–46.
124. Cao H, Hegele RA. Nuclear lamin A/C R482Q mutation in Canadian kindreds with Dunnigan-type familial partial lipodystrophy. Human molecular genetics 2000; 9(1):109–12.
125. Lanktree M, Cao H, Rabkin S, et al. Novel LMNA mutations seen in patients with familial partial lipodystrophy subtype 2 (FPLD2; MIM 151660). Clin Genet 2007; 71(2):183–6.
126. Agarwal AK, Garg A. A novel heterozygous mutation in peroxisome proliferator-activated receptor-gamma gene in a patient with familial partial lipodystrophy. The Journal of clinical endocrinology and metabolism 2002; 87(1):408–11.
127. Agostini M, Schoenmakers E, Mitchell C, et al. Non-DNA binding, dominant-negative, human PPARgamma mutations cause lipodystrophic insulin resistance. Cell Metab 2006; 4(4):303–11.
128. Al-Shali K, Cao H, Knoers N, et al. A single-base mutation in the peroxisome proliferator-activated receptor gamma4 promoter associated with altered in vitro expression and partial lipodystrophy. The Journal of clinical endocrinology and metabolism 2004; 89(11):5655–60.
129. Francis GA, Li G, Casey R, et al. Peroxisomal proliferator activated receptor-gamma deficiency in a Canadian kindred with familial partial lipodystrophy type 3 (FPLD3). BMC medical genetics 2006; 7:3.
130. Hegele RA, Cao H, Frankowski C, et al. PPARG F388L, a transactivation-deficient mutant, in familial partial lipodystrophy. Diabetes 2002; 51(12):3586–90.
131. Monajemi H, Zhang L, Li G, et al. Familial partial lipodystrophy phenotype resulting from a single-base mutation in deoxyribonucleic acid-binding domain of peroxisome proliferator-activated receptor-gamma. The Journal of clinical endocrinology and metabolism 2007; 92(5):1606–12.
132. Savage DB, Tan GD, Acerini CL, et al. Human metabolic syndrome resulting from dominant-negative mutations in the nuclear receptor peroxisome proliferator-activated receptor-gamma. Diabetes 2003; 52(4):910–7.
133. Hegele RA, Ur E, Ransom TP, et al. A frameshift mutation in peroxisome-proliferator-activated receptor-gamma in familial partial lipodystrophy subtype 3 (FPLD3; MIM 604367). Clinical genetics 2006; 70(4):360–2.
134. Li G, Leff T. Altered promoter recycling rates contribute to dominant-negative activity of human peroxisome proliferator-activated receptor-gamma mutations associated with diabetes. Molecular endocrinology Baltimore, Md 2007; 21(4):857–64.
135. San Millan JL, Corton M, Villuendas G, et al. Association of the polycystic ovary syndrome with genomic variants related to insulin resistance, type 2 diabetes mellitus, and obesity. The Journal of clinical endocrinology and metabolism 2004; 89(6):2640–6.
136. Escobar-Morreale HF, Villuendas G, Botella-Carretero JI, et al. Adiponectin and resistin in PCOS: a clinical, biochemical and molecular genetic study. Human reproduction (Oxford, England) 2006; 21(9):2257–65.
137. Xita N, Georgiou I, Chatzikyriakidou A, et al. Effect of adiponectin gene polymorphisms on circulating adiponectin and insulin resistance indexes in women with polycystic ovary syndrome. Clinical chemistry 2005; 51(2):416–23.
138. Waterworth DM, Bennett ST, Gharani N, et al. Linkage and association of insulin gene VNTR regulatory polymorphism with polycystic ovary syndrome. Lancet 1997; 349(9057):986–90.
139. Vankova M, Vrbikova J, Hill M, et al. Association of insulin gene VNTR polymorphism with polycystic ovary syndrome. Annals of the New York Academy of Sciences 2002; 967:558–65.
140. Powell BL, Haddad L, Bennett A, et al. Analysis of multiple data sets reveals no association between the insulin gene variable number tandem repeat element and polycystic ovary syndrome or related traits. The Journal of clinical endocrinology and metabolism 2005; 90(5):2988–93.
141. Sir-Petermann T, Perez-Bravo F, Angel B, et al. G972R polymorphism of IRS-1 in women with polycystic ovary syndrome. Diabetologia 2001; 44(9):1200–1.
142. Ehrmann DA, Tang X, Yoshiuchi I, et al. Relationship of insulin receptor substrate-1 and -2 genotypes to phenotypic features of polycystic ovary syndrome. The Journal of clinical endocrinology and metabolism 2002; 87(9):4297–300.
143. Ehrmann DA, Schwarz PE, Hara M, et al. Relationship of calpain-10 genotype to phenotypic features of polycystic ovary syndrome. The Journal of clinical endocrinology and metabolism 2002; 87(4):1669–73.
144. Haddad L, Evans JC, Gharani N, et al. Variation within the type 2 diabetes susceptibility gene calpain-10 and polycystic ovary syndrome. The Journal of clinical endocrinology and metabolism 2002; 87(6):2606–10.
145. Hara M, Alcoser SY, Qaadir A, et al. Insulin resistance is attenuated in women with polycystic ovary syndrome with the Pro(12)Ala polymorphism in the PPARgamma gene. The Journal of clinical endocrinology and metabolism 2002; 87(2): 772–5.
146. San Millan JL, Botella-Carretero JI, Alvarez-Blasco F, et al. A study of the hexose-6-phosphate dehydrogenase gene R453Q and 11beta-hydroxysteroid dehydrogenase type 1 gene 83557insA polymorphisms in the polycystic ovary syndrome. The Journal of clinical endocrinology and metabolism 2005; 90(7):4157–62.
147. Draper N, Powell BL, Franks S, et al. Variants implicated in cortisone reductase deficiency do not contribute to susceptibility to common forms of polycystic ovary syndrome. Clinical endocrinology 2006; 65(1):64–70.
148. Kahsar-Miller M, Azziz R, Feingold E, et al. A variant of the glucocorticoid receptor gene is not associated with adrenal androgen excess in women with polycystic ovary syndrome. Fertility and sterility 2000; 74(6):1237–40.
149. Milner CR, Craig JE, Hussey ND, et al. No association between the -308 polymorphism in the tumour necrosis factor alpha (TNFalpha) promoter region and polycystic ovaries. Molecular human reproduction 1999; 5(1):5–9.

150. Korhonen S, Romppanen EL, Hiltunen M, et al. Lack of association between C-850T polymorphism of the gene encoding tumor necrosis factor-alpha and polycystic ovary syndrome. Gynecological endocrinology 2002; 16(4):271–4.
151. Walch K, Grimm C, Zeillinger R, et al. A common interleukin-6 gene promoter polymorphism influences the clinical characteristics of women with polycystic ovary syndrome. Fertility and sterility 2004; 81(6):1638–41.
152. Soderlund D, Canto P, Carranza-Lira S, et al. No evidence of mutations in the P450 aromatase gene in patients with polycystic ovary syndrome. Human reproduction (Oxford, England) 2005; 20(4):965–9.
153. Urbanek M, Legro RS, Driscoll DA, et al. Thirty-seven candidate genes for polycystic ovary syndrome: strongest evidence for linkage is with follistatin. Proceedings of the National Academy of Sciences of the United States of America 1999; 96(15):8573–8.
154. Xita N, Tsatsoulis A, Chatzikyriakidou A, et al. Association of the (TAAAA)n repeat polymorphism in the sex hormone-binding globulin (SHBG) gene with polycystic ovary syndrome and relation to SHBG serum levels. The Journal of clinical endocrinology and metabolism 2003; 88(12):5976–80.
155. Cousin P, Calemard-Michel L, Lejeune H, et al. Influence of SHBG gene pentanucleotide TAAAA repeat and D327N polymorphism on serum sex hormone-binding globulin concentration in hirsute women. The Journal of clinical endocrinology and metabolism 2004; 89(2):917–24.
156. Meirhaeghe A, Cottel D, Amouyel P, et al. Lack of association between certain candidate gene polymorphisms and the metabolic syndrome. Molecular genetics and metabolism 2005; 86(1–2):293–9.
157. Frederiksen L, Brodbaek K, Fenger M, et al. Comment: studies of the Pro12Ala polymorphism of the PPAR-gamma gene in the Danish MONICA cohort: homozygosity of the Ala allele confers a decreased risk of the insulin resistance syndrome. The Journal of clinical endocrinology and metabolism 2002; 87(8):3989–92.
158. Korhonen S, Heinonen S, Hiltunen M, et al. Polymorphism in the peroxisome proliferator-activated receptor-gamma gene in women with polycystic ovary syndrome. Human reproduction (Oxford, England) 2003; 18(3):540–3.
159. Orio F, Jr., Matarese G, Di Biase S, et al. Exon 6 and 2 peroxisome proliferator-activated receptor-gamma polymorphisms in polycystic ovary syndrome. The Journal of clinical endocrinology and metabolism 2003; 88(12):5887–92.
160. Lee EJ, Yoo KJ, Kim SJ, et al. Single nucleotide polymorphism in exon 17 of the insulin receptor gene is not associated with polycystic ovary syndrome in a Korean population. Fertility and sterility 2006; 86(2):380–4.
161. Siegel S, Futterweit W, Davies TF, et al. A C/T single nucleotide polymorphism at the tyrosine kinase domain of the insulin receptor gene is associated with polycystic ovary syndrome. Fertility and sterility 2002; 78(6):1240–3.
162. Zawadski JK, Dunaif A. Diagnostic Criteria for polycystic ovary syndrome: towards a rational approach. In: Dunaif A GJ, Haseltine FP, Merriam GR ed. Polycystic ovary syndrome. Boston: Blackwell Scientific Publications; 1992:377–84.
163. Revised 2003 consensus on diagnostic criteria and long-term health risks related to polycystic ovary syndrome (PCOS). Human reproduction (Oxford, England) 2004; 19(1):41–7.

Chapter 6
The Genetics of Polycystic Ovary Syndrome

Brad Eilerman, Marzieh Salehi, and Yaron Tomer

6.1 Introduction

Polycystic ovary syndrome is one of the most common endocrine disorders in women, affecting up to 7% of women of reproductive age. It is characterized by chronic anovulation, hyperandrogenemia, and often obesity [1]. Key reproductive features of PCOS are disordered gonadotropin secretion [2], elevated ovarian and adrenal androgen production [3], and frequently polycystic ovaries. Women with PCOS have profound insulin resistance as well as beta cell dysfunction, regardless of obesity and glucose tolerance status [4].

While the etiology of PCOS is not fully understood, it is believed to result from an interplay between genetic and epigenetic factors. Indeed, there is well-documented familial aggregation of PCOS that provides evidence for a genetic susceptibility to the disorder [5]. Earlier studies have suggested an autosomal dominant [6] or X-linked mode of inheritance [7]. However, these very early studies were underpowered failing to examine enough first-degree relatives and lacking a clear phenotype definition, except in women of reproductive age. Studies on monozygotic and dizygotic twin sisters from the Netherlands twin registry showed a heritability of 0.7 with a correlation of 0.7 and 0.4 between monozygotic and dizygotic twins, respectively. These data strongly suggest that PCOS has complex heritability with at least several major susceptibility genes [8].

Reproductive phenotype of hyperandrogenemia clusters in PCOS families [5, 7, 9]. About 50% of sisters of women with PCOS are hyperandrogenic, half of which have normal menstrual cycles (hyperandrogenism only) as opposed to the other half who have irregular menstrual cycles (classic PCOS) [5]. Likewise, one family study in a different population demonstrated an increased serum androgen concentration in sisters and mothers of women with PCOS [10]. Another large family study of male relatives of women with PCOS showed elevated dehydroepiandrosterone sulfate (DHEAS) levels that correlated with DHEAS levels in their counterpart sisters, suggesting a heritable defect in steroidogenesis [11]. Insulin resistance, the cardinal metabolic complication of PCOS, is also more common in brothers of PCOS patients [12, 13] and in sisters of women with PCOS [10, 14, 15].

In the last decade, more than 100 genes have been examined for association with PCOS, and yet no gene or genes are universally accepted as the major contributor to the heritability of PCOS, albeit some genes/loci have been reproduced in several studies. Most studies have utilized the candidate gene approach targeting loci involved in different pathogenetic pathways, such as steroid hormone biosynthesis/action, gonadotropin synthesis/action, insulin secretion/action, and obesity and energy regulation. Given that the pathogenesis of PCOS, particularly the cause-and-effect relationship between insulin resistance and hyperandrogenemia, is not fully understood, the candidate gene approach has the limitation of missing possible genes that can contribute to PCOS by other mechanisms.

The role of androgen exposure early in life adds additional complexity to the heritability of PCOS. Androgen excess or increased GNRH release can reproduce the reproductive phenotype of PCOS [16], and, therefore, in

Y. Tomer (✉)
Division of Endocrinology, University of Cincinnati college of Medicine, The Vontz Center for Molecular Studies, Cincinnati, OH 45267, USA
e-mail: tomery@UCMAIL.UC.EDU

N.R. Farid, E. Diamanti-Kandarakis (eds.), *Diagnosis and Management of Polycystic Ovary Syndrome*,
DOI 10.1007/978-0-387-09718-3_6,

general hyperandrogenemia is considered the dominant phenotypic trait in PCOS [17]. Recognizing permanent ovarian hyperandrogenism as well as elevated LH and increased responses to GnRH in some women who were exposed to increased androgen production earlier in their life due to congenital adrenal hyperplasia suggested that early exposure to androgen may have a long-term programing effect [18]. A recent experiment, using animal models (female rhesus monkey), demonstrated that in utero testosterone exposure could replicate PCOS-like syndrome, characterized by insulin secretion abnormality, hypersecretion of LH, and in obese animals, hyperandrogenic anovulation [19]. It is possible that early excess of androgen can lead to permanent changes in gene expression causing the long-term consequences of PCOS. Thus, epigenetic factors, such as early exposure to androgens may play a significant role in the transmission of the PCOS trait.

6.2 Methods for Identifying PCOS Genes

The two basic methods for mapping complex disease genes, such as PCOS, are linkage and association studies. Both of these methods can be applied to candidate genes or to the entire human genome.

6.2.1 Linkage and Association

Linkage: The principle of linkage analysis is based on the fact that if two genes or markers are close together on a chromosome, they will co-segregate because the likelihood that a recombination will occur between them during meiosis is low. Therefore, if a tested marker is close to a disease-susceptibility gene, its alleles will co-segregate with the disease in families. The LOD (logarithm of odds) score is the measure of the likelihood of linkage between a disease and a genetic marker [20]. The LOD score is the base-10 logarithm of the odds ratio in favor of linkage. The classical linkage tests are model based (parametric), i.e., different modes of inheritance and penetrance have to be tested when calculating the likelihood of linkage [21]. In complex diseases, the mode of inheritance is often unknown and, therefore, model-independent methods (non-parametric) have also been widely used [22]. One such method is sib-pair analysis [22]. In this method, siblings that are both affected by the disease being studied are tested for sharing of alleles at a marker locus. By random chance alone, the sibs would be expected to share one allele about 50% of the time and two alleles 25% of the time. If affected sib-pairs share a significantly higher than expected proportion of alleles at the marker locus, this suggests that the region containing the marker locus also contains the disease gene. According to well-accepted guidelines, in complex diseases, a LOD score of >1.9 is suggestive of linkage, and a LOD score of >3.3 indicates significant linkage in studies using the parametric approach. For non-parametric sib-pair studies the cutoff LOD scores are higher [23]. Linkage is confirmed if evidence for linkage is replicated in two or more separate datasets [23]. Conversely, a LOD score lower than –2.0 has been used to exclude linkage.

Association: Linkage studies are excellent for screening the whole genome for major genes/loci. However, they have limited resolution (~ 2–3 million base pairs [Mbp]) [24]. Association studies are more sensitive than linkage studies and may detect minor susceptibility genes contributing < 5% of the total genetic contribution to a disease [25]. Association analyses are performed by comparing the frequency of the allele studied (e.g., HLA-DR3) in unrelated patients and in unrelated, ethnically matched controls. If the allele tested is associated with the disease, it will appear significantly more frequently in patients than in controls. The probability of having the disease in an individual positive for the allele compared with an individual negative for the allele is estimated by the odds ratio (OR) [26]. There are at least two possible explanations for the existence of an association between an allele and a disease: (1) the associated allele itself is the genetic variant causing an increased risk for the disease; (2) the associated allele itself is not causing the disease but rather a gene in linkage disequilibrium with it [27]. Linkage disequilibrium exists when chromosomes with the mutant allele at the disease locus carry certain marker alleles more often than expected (see below).

The population-based association method may produce spurious associations if the patients and controls are not accurately matched ("population stratification") [28]. Therefore, additional association tests have been developed which are family based and use an internal control group from within each family, thus avoiding the necessity to match patients and controls altogether. The most widely used family-based association test is the transmission disequilibrium test (TDT) [28]. The TDT is based on comparison of parental marker alleles which are transmitted and those which are not transmitted to affected children.

6.2.2 Markers Used in Linkage and Association Studies

Microsatellites: Microsatellites are regions in the genome that are composed of short sequence repeats, most commonly two-base (e.g., CA) repeats [29]. Microsatellite loci are highly polymorphic (i.e., have many alleles) because the number of repeats in each individual is variable. Moreover, they are uniformly distributed throughout the genome at distances of less than 1 million base pairs [29].The main advantage of microsatellites is that in contrast to single nucleotide polymorphisms (SNPs) which are bi-allelic, they have several alleles. This makes them highly informative, especially in linkage studies. Therefore, microsatellites serve as excellent markers in whole genome linkage studies.

Single nucleotide polymorphisms (SNPs): SNPs are single base pair positions in genomic DNA at which different sequence alternatives (alleles) exist in normal individuals. In humans, most SNPs are di-allelic (reviewed in [30]). SNPs are very abundant, and their frequency is about less than one SNP per 1000 bp [31]. Since SNPs are less informative than microsatellites, more SNPs are needed than microsatellites to screen a locus or the entire human genome. However, since SNPs are much more abundant and closely spaced than microsatellites, they are ideal for fine mapping genes in linked regions using association studies.

6.2.3 Candidate Gene Analysis

Candidate genes are of known sequence and location which by virtue of their physiological functions may be involved in disease pathogenesis. For example, mutations in the glucokinase genes were found to be the cause of maturity onset diabetes of the young (MODY) 2 [32]. This gene was tested because its function in the glucose-sensing mechanism made it a candidate gene for MODY 2 [32]. Since the phenotype of PCOS manifests by androgen excess and insulin resistance, potential candidate genes for PCOS include the genes controlling the ovarian steoidogenic biosynthetic pathways, as well as the insulin-signalling pathway genes.

6.2.4 Genome-Wide Screens

A more powerful approach is to screen the whole human genome for linkage or association with a disease without any assumptions on disease pathogenesis [33, 34]. Whole genome screening is performed by testing a panel of markers which span the entire human genome for linkage/association with a disease in a given dataset.

Whole genome linkage studies in families: Here, a panel of markers, spanning the entire human genome at distances of approximately 10 cM (about 10 Mbp), are tested for linkage with a disease in a dataset of families. If one or more of the markers shows evidence for linkage with the disease, these regions may harbor susceptibility genes for the disease studied. These linked regions can then be fine mapped and the genes identified (see below). Whole genome linkage studies have been successful in identifying complex disease genes such as the NOD2 gene in Crohn's disease [35] and the thyroglobulin gene in thyroid autoimmunity [36]. However, since only major susceptibility genes can be identified by linkage and less influential genes cannot, whole genome association studies were needed.

Genome-wide association studies: Until recently, genome-wide association studies were not feasible because reliable markers spanning the entire human genome at short intervals were not available. Genome-wide association studies became a reality with the publication of the HapMap of the human genome. The HapMap project genotyped about one million SNPs spanning the entire human genome, at average intervals of 5 Kb, in four populations – Africans, Caucasians, Chinese, and Japanese – and tested them for haplotypes and linkage disequilibrium (LD). SNP haplotypes are specific combinations of alleles of SNPs that located on the same chromosome. Linkage disequilibrium (LD) is the non-random association of alleles (e.g., HLA-B8 and DR3 are in LD and are frequently inherited together). The findings of the HapMap project were remarkable. The HapMap project demonstrated that approximately 80% of the human genome is made of LD blocks [37]. In each block, the SNPs are in tight LD and certain haplotypes are preferred. The significance of the HapMap project is that it now allows us to identify complex disease genes using tagSNPs. TagSNPs are representative SNPs from LD blocks. If a tagSNP shows association with disease, it indicates that the gene predisposing to the disease is most likely located within the same block as the tagSNP. This makes fine mapping of linked regions much easier. Moreover, tagSNPs can now be used to screen the entire human genome. To screen the entire human genome at least 500,000 tagSNPs are necessary in order to have a dense-enough SNP coverage. This creates a problem of multiple testing as 500,000 independent tests are being performed. A simple Bonferroni correction would require a genome-wide significance cutoff p-value of 1×10^{-7}[34]. However, this approach may miss true positive associations that do not result in such a low p-value. Despite these difficulties, several replicated genes have been identified recently using genome-wide association studies, e.g., type 2 diabetes [38].

6.3 Genes Associated with PCOS

Many genes have been explored as candidates for association with PCOS. The observed pathophysiology of PCOS served as the basis for gene discovery. While new genes continue to be tested, a cluster of candidate genes have attracted the most research.

6.3.1 Genes Associated with Sex Hormone Regulation

6.3.1.1 FBN3

Function: Codes for *fibrillin 3*, an extracellular architectural protein.

Genetic studies: Early gene mapping identified a PCOS susceptibility locus near a dinucleotide repeat marker in 19p13.2 (D19S884) [9, 39, 40]. This locus is notable due to its proximity to the insulin receptor. Further genetic analysis of 1723 individuals in 412 families with 412 index cases and 43 affected sisters of predominantly European origin was performed [9]. Of the 53 variants tested, D19S884 within intron 55 of the fibrillin-3 showed the strongest evidence of association with PCOS ($p=0.0037$).

Contribution to PCOS: While near the insulin receptor gene on chromosome 19, the precise role of fibrillin-3 in PCOS is yet unknown. Independent of obesity, analysis of the carriers of the A8 allele demonstrated higher levels of fasting insulin (17 ± 11 μU/ml A8 (+) vs. 12 ± 4 μU/ml A8 (−); $P=0.008$) with an odds ratio (OR) of 1.44. HOMA IR was also elevated in carriers of the A8 allele (1.94 ± 1.1 A8(+) vs. 1.49 ± 0.55 A8(−); $P=0.02$). Women carrying with A8 allele without PCOS did not demonstrate these metabolic changes. Moreover, brothers of PCOS patients carrying the A8 allele demonstrated higher fasting levels of proinsulin and proinsulin/insulin ratio [41]. The role of fibrillin-3 in PCOS is thought to be rooted in the role of fibrillins in the regulation of the TGFβ family genes, including activin, inhibin, and follistatin [41]. Moreover, fibrillin-3 knockout mice have increased islet cell mass and increased insulin sensitivity [42].

6.3.1.2 SHBG

Function: Codes for *sex hormone binding globulin*, a glycoprotein which is secreted by the liver and binds sex hormones.

Genetic studies: Xita et al. analyzed alleles of a (TAAAA)n repeat in the SHBG gene. Individuals with PCOS demonstrated a statistically significant higher rate of longer repeats compared to women without PCOS. No difference was observed comparing lean women with PCOS and obese women with PCOS. Additionally, lower SHBG levels were observed in individuals carrying the longer repeats [43]. However, Urbanek et al. found no association of PCOS with SHBG levels in a large analysis of 37 candidate genes [9].

Contribution to PCOS: SHBG levels are frequently low in women with PCOS, and it is possible that the long (TAAAA)n repeats contribute to the low SHBG levels. However, these results need to be replicated. Moreover, hyperinsulinemia is known to suppress SHBG in the liver and increase systemic free androgens.

6.3.1.3 The AR Gene

Function: Codes for the *X-linked androgen receptor gene*

Genetic studies: The androgen receptor gene contains polymorphic CAG trinucleotide repeat encoding a poly-glutamine in the N-terminal domain. In one study, 91 patients with clinically diagnosed PCOS were compared to 112 women with proven fertility and normal menses [44]. CAG repeat length was measured in affected women with high testosterone, low/normal testosterone, and control group. A statistically significantly association was found between carriage of the short CAG repeats and a phenotype of anovulatory PCOS with low testosterone levels ($P = 0.004$).

Contribution to PCOS: A hyperandrogenic state is a cardinal feature of PCOS. If this association is confirmed, it may suggest that AR polymorphisms may contribute to the phenotype of PCOS with normal testosterone levels.

6.3.1.4 CYP21

Function: Codes for *adrenal steroid 21-hydroxylase,* responsible for the conversion of pogesterone to deoxycorticosterone and 17-hydroxyprogesterone to 11-deoxycortisol.

Genetic studies: Escobar-Morreale et al. analyzed 40 hirsute women for association with mutations of the CYP21 gene [45]. Eight hirsute patients demonstrated were heterozygote carriers of CYP21 mutations versus one control. Of the carrier women, four of the hirsute women demonstrated normal 17-hydroxyprogesterone levels both at baseline and with ACTH stimulation, suggesting a PCOS-like phenotype without the full features of non-classical congenital adrenal hyperplasia (CAH). Witchel and Aston published a small study of 30 adolescent females with hyperandrogenism and suggested an increased frequency of carriage of CYP21 mutations compared to healthy controls [46]. They concluded that missense CYP21 mutation carriers had a PCOS phenotype while nonsense mutations showed the non-classical CAH phenotype. However, a follow up study of 109 women with PCOS and 95 controls showed no association [47].

Contribution to PCOS: Decreased or absent activity of the adrenal steroid 21-hydroxylase is the cause of non-classical CAH. There is some evidence that heterozygosity of CYP21 mutations may lead to increased adrenal androgens without the total CAH phenotype [48]. However, it is possible that some cases of CAH may be misdiagnosed as PCOS, but it is unlikely that CYP21 polymorphisms have a major contribution to PCOS.

6.3.1.5 Dopamine D3 Receptor

Function: Encodes for the dopamine receptor D_3 which inhibits adenylyl cyclase through inhibitory G-proteins. D3 receptors are involved in regulation of GnRH and prolactin genes.

Genetic studies: Legro et al. found an association of PCOS with homozygosity for a particular allele (the "2 allele") of the D3 Dopamine receptor in Latino women [49]. These patients demonstrated very irregular periods, frequent anovulation, as well as higher testosterone levels compared to women without homozygosity for the 2 allele. Moreover, patients with homozygous 2 allele required higher doses of clomiphene to induce ovulation. A later study examined non-Hispanic Caucasian women in the southeastern United States and did not find association of PCOS with this variant [50].

Contribution to PCOS: Involvement of dopamine in the pathophysiology of PCOS is rooted in two main factors. First, women with PCOS characteristically have elevated LH secretion which is suppressible with dopamine [51]. Secondly, mild prolactinemia is seen in up to one third of women with PCOS [52]. Both these factors could be caused by a relative deficiency of dopamine or dopamine activity in women with PCOS. However, the association with the D3 receptor polymorphism and the effects of the 2 allele on the receptor function have to be confirmed before this mechanism can be implicated in the heritability of PCOS.

6.3.1.6 FSH-Beta

Function: Codes for the beta subunit of follicle stimulating hormone.

Genetic studies: Tong et al. studied 135 Chinese women with PCOS and 105 control subjects for polymorphisms or mutations in exons 2 and 3 of the FSHβ gene [53]. No missense mutations were identified, but a T to C substitution was identified in exon 3. The CC genotype was significantly more frequent in PCOS patients (12.6%) than in the control group (3.8%). Moreover, this allele was found more frequently in women with obesity and PCOS than in those with PCOS without obesity.

Contribution to PCOS: Administration of exogenous FSH has been demonstrated to restore follicular growth, selection, and ovulation in some patients with PCOS [54]. Additionally, suppression of FSH by follistatin, a regulatory protein, in transgenic mice led to arrested folliculogenesis [55]. Both of these factors suggest that abnormalities in the FSH gene may contribute to the etiology of PCOS. However, these association data have to be replicated.

6.3.2 Genes Associated with Insulin Resistance

6.3.2.1 CAPN10

Function: Codes for *Calpain-10*, a calcium-dependent cysteine protease. Whole genome scan in type 2 diabetes showed an association of CAPN10 variants with type 2 diabetes and insulin resistance [59].

Genetic studies: Haddad et al. studied four SNPs in the CAPN10 gene in 146 parent–offspring trios, 185 unrelated PCOS cases, and 525 control subjects of European ancestry [56]. One common variant showed a modest association in the family based transmission disequilibrium test (TDT), but not in the case-control study. Thus, an association between CAPN10 and PCOS is not confirmed.

Contribution to PCOS: Insulin resistance is considered a major feature of the pathogenesis of polycystic ovarian syndrome. Calpain-10 is associated with insulin resistance and thus is a strong candidate gene for PCOS. However, so far the data does not support a major effect of CAPN10 on the etiology of PCOS.

6.3.2.2 IGF2

Function: Codes for insulin-like growth factor 2, a protein hormone with structural similarity to insulin.

Genetic studies: San Millan et al. evaluated 15 candidate genes involved insulin resistance, obesity, and/or type 2 diabetes in patients with PCOS. There was a significant association of between the GG genotype of the ApaI variant of the IGF2 gene and PCOS (62.9% vs. 38.1%; P=0.018) [57].

Contribution to PCOS: The variant of the IGF2 gene associated with PCOS patients may lead to increased IGF2 expression. IGF2 has been demonstrated to stimulate adrenal and ovarian androgen secretion which could contribute to the pathogenesis of PCOS.

6.3.2.3 IRS1 and IRS2

Function: Code for insulin receptor substrates 1 and 2; these are postreceptor proteins involved with insulin gene signal transduction.

Genetic studies: El Mkadem et al. sequenced the IRS-1 and IRS-2 genes in Caucasian women with PCOS of European extraction [58]. Insulin resistance was measured via the homeostasis model assessment index for insulin resistance. No mutations were discovered, but an association was found between the Gly972Arg polymorphism of IRS-1 and the Gly1057Arg polymorphism of IRS-2 and insulin resistance.

Contribution to PCOS: PCOS is associated with insulin resistance which could be caused by downstream proteins involved in the insulin gene signal transduction. Altered expression of IRS1 and IRS2 may lead to the insulin resistance which features prominently in the pathophysiology of polycystic ovarian syndrome. However, the association of the IRS-1 and IRS-2 genes with PCOS has to be confirmed, as well as the effects of these variants on gene function and/or expression.

6.4 Conclusion

PCOS is a heterogeneous disorder that can be viewed as a final common pathway of a number of endocrinologic abnormalities in hormone release, receptor activity, and postreceptor action. It is clear that this is a complex disease that is caused by the combined effects of multiple susceptibility genes and environmental triggers. There are now solid epidemiologic data to support an important genetic contribution to the development of PCOS, and in the past decade several loci and genes have shown evidence for association with PCOS. The PCOS susceptibility genes/loci tested so far can be divided into two broad groups: (1) genes associated with sex hormone regulation and (2) genes associated with insulin resistance. So far the FBN3 gene shows the strongest evidence for association with PCOS. However, it is clear that additional genes must contribute to the genetic susceptibility to PCOS, as well as to the different phenotypes of PCOS, disease severity, and, possibly, response to therapy. With the completion of landmark projects in human genetics including the human genome project and the HapMap project and the mapping of most of the single nucleotide polymorphisms in humans, additional PCOS susceptibility genes will likely be identified in the near future. This will hopefully lead to targeted treatments based on the mechanisms of each individual's specific phenotype.

References

1. Ehrmann DA. Polycystic ovary syndrome – Reply. New England Journal of Medicine 2005; 352(26):2757.
2. Mansfield R, Galea R, Brincat M, Hole D, Mason H. Metformin has direct effects on human ovarian steroidogenesis. Fertility and Sterility 2003; 79(4):956–962.
3. Rosenfield RL. Ovarian and adrenal function in polycystic ovary syndrome. Endocrinology and Metabolism Clinics of North America 1999; 28(2):265–293.
4. Dunaif A. Insulin resistance in women with polycystic ovary syndrome. Fertility and Sterility 2006; 86:S13–S14.
5. Legro RS, Driscoll D, Strauss JF, Fox J, Dunaif A. Evidence for a genetic basis for hyperandrogenemia in polycystic ovary syndrome. Proceedings of the National Academy of Sciences of the United States of America 1998; 95(25):14956–14960.
6. Cooper HE, Spellacy WN, Prem KA, Cohen WD. Hereditary factors in the Stein-Leventhal syndrome. American Journal of Obstetrics and Gynecology 100, 371–387. 1968. Ref Type: Generic
7. Ferriman D, Purdie AW. The inheritance of polycystic ovarian disease and a possible relationship to premature balding. Clinical Endocrinology 11, 291–300. 1979. Ref Type: Generic
8. Vink JM, Sadrzadeh S, Lambalk CB, Boomsma DI. Heritability of polycystic ovary syndrome in a Dutch twin-family study. Journal of Clinical Endocrinology and Metabolism 2006; 91(6):2100–2104.
9. Urbanek M, Legro RS, Driscoll DA, Azziz R, Ehrmann DA, Norman RJ et al. Thirty-seven candidate genes for polycystic ovary syndrome: strongest evidence for linkage is with follistatin. Proceedings of the National Academy of Sciences of the United States of America 1999; 96(15):8573–8578.
10. Yildiz BO, Yarali H, Oguz H, Bayraktar M. Glucose intolerance, insulin resistance, and hyperandrogenemia in first degree relatives of women with polycystic ovary syndrome. Journal of Clinical Endocrinology and Metabolism 2003; 88(5): 2031–2036.
11. Legro RS, Kunselman AR, Demers L, Wang SC, Bentley-Lewis R, Dunaif A. Elevated dehydroepiandrosterone sulfate levels as the reproductive phenotype in the brothers of women with polycystic ovary syndrome. Journal of Clinical Endocrinology and Metabolism 2002; 87(5):2134–2138.
12. Kaushal R, Parchure N, Bano G, Kaski JC, Nussey SS. Insulin resistance and endothelial dysfunction in the brothers of Indian subcontinent Asian women with polycystic ovaries. Clinical Endocrinology 2004; 60(3):322–328.
13. Sam S, Coviello AD, Sung YA, Legro RS, Dunaif A. Metabolic Phenotype in the Brothers of Women with Polycystic Ovary Syndrome. Diabetes Care 2008; 31(6):1237–41.
14. Sam S, Legro RS, Bentley-Lewis R, Dunaif A. Dyslipidemia and metabolic syndrome in the sisters of women with polycystic ovary syndrome. Journal of Clinical Endocrinology and Metabolism 2005; 90(8):4797–4802.

15. Diamanti-Kandarakis E, Alexandraki K, Bergiele A, Kandarakis H, Mastorakos G, Aessopos A. Presence of metabolic risk factors in non-obese PCOS sisters: Evidence of heritability of insulin resistance. Journal of Endocrinological Investigation 2004; 27(10):931–936.
16. Franks S, Gharani N, Waterworth D, Batty S, White D, Williamson R et al. The genetic basis of polycystic ovary syndrome. Human Reproduction 1997; 12(12):2641–2648.
17. Azziz R, Carmina E, Dewailly D, Diamanti-Kandarakis E, Escobar-Morreale HF, Futterweit W et al. Criteria for defining polycystic ovary syndrome as a predominantly hyperandrogenic syndrome: An Androgen Excess Society guideline. Journal of Clinical Endocrinology and Metabolism 2006; 91(11):4237–4245.
18. Barnes RB, Rosenfield RL, Ehrmann DA, Cara JF, Cuttler L, Levitsky LL et al. Ovarian Hyperandrogynism As A Result of Congenital Adrenal Virilizing Disorders – Evidence for Perinatal Masculinization of Neuroendocrine Function in Women. Journal of Clinical Endocrinology and Metabolism 1994; 79(5):1328–1333.
19. Abbott DH, Dumesic DA, Eisner JR, Colman RJ, Kemnitz JW. Insights into the development of polycystic ovary syndrome (PCOS) from studies of prenatally androgenized female rhesus monkeys. Trends in Endocrinology and Metabolism 1998; 9(2):62–67.
20. Ott J. Analysis of human genetic linkage. Third ed. Baltimore: Johns Hopkins University Press, 1999.
21. Greenberg DA, Abreu PC. Determining trait locus position from multipoint analysis: Accuracy and power of three different statistics. Genetic Epidemiology 2001; 21:299–314.
22. Risch N. Linkage strategies for genetically complex traits. II. The power of affected relative pairs. American Journal of Human Genetics 1990; 46(2):229–241.
23. Lander E, Kruglyak L. Genetic dissection of complex traits: guidelines for interpreting and reporting linkage results. Nature Genetics 1995; 11:241–247.
24. Greenberg DA. Linkage analysis of "necessary" loci versus "susceptibility" loci. American Journal of Human Genetics 1993; 52:135–143.
25. Risch N, Merikangas K. The future of genetic studies of complex human diseases. Science 1996; 273:1516–1517.
26. Woolf B. On estimating the relation between blood group and disease. American Journal of Human Genetics 1955; 19: 251–253.
27. Hodge SE. What association analysis can and cannot tell us about the genetics of complex disease. American Journal of Human Genetics 1994; 54:318–323.
28. Spielman RS, McGinnis RE, Ewens WJ. Transmission test for linkage disequilibrium: the insulin gene region and insulin-dependent diabetes mellitus. American Journal of Human Genetics 1993; 52:506–516.
29. Weber JL. Human DNA polymorphisms based on length variations in simple- sequence tandem repeats. Genome Analysis 1990; 1:159–181.
30. Brookes AJ. The essence of SNPs. Gene 1999; 234(2):177–186.
31. Laan M, Paabo S. Mapping genes by drift-generated linkage disequilibrium. American Journal of Human Genetics 1998; 63(2):654–656.
32. Froguel P, Zouali H, Vionnet N, Velho G, Vaxillaire M, Pharm D et al. Familial hyperglycemia due to mutations in glucokinase. Definition of a subtype of diabetes mellitus. The New England Journal of Medicine 1993; 328:697–702.
33. Davies JL, Kawauchi Y, Bennet ST, Copeman JB, Cordell HJ, Pritchard LE et al. A genome-wide search for human type1 diabetes susceptibility genes. Nature 1994; 371:130–136.
34. Hunter DJ, Kraft P. Drinking from the fire hose–statistical issues in genomewide association studies. The New England Journal of Medicine 2007; 357(5):436–439.
35. Hugot JP, Chamaillard M, Zouali H, Lesage S, Cezard JP, Belaiche J et al. Association of NOD2 leucine-rich repeat variants with susceptibility to Crohn's disease. Nature 2001; 411:599–603.
36. Ban Y, Greenberg DA, Concepcion E, Skrabanek L, Villanueva R, Tomer Y. Amino acid substitutions in the thyroglobulin gene are associated with susceptibility to human and murine autoimmune thyroid disease. Proceedings of the National Academy of Sciences of the United States of America 2003; 100:15119–15124.
37. Altshuler D, Brooks LD, Chakravarti A, Collins FS, Daly MJ, Donnelly P. A haplotype map of the human genome. Nature 2005; 437(7063):1299–1320.
38. Frayling TM. Genome-wide association studies provide new insights into type 2 diabetes aetiology. Nature Reviews. Genetics 2007; 8(9):657–662.
39. Tucci S, Futterweit W, Concepcion ES, Greenberg DA, Villanueva R, Davies TF et al. Evidence for association of polycystic ovary syndrome in caucasian women with a marker at the insulin receptor gene locus. The Journal of Clinical Endocrinology and Metabolism 2001; 86(1):446–449.
40. Urbanek M, Woodroffe A, Ewens KG, Diamanti-Kandarakis E, Legro RS, Strauss JF, III et al. Candidate gene region for polycystic ovary syndrome on chromosome 19p13.2. The Journal of Clinical Endocrinology and Metabolism 2005; 90(12): 6623–6629.
41. Urbanek M, Sam S, Legro RS, Dunaif A. Identification of a Polycystic ovary syndrome susceptibility variant in fibrillin-3 and association with a metabolic phenotype. Journal of Clinical Endocrinology and Metabolism 2007; 92(11):4191–4198.
42. Mukherjee A, Sidis Y, Mahan A, Raher MJ, Xia Y, Rosen ED et al. FSTL3 deletion reveals roles for TGF-beta family ligands in glucose and fat homeostasis in adults. Proceedings of the National Academy of Sciences of the United States of America 2007; 104(4):1348–1353.

43. Xita N, Tsatsoulis A, Chatzikyriakidou A, Georgiou I. Association of the (TAAAA)n repeat polymorphism in the sex hormone-binding globulin (SHBG) gene with polycystic ovary syndrome and relation to SHBG serum levels. Journal of Clinical Endocrinology and Metabolism 2003; 88(12):5976–5980.
44. Mifsud A, Ramirez S, Yong EL. Androgen receptor gene CAG trinucleotide repeats in anovulatory infertility and polycystic ovaries. Journal of Clinical Endocrinology and Metabolism 2000; 85(9):3484–3488.
45. Escobar-Morreale HF, Sanchon R, Millan JLS. A prospective study of the prevalence of nonclassical congenital adrenal hyperplasia among women presenting with hyperandrogenic symptoms and signs. Journal of Clinical Endocrinology & Metabolism 2008; 93(2):527–533.
46. Witchel SF, Aston CE. The role of heterozygosity for CYP21 in the polycystic ovary syndrome. Journal of Pediatric Endocrinology & Metabolism 2000; 13:1315–1317.
47. Witchel SF, Kahsar-Miller M, Aston CE, White C, Azziz R. Prevalence of CYP21 mutations and IRS1 variant among women with polycystic ovary syndrome and adrenal androgen excess. Fertility and Sterility 2005; 83(2):371–375.
48. Deneux C, Tardy V, Dib A, Mornet E, Billaud L, Charron D et al. Phenotype-genotype correlation in 56 women with non-classical congenital adrenal hyperplasia due to 21-hydroxylase deficiency. Journal of Clinical Endocrinology and Metabolism 2001; 86(1):207–213.
49. Legro RS, Muhleman DR, Comings DE, Lobo RA, Kovacs BW. A Dopamine D-3 Receptor Genotype Is Associated with Hyperandrogenic Chronic Anovulation and Resistant to Ovulation Induction with Clomiphene Citrate in Female Hispanics. Fertility and Sterility 1995; 63(4):779–784.
50. Kahsar-Miller M, Boots LR, Azziz R. Dopamine D-3 receptor polymorphism is not associated with the polycystic ovary syndrome. Fertility and Sterility 1999; 71(3):436–438.
51. Marshall JC, Eagleson CA. Neuroendocrine aspects of polycystic ovary syndrome. Endocrinology and Metabolism Clinics of North America 1999; 28(2):295–324.
52. Lechin F, van der Dijs B. Neuroendocrine profiling in PCOS. Fertility and Sterility 2004; 82(3):765–766.
53. Tong Y, Liao WX, Roy AC, Ng SC. Association of Accl polymorphism in the follicle-stimulating hormone beta gene with polycystic ovary syndrome. Fertility and Sterility 2000; 74(6):1233–1236.
54. Franks S, Mason H, Willis D. Follicular dynamics in the polycystic ovary syndrome. Molecular and Cellular Endocrinology 2000; 163(1–2):49–52.
55. Liao WX, Roy AC, Ng SC. Preliminary investigation of follistatin gene mutations in women with polycystic ovary syndrome. Molecular Human Reproduction 2000; 6(7):587–590.
56. Haddad L, Evans JC, Gharani N, Robertson C, Rush K, Wiltshire S et al. Variation within the type 2 diabetes susceptibility gene calpain-10 and polycystic ovary syndrome. Journal of Clinical Endocrinology and Metabolism 2002; 87(6):2606–2610.
57. San Millan JL, Corton M, Villuendas G, Sancho J, Peral B, Escobar-Morreale HF. Association of the polycystic ovary syndrome with genomic variants related to insulin resistance, type 2 diabetes mellitus, and obesity. Journal of Clinical Endocrinology and Metabolism 2004; 89(6):2640–2646.
58. El Mkadem SA, Lautier C, Macari F, Mechaly I, Renard E, Cros G et al. Combined defects in IRS-1 and IRS-2 genes me associated with insulin resistance in polycystic ovary syndrome. Diabetes 1999; 48:A436.
59. Horikawa Y, Oda N, Cox NJ, et al. Genetic variation in the gene encoding calpain-10 is associated with type 2 diabetes mellitus. Nat Genetics 2000; 26:163–175.

Chapter 7
Uterine Origins and Evolution in Childhood

Agathocles Tsatsoulis and Nectaria Xita

7.1 Introduction

Hyperandrogenism appears to present the fundamental manifestation of PCOS, probably driven by an inherent hyperandrogenic activity of the ovarian theca cells [1]. A number of molecular studies have shown that ovarian theca cells in women with PCOS are more efficient at converting androgenic precursors to testosterone than normal theca cells due to increased activity of multiple steroidogenic enzymes in PCOS theca cells [2, 3] This hyperandrogenic activity of theca cells in PCOS persists despite many passages in cell culture, indicating that it is an intrinsic property of these cells [2]. The metabolic trait of central adiposity and features of the metabolic syndrome, including insulin resistance and hyperinsulinemia, characterizing PCOS, further exaggerate the hyperandrogenic phenotype [1].

PCOS usually becomes clinically manifest during adolescence along with maturation of the hypothalamic–pituitary–gonadal axis [4]. However, recent evidence suggests that the natural history of PCOS may originate in very early development, supporting the developmental origin hypothesis for PCOS [5]. It is well known that alterations in the nutritional and endocrine milieu during fetal development can result in permanent structural and functional changes, predisposing an individual to metabolic and cardiovascular disease in adult life [6]. According to the developmental origin hypothesis, the development of PCOS is a linear process with its origins in intrauterine life, induced by androgen excess, and expressed during adolescence and adulthood [5].

In this chapter, the developmental origin hypothesis of PCOS is explored in the light of clinical and experimental animal research. The potential mechanisms that may be linked to prenatal androgen excess are also discussed. Lastly, the potential phenotypes of PCOS in childhood associated with low birth weight are also described.

7.2 Prenatal Androgen Excess – Evidence for the Fetal Origins of PCOS

Evidence from clinical observations and experimental animal research suggests that fetal exposure to androgen excess may program in utero the development of PCOS traits that are expressed in adulthood. Further evidence comes from longitudinal observations of girls with low birth weight that follow a path through postnatal catch-up weight gain, amplified adrenarche, and ovarian hyperandrogenism in adolescence. This pathway is strongly related to central adiposity and insulin resistance, and has been thought of as the hyperinsulinemic pathway to PCOS as opposed to the hyperandrogenic pathway suggested above [7]. It is likely, however, that both pathways have a common origin in intrauterine life as discussed below.

A. Tsatsoulis (✉)
Professor of Medicine/Endocrinology, Department of Endocrinology, University of Ioannina, Ioannina, 45110, Greece
e-mail: atsatsou@uoi.gr

N.R. Farid, E. Diamanti-Kandarakis (eds.), *Diagnosis and Management of Polycystic Ovary Syndrome*,
DOI 10.1007/978-0-387-09718-3_7, © Springer Science+Business Media, LLC 2009

7.2.1 Clinical Observations

The developmental origin hypothesis of PCOS emerged following astute clinical observations in women with congenital virilizing disorders. Women with classical congenital adrenal hyperplasia from 21-hydroxylase deficiency and rare cases of women with congenital adrenal virilizing tumors are exposed to excess adrenal androgens during intrauterine life and, despite the normalization of androgen excess with treatment, manifest a PCOS-like syndrome in adult life including functional ovarian hyperandrogenism, LH hypersecretion, anovulatory cycles, and polycystic ovarian morphology, as well as, central adiposity and insulin resistance [8, 9].

Similar PCOS traits have also been reported recently for girls with congenital P450 oxidoreductase deficiency who are exposed to excess adrenal androgens in prenatal life but not after birth [10]. Additional experiments of nature associated with prenatal androgenization in humans are women with rare loss-of-function mutations of P450 aromatase *(CYP19)* gene or the *SHBG* gene. Such patients are reported to develop features of PCOS in adult life [11, 12]. Therefore, androgen excess during early life might provide a crucial hormonal insult that is necessary for the developmental programing of PCOS.

7.2.2 Experimental Animal Research

An appropriate animal model to study the reproductive and metabolic outcomes of fetal programing by androgen excess is the prenatally androgenized female rhesus monkey, since it shares similar chronological patterns of reproductive function and growth with humans [13]. Studies using this animal model have convincingly shown that a PCOS-like phenotype can be produced by injecting pregnant rhesus monkeys carrying female fetuses with testosterone propionate achieving circulating testosterone levels in female fetuses similar to those normally found in male fetuses [14].

Prenatal testosterone excess in female rhesus monkeys leads to reproductive, neuroendocrine, and metabolic disruptions, resulting in phenotypes mimicking that of women with polycystic ovary syndrome (PCOS). Thus, prenatally testosterone-treated adult female monkeys exhibit basal hyperandrogenemia with exaggerated androgen response to hCG stimulation, as well as ACTH-stimulated adrenal androgen secretion indicating the development of functional ovarian and adrenal hyperandrogenism, respectively [15, 16]. In addition, they have a tenfold increase in the risk of anovulation with 40–50% fewer menstrual cycles than normal females [13]. Moreover, they have enlarged polyfollicular ovaries resembling the morphology of polycystic ovaries seen in PCOS women [5]. (see Chapter 3)

Furthermore, prenatally androgenized female monkeys exhibit neuroendocrine dysregulation with LH excess and increased LH responsiveness to exogenous GnRH suggestive of enhanced hypothalamic GnRH release and/or increased pituitary sensitivity to GnRH [17, 18]. Interestingly, this neuroendocrine dysfunction is manifested only in early gestation-treated animals than in late gestation, indicating that the timing of fetal androgen excess may be important for the expression of this PCOS phenotype [17, 18]. Diminished sex steroid negative feedback on LH may explain the increased pulsatile LH secretion. This defect promotes excessive LH feed-forward drive with subsequent excessive ovarian androgen production as well as relative FSH deficiency that contribute to ovulatory dysfunction.

In addition to its impact on the reproductive endocrine axis, prenatal androgenized female rhesus monkeys selectively deposit fat intra-abdominally and exhibit impaired insulin secretion or action in ways that resemble those of PCOS women, depending on whether the androgen excess occurred during early or late gestation [19–21]. Thus, early testosterone-treated females have increased visceral fat, impaired insulin secretion, and liberate more fatty acids than controls [19, 22]. On the other hand, late testosterone-treated monkeys have increased total body fat and non-visceral abdominal fat and show reduced insulin sensitivity with preservation of insulin secretion compared to control females [20]. Both early and late treated female monkeys preferentially accumulate visceral fat with increasing weight and have an increased risk of diabetes [21]. Interestingly, adult male monkeys exposed to excess androgens in utero may also develop defects in insulin secretion and action in a similar way to female counterparts [23].

A similar PCOS-like reproductive and metabolic outcome has been reported in the prenatally androgenized sheep and rats, providing convincing evidence that fetal androgen excess programs not only the reproductive phenotype but also the metabolic traits of PCOS [24–27].

7.2.3 Potential Origin of Prenatal Androgen Excess in Humans

The potential sources of excess androgens during intrauterine life to account for fetal programing of PCOS in humans are not clearly known and remain an issue for further research. Normally, the female fetus is protected in utero from maternal androgens, or androgens from other source, by the increased placental sex hormone-binding globulin (SHBG) that binds the androgens and the placental aromatase activity that converts them to estrogens. However, this buffering effect may be overcome if either the production of SHBG or the aromatase activity is lower than normal due to genetic or other influences. In a similar way, the fetus is protected from excess maternal glucocorticoids by the feto-placental 11β-hydroxysteroid dehydrogenase type 2 (11β – HSD2), which catalyses the metabolism of active cortisol to inactive cortisone [28]. Theoretically, therefore, exposure of the female fetus to gestational hyperandrogenism may occur due to increased maternal or endogenous fetal androgen production, and decreased placental SHBG or aromatase activity.

The possible role of PCOS itself as a cause for gestational hyperandrogenism was evaluated by Sir-Petermann et al. [29]. Pregnant PCOS women were found to have higher concentrations of androgens than normal pregnant women, thus potentially exposing their unborn daughters to elevated androgen levels in utero. The origin of the androgen excess during pregnancy in PCOS women is uncertain, but it could be due to increase in androgen production by the maternal theca interstitial cells stimulated by hCG or insulin levels which are significantly increased during pregnancy in PCOS women. In this respect, the same investigators also reported that after delivery, androstenedione levels and ovarian volume of PCOS patients were increased, suggesting that their ovaries were persistently stimulated during pregnancy [30].

In addition, the human placenta expresses 17β-hydroxysteroid dehydrogenase (17β-HSD), aromatase, as well as 3β–hydroxysteroid dehydrogenase (3β-HSD), and it can therefore synthesize androstenedione from adrenal or ovarian DHEAS and can undertake the onward synthesis of both testosterone and estradiol [31, 32]. Normally, maternal androgens or androgens produced in the placenta are rapidly converted to estrogens by the activity of the placental aromatase, and therefore, they probably contribute only slightly to gestational hyperandrogenism. However, when the aromatase activity is inhibited, these androgens could be increased.

Insulin has been shown to inhibit aromatase activity in human cytotrophoblasts and stimulate 3β-HSD activity [33, 34]. This could be a mechanism to explain, in part, the high androgen levels observed in these patients during gestation. In addition, hyperinsulinemia is also known to reduce SHBG production [35]. Therefore, in pregnant PCOS women with hyperinsulinemia, the combination of excess androgen production and the associated low aromatase activity and SHBG production could conceivably contribute to excess androgen exposure of their female offspring.

Besides insulin, genetic factors may also contribute to decreased aromatase activity and SHBG levels. Recently, a study indicated that a short microsatellite (TTTA)n repeat allele in the fourth intron of the *CYP19* gene is associated with elevated androgens, perturbed regulation of the hypothalamic–pituitary–adrenal axis, and abdominal obesity among premenopausal women from the general population [36]. With regard to SHBG, a (TAAAA)n pentanucleotide repeat polymorphism at the promoter of the human *SHBG* gene has been described and reported to influence its transcriptional activity in vitro [37]. We have recently shown in a case-control study an association between the (TAAAA)n polymorphism of the *SHBG* gene and PCOS among Greek women [38]. In particular, women with PCOS were more frequently carriers of longer (TAAAA)n alleles compared to controls. Furthermore, carriers of the longer allele genotypes had lower SHBG levels and higher free androgen index than those with shorter alleles (Fig. 7.1). Similar findings were reported among French women with hirsutism [39].

Studying the combined effect of *CYP19(TTTA)n* and *SHBG(TAAAA)N* polymorphisms, we found that women with PCOS had the combination of long *SHBG(TAAAA)n*-short *CYP19(TTTA)n* alleles more frequently,

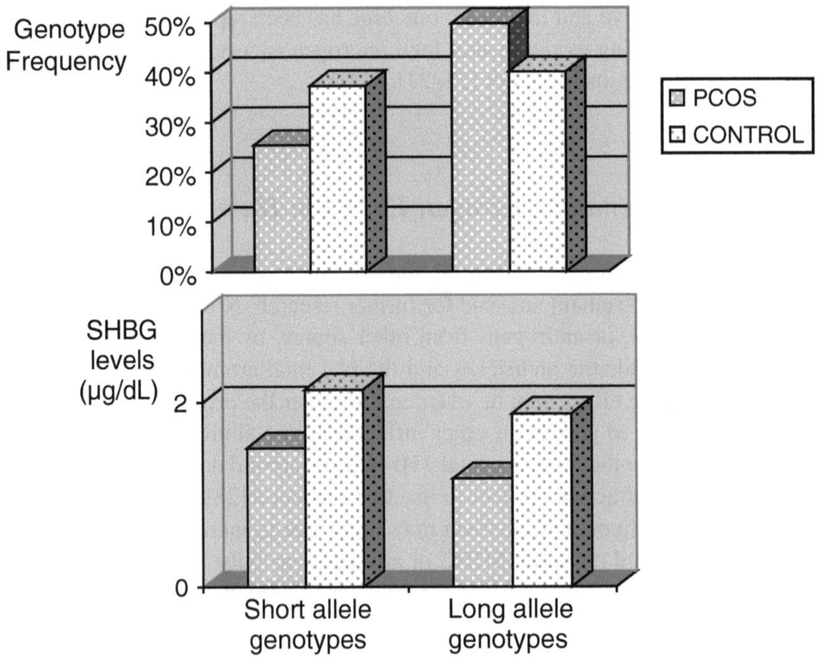

Fig. 7.1 *Upper panel*: frequency of SHBG(TAAAA)n genotypes, grouped in short and long allele genotypes, show significant differences between PCOS and controls (p = 0.009). *Lower panel*: correlation of (TAAAA)n genotypes with SHBG levels. PCOS women with long allele genotypes have lower SHBG levels, compared to women with short allele genotypes (p = 0.002)

compared to control women, a difference that was close to being significant (p = 0.07). More importantly, PCOS women who were carriers of the above genotype combination had a higher androgenic profile compared to patients with other genotype combinations [40]. Those individuals with genetically determined low SHBG levels and aromatase activity may be exposed to higher free androgen levels throughout life, but more importantly, during fetal life when programing of the differentiating target tissues takes place.

Although it is thought that the human fetal ovary is quiescent in terms of sex steroid production, it is possible that genetic or other factors may influence the steroidogenic activity in utero in response to hCG or during infancy by the burst of gonadotropin secretion resulting in a hyperandrogenic fetal ovary [41, 42]. Maternal hyperinsulinemia may induce excessive placental hCG production leading to fetal ovarian hyperplasia and hyperandrogenism [41]. A hyperandrogenic adrenal cortex may also contribute to ovarian androgen production, since fetal ovaries are able to convert steroid precursors to functional ovarian androgens [43].

Furthermore, a recent study suggested that unlike the norm in the adult, where testosterone production is often inhibited by cortisol, in the fetus there is a positive link between the two [44]. Thus, fetal testosterone correlated positively with both fetal cortisol and maternal testosterone concentrations [44]. These findings indicate that some of the factors that cause raised cortisol levels during fetal life, for example, fetal stress may also cause increase in testosterone. Whether fetal androgen production is sufficient to contribute to the fetal endocrine milieu remains to be studied.

7.2.4 Plausible Biological Mechanisms

Fetal programing of PCOS by androgen excess may be related to the phenomenon of sexually dimorphic programing of tissues. Normally, sexually dimorphic traits are programed during the neonatal period by the burst of gonadotropin and sex-steroid secretion in both sexes [45]. Such developmental programing in the female may occur in prenatal life, under the influence of androgen excess, and be directed toward a more masculine phenotype with regard to reproductive, neuroendocrine, and metabolic traits.

In the reproductive context, it is likely that the structural and functional phenotype of PCOS theca cells is programed during differentiation by the altered intrauterine sex-steroid milieu. This notion is supported by reports on the phenotype of the aromatase knockout female mice in which the androgen to estrogen ratio is altered in favor of androgen excess, and this may influence the differentiation of the ovarian theca cells toward a male-type phenotype. Indeed, the ovaries of these mice exhibit an increased interstitium with the presence of theca cells morphologically resembling Leydig cells [46].

Secondly, the pattern of hypothalamic GnRH pulsatility is different between the sexes, being more frequent in the male (and PCOS women) and resulting in LH hypersecretion relative to FSH [47]. This functional neuroendocrine dimorphism is partly related to androgen-dependent decrease in GnRH pulse generator sensitivity to the negative feedback action of sex steroids [48]. Thus, it is possible that androgen excess during fetal life may program a male-type pattern of pulsatile GnRH secretion. Of course, the resulting abnormality in gonadotropin secretion (increase in the LH to FSH ratio) would further contribute to ovarian hyperandrogenism, establishing a vicious cycle that promotes the progress toward the adult PCOS phenotype.

Furthermore, an important metabolic trait of PCOS that may also be programed in utero is visceral fat deposition associated with insulin resistance and hyperinsulinism. Since body fat distribution in humans is sexually dimorphic, the central adiposity in PCOS may, in part, reflect an android pattern of fat distribution programed at a time of tissue differentiation. Indeed, exposure to androgen excess from early life may contribute to the differences in gene and protein expression that have recently been reported in visceral fat biopsies obtained from obese women with or without PCOS [49].

The molecular mechanisms underlying the programing of the above endocrine and metabolic traits of PCOS by androgens are not known. Androgens produced during differentiation may act as potent gene transcription factors and induce other critical transcription factors that may permanently alter gene expression. An interesting hypothesis is the involvement of epigenetic mechanisms in the fetal programing of PCOS [50]. Epigenetic modification of gene expression through DNA methylation or histone modification has been described in the programing of metabolic syndrome by maternal nutrition [51]. Moreover, in a number of diseases with fetal origin, besides epigenetic abnormality in the offspring, there is also evidence for epigenetic inheritance, which is non-genomic transmission of environmentally induced abnormality across several generations [52]. Whether epigenetic inheritance with intergenerational effect is also implicated for the familiar clustering of PCOS is a point that needs further investigation.

7.3 Prenatal Growth and PCOS

Fetal growth restriction may also be related to prenatal exposure to androgen excess. A study based on a random selection of pregnant women reported that endogenous maternal circulating androgen levels were negatively associated with birth size of the offspring [53]. Furthermore, Sir-Petermann et al. reported a high prevalence of small for gestational age births in PCOS mothers compared with control pregnancies while the prevalence of large for gestational age births were the same in both groups [54]. This association between low birth weight and PCOS cannot be attributed to pregnancy complications, and it seems to be more related to the PCOS condition of the mother. Maternal testosterone may modify energy homeostasis and thus decrease nutrient supplies to the placenta and fetus. Testosterone may affect newborn size by modifying placental function and reducing the capacity for transport of nutrients to the fetus, or it may cross the placenta and exert a direct effect on fetal growth and/or energy homeostasis.

Low birth weight for gestational age, in turn, has been associated with precocious pubarche and functional ovarian hyperandrogenism in adolescence in a Spanish population of girls [55]. Even in normal children, there appears to be a relationship between birth weight, postnatal growth rate, and onset of adrenarche with the highest DHEAS concentrations to be found among the lowest birth weight children with the highest rate of postnatal weight gain [56] One French study reported confirmatory results, while no association between low birth weight and precocious pubarche was found in another smaller Parisian cohort [57, 58].

Postmenarcheal follow-up of Spanish girls with exaggerated adrenarche revealed that 52% were not hyperandrogenic, whereas 25% had the PCOS type of functional ovarian hyperandrogenism without hyperinsulinemia, and 23% had both hyperandrogenism and hyperinsulinemia [55]. The birth weight of these successive groups was 0.25, 1.0, and 2.0 SD below average. Thus, increasing degrees of intrauterine growth restriction appeared to be associated with successively increasing risk for premature pubarche, PCOS, and hyperinsulinemia. This is one pathway leading to PCOS, and it seems that premature pubarche and PCOS were likewise consequences of low birth weight-related insulin resistance [59]. However, follow-up of birth cohorts in other populations has not found a relationship of low birth weight to PCOS [60–62]. On the contrary, heavy babies from overweight mothers developed PCOS [60]. As a conclusion, although low birth weight predisposes to insulin resistance, it

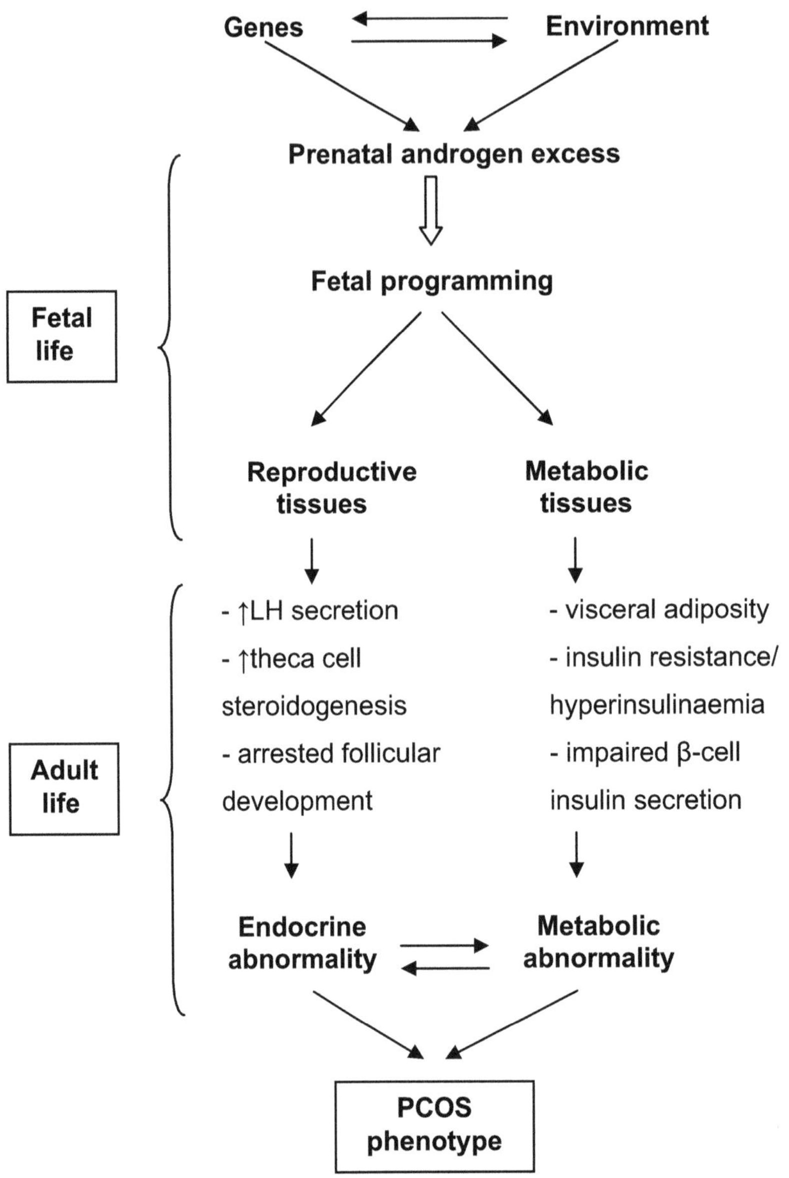

Fig. 7.2 Programing of PCOS phenotypes by prenatal androgen excess

appears to pose a risk for PP and PCOS in some but not all populations studied to date reflecting the heterogeneity of PCOS phenotypes.

7.4 Pubarche and PCOS

The link between premature adrenarche and subsequent risk of ovarian hyperandrogenism has been established over the past years suggesting that premature adrenarche may be a forerunner of PCOS. Ibanez et al. described a correlation between androgen levels at the time of premature pubarche and the development of PCOS in adult life [63]. Girls with premature adrenarche appear to carry 15–20% risk of developing PCOS, and the risk is relatively higher in those with exaggerated adrenarche [63]. The correlation between androgen levels with premature pubarche and the development of the PCOS type of ovarian dysfunction during adolescence is compatible with the concept that ovarian and adrenal dysfunction of PCOS represent an inborn dysregulation of steroidogenesis.

There appear to be two groups of adolescent girls with PCOS. In one group, premature pubarche precedes PCOS, while in the second group, symptoms typical of PCOS develop during or after adolescence. Prior to gonadarche, adrenal androgen secretion accounts for most of the circulating androgens. Upon gonadarche with increased gonadotropin secretion, ovarian androgen secretion increases. Hence, girls in whom premature pubarche precedes, PCOS presumably have a component of adrenal hyperandrogenism that persists and may be exacerbated by the onset of gonadarche. Among girls who develop PCOS during the adolescent years, the relative proportions of ovarian vs. adrenal contributions to the androgen excess are likely to be more variable [64].

Furthermore, peripubertal obesity has been proposed to predispose to PCOS since it has been associated with subclinical increase in testosterone that normalizes with weight loss [65, 66]. Adipose tissue is a major site for the formation of testosterone from circulating precursors [67]. In adults, androgen excess inhibits progestin negative feedback resulting in increased LH secretion, which in turn enhances ovarian androgen production and leads to PCOS [66].

7.5 Conclusion

In summary, fetal programing of PCOS by androgen excess may be related to sexually dimorphic programing of tissues during intrauterine life leading to the development of the PCOS phenotypes in adult life (Fig. 7.2). The underlying molecular mechanisms implicated in this process remain to be elucidated by further research. This may open new avenues for the possible intervention at the critical period of prenatal life to prevent PCOS occurrence.

References

1. Azziz R, Carmina E, Dewailly B, et al. Positions statement: criteria for defining polycystic ovary syndrome as a predominantly hyperandrogenic syndrome: an Androgen Excess Society guideline. J Clin Endocrinol Metab 2006; 91:4237–4245.
2. Nelson VL, Legro RS, Strauss JF 3rd, et al. Augmented androgen production is a stable steroidogenic phenotype of propagated theca cells from polycystic ovaries. Mol Endocrinol 1999; 13:946–957.
3. Nelson VL, Qin Kn KN, Rosenfield RL, et al. The biochemical basis for increased testosterone production in theca cells propagated from patients with polycystic ovary syndrome. J Clin Endocrinol Metab 2001; 86:5925–5933.
4. Franks S. Adult polycystic ovary syndrome begins in childhood. Best Pract Res Clin Endocrinol Metab 2002; 16:263–272.
5. Abbott DH, Dumesic DA, Franks S. Developmental origin of polycystic ovary syndrome-a hypothesis. J Endocrinol 2002; 174:1–5.
6. Barker DJ. In utero programming of chronic disease. Clin Sci 1998; 95:115–128.
7. Ibanez L, Potau N, Francois I, et al. Precocious pubarche, hyperinsulinism, and ovarian hyperandrogenism in girls: relation to reduced fetal growth. J Clin Endocrinol Metab 1998; 83:3558–3562.

8. Hague WM, Adams J, Rodda C, et al. The prevalence of polycystic ovaries in patients with congenital adrenal hyperplasia and their close relatives. Clin Endocrinol 1990; 33:501–510.
9. Barnes RB, Rosenfield RL, Ehrmann DA et al. Ovarian hyperandrogenism as a result of congenital adrenal virilizing disorders: evidence for perinatal masculinization of neuroendocrine function in women. J Clin Endocrinol Metab 1994; 79:1328–1333.
10. Miller WL. P450 oxidoreductase deficiency: a new disorder of steroidogenesis with multiple clinical manifestations. Trends Endocrinol Metab 2004; 15:311–315.
11. Morishima A, Grumbach MM, Simpson ER, et al. Aromatase deficiency in male and female siblings caused by a novel mutation and the physiological role of estrogens. J Clin Endocrinol Metab 1995; 80:3689–3698.
12. Hogeveen KN, Cousin P, Pugeat M et al. Human sex hormone-binding globulin variants associated with hyperandrogenism and ovarian dysfunction. J Clin Invest 2002; 109:973–981.
13. Abbott DH, Dumesic DA, Eisner JR, et al. The prenatally androgenized female rhesus monkey as a model for polycystic ovarian syndrome. In: Azziz R, Nestler JE, Dewailly D (eds). Androgen Excess Disorders in Women. Philadelphia, PA, Lippincott-Raven Press, 1997 pp. 369–382.
14. Eisner JR, Barnett MA, Dumesic DA, et al. Ovarian hyperandrogenism in adult female rhesus monkeys exposed to prenatal androgen excess. Fertil Steril 2002; 77:167–172.
15. Zhou R, Bird IM, Dumesic DA, et al. Adrenal hyperandrogenism is induced by fetal androgen excess in a rhesus monkey model of polycystic ovary syndrome. J Clin Endocrinol Metab 2005; 90:6630–6637.
16. Abbott DH, Dumesic DA, Eisner JR, et al. Insights into the development of PCOS from studies of prenatally androgenized female rhesus monkeys. Trends Endocrinol Metab 1998; 9:62–67.
17. Dumesic DA, Abbott DH, Eisner JR, et al. Prenatal exposure of female rhesus monkeys to testosterone propionate increases serum luteinizing hormone levels in adulthood. Fertil Steril 1997; 67:155–163.
18. Steiner RA, Clifton DK, Spies HG, et al. Sexual differentiation and feedback control of luteinizing hormone secretion in the rhesus monkey. Biol Reprod 1976; 15:206–212.
19. Eisner JR, Dumesic DA, Kemnitz JW, et al. Increased adiposity in female rhesus monkeys exposed to androgen excess during early gestation. Obes Res 2003; 11:279–286.
20. Bruns CM, Baum ST, Colman RJ, et al. Prenatal androgen excess negatively impacts body fat distribution in a nonhuman primate model of polycystic ovary syndrome (PCOS). Int J Obesity 2007; 31:1579–1585.
21. Eisner JR, Dumesic DA, Kemnitz JW, et al. Timing of prenatal androgen excess determines differential impairment in insulin secretion and action in adult female rhesus monkeys. J Clin Endocrinol Metab 2000; 85:1206–1210.
22. Zhou R, Bruns CM, Bird IM, et al. Pioglitazone improves insulin action and normalizes menstrual cycles in a majority of prenatally androgenized female rhesus monkeys. Reprod Toxicol 2007; 23:438–448.
23. Bruns CM, Baum ST, Colman RJ, et al. Insulin resistance and impaired insulin secretion in prenatally androgenized male rhesus monkeys. J Clin Endocrinol Metab 2004; 89:6218–6223.
24. Barraclough CA, Gorski RA. Evidence that the hypothalamus is responsible for androgen-induced sterility in the female rat. Endocrinology 1961; 68:68–79.
25. Vom Saal FS, Bronson FH. Sexual characteristics of adult female mice are correlated with their blood testosterone levels during prenatal development. Science 1980; 208:597–599.
26. Padmanabhan V, Evans N, Taylor JA, et al. Prenatal exposure to androgens leads to the development of cystic ovaries in the sheep. Biol Reprod 1998; 56(Suppl 1): 194.
27. Recabarren SE, Padmanabhan V, Codner E, et al. Postnatal developmental consequences of altered insulin sensitivity in female sleep treated prenatally with testosterone. Am J Physiol Endocrinol Metab 2005; 289:E801–E806.
28. Benediktsson R, Calder AA, Edwards CR, et al. Placental 11beta-hydroxysteroid dehydrogenase: a key regulator of fetal glucocorticoid exposure. Clin Endocrinol 1997; 46:161–166.
29. Sir-Petermann T, Maliqueo M, Angel B, et al. Maternal serum androgens in pregnant women with polycystic ovarian syndrome: possible implications in prenatal androgenization. Hum Reprod 2002; 17:2573–2579.
30. Sir-Petermann T, Devoto L, Maliqueo M, et al. Resumption of ovarian function during lactational amenorrhoea in breastfeeding women with polycystic ovarian syndrome: endocrine aspects. Hum Reprod 2001; 16:1603–1610.
31. Takeyama J, Sasano H, Suzuki T, et al. 17beta-hydroxysteroid dehydrogenase types 1 and 2 in human placenta: an immunohistochemical study with correlation to placental development. J Clin Endocrinol Metab 1998; 83:3710–3715.
32. Mason JI, Ushijima K, Doody KM, et al. Regulation of expression of the 3beta-hydroxysteroid dehydrogenase of human placenta and fetal adrenal. J Steroid Biochem Mol Biol 1993; 47:151–159.
33. Nestler JE. Modulation of aromatase and P450 cholesterol side-chain cleavage enzyme activities of human placental cytotrophoblasts by insulin and insulin-like growth factor I. Endocrinology 1987; 121:1845–1852.
34. Nestler JE. Insulin and insulin-like growth factor-I stimulate the 3 betahydroxysteroid dehydrogenase activity of human placental cytotrophoblasts. Endocrinology 1989; 125:2127–2133.
35. Nestler JE, Powers LP, Matt DW et al. A direct effect of hyperinsulinemia on serum sex hormone-binding globulin levels in obese women with the polycystic ovary syndrome. J Clin Endocrinol Metab 1991; 72:83–89.
36. Baghaei F, Rosmond R, Westberg L, et al. The CYP19 gene and associations with androgens and abdominal obesity in premenopausal women. Obes Res 2003; 11:578–585.
37. Hogeveen KN, Talikka M, Hammond GL. Human sex hormone-binding globulin promoter activity is influenced by a (TAAAA)n repeat element within an Alu sequence. J Biol Chem 2001; 276:36383–36390.

38. Xita N, Tsatsoulis A, Chatzikyriakidou A, et al. Association of the (TAAAA)n repeat polymorphism in the sex hormone-binding globulin (SHBG) gene with polycystic ovary syndrome and relation to SHBG serum levels. J Clin Endocrinol Metab 2003; 88:5976–5980.
39. Cousin P, Calemard-Michel L, Lejeuve H, et al. Influence of SHBG gene pentanucleotide TAAAA repeat and D327N polymorphism on serum sex hormone-binding globulin concentrations in hirsute women. J Clin Endocrinol Metab 2004; 89:917–924.
40. Xita N, Georgiou I, Lazaros L, et al. The synergistic effect of sex hormone-binding globulin and aromatase genes on polycystic ovary syndrome phenotype. Eur J Endocrinol 2008; 158:861–865.
41. Barbieri RL, Saltzman DH, Torday JS, et al. Elevated concentrations of the beta-subunit of human chorionic gonadotropin and testosterone in the amniotic fluid of gestations of diabetic mothers. Am J Obstet Gynecol 1986; 154:1039–1043.
42. Beck-Peccoz P, Padmanabhan V, Baggiani AM, et al. Maturation of hypothalamic–pituitary–gonadal function in normal human fetuses: circulating levels of gonadotropins, their common alpha-subunit and free testosterone, and discrepancy between immunological and biological activities of circulating follicle-stimulating hormone. J Clin Endocrinol Metab 1991; 73: 525–532.
43. Bonser J, Walker J, Purohit A, et al. Human granulosa cells are a site of sulphatase activity and are able to utilize dehydroepiandrosterone sulphate as a precursor for oestradiol production. J Endocrinol 2000; 167:465–471.
44. Gitau R, Adams D, Fisk NM, et al. Fetal plasma testosterone correlates positively with cortisol. Arch Dis Child Fetal Neonotal Ed 2005; 90: F166–F169.
45. Soder O. Sexual dimorphism of gonadal development Best Pract Res Clin Endocrinol Metab 2007; 21:381–391.
46. Britt KL, Findlay JK. Estrogen actions in the ovary revisited. J Endocrinol 2002; 175:269–276.
47. Ehrmann DA. Polycystic ovary syndrome. N Engl J Med 2005; 352:1223–1236.
48. Apter D, Butzow T, Laughlin GA, et al. Accelerated 24-hour luteinizing hormone pulsatile activity in adolescent girls with ovarian hyperandrogenism: relevance to the developmental phase of polycystic ovarian syndrome. J Clin Endocrinol Metab 1994; 74:119–125.
49. Corton M, Botella-Carretero JI, Benguria A, et al. Differential gene expression profile in omental adipose tissue in women with polycystic ovary syndrome. J Clin Endocrinol Metab 2007; 92:328–337.
50. Li Z, Huang H. Epigenetic abnormality: a possible mechanism underlying the fetal origin of polycystic ovary syndrome. Med Hypotheses 2008; 70:638–642.
51. Gluckman PD, Hanson MA. The developmental origins of the metabolic syndrome. Trends Endocrinol Metab 2004; 15: 183–187.
52. Waterland RA, Michels KB. Epigenetic epidemiology of the developmental origins hypothesis. Annu Rev Nutr 2007; 27: 363–388.
53. Carlsen SM, Jacobsen G, Romundstad P. Maternal testosterone levels during pregnancy are associated with offspring size at birth. Eur J Endocrinol 2006; 155:365–370.
54. Sir-Petermann T, Hitchsfeld C, Maliqueo M, et al. Birth weight in offspring of mothers with polycystic ovarian syndrome. Hum Reprod 2005; 20:2122–2126.
55. Ibanez L, Potau N, Francois I, et al. Precocious pubarche, hyperinsulinism, and ovarian hyperandrogenism in girls: relation to reduced fetal growth. J Clin Endocrinol Metab 1998; 83:3558–3562.
56. Ong KK, Potau N, Petry CJ, et al. Opposing influences of prenatal and postnatal weight gain on adrenarche in normal boys and girls. J Clin Endocrinol Metab 2004; 89:2647–2651.
57. Charkaluk ML, Trivin C, Brauner R. Premature pubarche as an indicator of how body weight influences the onset of adrenarche. Eur J Pediatr 2004; 163:89–93.
58. Meas T, Chevenne D, Thibaud E, et al. Endocrine consequences of premature pubarche in post-pubertal Caucasian girls. Clin Endocrinol 2002; 57:101–106.
59. Barker DJ, Eriksson JG, Forsen T, et al. Fetal origins of adult disease: strength of effects and biological basis. Int J Epidemiol 2002; 31:1235–1239.
60. Cresswell JL, Barker DJ, Osmond C, et al. Fetal growth, length of gestation, and polycystic ovaries in adult life. Lancet 1997; 350:1131–1135.
61. Laitinen J, Taponen S, Martikainen H, et al. Body size from birth to adulthood as a predictor of self-reported polycystic ovary syndrome symptoms. Int J Obes Relat Metab Disord 2003; 27:710–715.
62. Michelmore K, Ong K, Mason S, et al. Clinical features of women with polycystic ovaries: relationships to insulin sensitivity, insulin gene VNTR and birth weight. Clin Endocrinol 2001; 55:439–446.
63. Ibanez L, Potau N, Virdis R, et al. Postpubertal outcome in girls diagnosed of premature pubarche during childhood: increased frequency of functional ovarian hyperandrogenism. J Clin Endocrinol Metab 1993; 76:1599–1603.
64. Witchel SF. Puberty and polycystic ovary syndrome. Mol Cell Endocrinol 2006; 254–255:146–153.
65. Reinehr T, de Sousa G, Roth CL, et al. Androgens before and after weight loss in obese children. J Clin Endocrinol Metab 2005; 90:5588–5595.
66. McCartney CR, Prendergast KA, Chhabra S, et al. The association of obesity and hyperandrogenemia during the pubertal transition in girls: obesity as a potential factor in the genesis of postpubertal hyperandrogenism. J Clin Endocrinol Metab 2006; 91:1714–1722.
67. Kershaw EE, Flier JS. Adipose tissue as an endocrine organ J Clin Endocrinol Metab 2004; 89:2548–2556.

Part III
Consequences

Chapter 8
Hyperandrogenism in PCOS

Neoklis A. Georgopoulos , Eleni Kandaraki, and Dimitrios Panidis

8.1 Introduction

In women with polycystic ovary syndrome (PCOS), hyperandrogenism is clinically manifested by hirsutism, acne and androgenic alopecia, and it contributes to chronic anovulation and menstrual dysfunction. Biochemically, hyperandrogenism is established by elevated circulating levels of serum total or unbound testosterone, androstenedione and an increased free androgen index (FAI). In prospective studies, hyperandrogenism appears to affect about 1 in 10 women of reproductive age [1], although racial differences or the selection criteria of patients can increase its prevalence up to 30% [2].

8.2 Clinical Evaluation of Hyperandrogenism

8.2.1 Hirsutism

Hirsutism in women is defined as the growth of terminal hair in an adult male distribution. Terminal hairs are pigmented, coarse and greater than 1 cm in length. Common presentations are excess facial hair (especially the upper lip and chin), hair on the chest between the breasts and hair on the lower abdomen. Excessive terminal hair affecting only the lower legs and forearms does not constitute hirsutism as these areas are normally covered by a mixture of terminal and vellus hairs [3]. Hirsutism is usually of benign aetiology and must be differentiated from virilisation, which includes increased muscle mass and libido, breast atrophy, clitoromegaly and deepening of the voice. Hirsutism is affected by familial and racial factors.

Hirsutism has frequently been used as the primary clinical indicator of androgen excess. A score has been validated to reflect the extent of hirsutism by Ferriman–Gallwey [4]. The total score is obtained by adding up the scores in each one of nine different body areas. The buttocks/perineum, sideburn and neck areas greatly contributed to the total hirsutism score, rather than the upper part of the body (arm, back and abdomen) [5]. However, although hirsutism is an important clinical sign, and often particularly distressing for patients, its assessment is often very subjective and is partially racially determined.

Hirsutism in PCOS reflects androgen excess, predominantly local dihydrotestosterone. The dermal papillae express androgen receptors that directly influence the size of the hair follicle and hence the hair produced. PCOS is by far the most common cause of hirsutism. Excess body and facial hair may occur alone or in combination with other symptoms of hyperandrogenemia, like cycle irregularity, acne and male-pattern alopecia. Obesity and hyperinsulinaemia exacerbate the clinical appearance of hirsutism.. The presence of signs of severe hyperandrogenism such as clitoromegaly, severe male-pattern balding and masculinization of the body should point towards the need to exclude an androgenic tumor, congenital adrenal hyperplasia (CAH),

N.A. Georgopoulos (✉)
Department of Obstetrics and Gynecology, Division of Reproductive Endocrinology, Patras Medical School, Greece
e-mail: neoklisg@hol.gr

N.R. Farid, E. Diamanti-Kandarakis (eds.), *Diagnosis and Management of Polycystic Ovary Syndrome*,
DOI 10.1007/978-0-387-09718-3_8,

or HAIR-AN syndrome (hyperandrogenism, insulin resistance, acanthosis nigricans), the latter being a subphenotype of polycystic ovary syndrome characterized by acne, obesity, hirsutism and acanthosis nigricans. In PCOS the ovary rather than the adrenals is the principal source of androgen excess, hence these patients benefit from treatment targeted at pituitary FSH and LH suppression. Most women with PCOS report symptoms dating from puberty, with a gradual worsening over time and usually accompanied by an increase in body weight.

A sudden development of hirsutism is suggestive of more worrying pathology such as Cushing's syndrome or an androgen-secreting tumour, particularly in the presence of virilisation [6].

8.2.2 *Acne*

Acne is an inflammatory disorder of the hair follicle and its associated sebaceous and apocrine gland. Androgens have a direct effect on sebaceous glands, increasing both gland cell division and sebum production. Still, unlike androgenic alopecia and hirsutism, the principal problem for women with acne is an increased sebaceous secretion and serum androgen levels are often not raised. Acne is a reasonable indicator of hyperandrogenism, although studies are somewhat conflicting regarding the exact prevalence of androgen excess in these patients [7, 8]. Still, acne is by any means less frequent than hirsutism as the sole clinical manifestation of androgen excess, affecting between 20–40% of patients without hirsutism and menstrual irregularities [3, 4]. In a large series of PCOS, women (4.6%) had only acne, while hirsutism was associated with acne in 12.6% of patients [8]. Increased androsterone metabolism has been shown to be specifically related to acne both in normoandrogenic and in hyperandrogenic women [9].

8.2.3 *Male-Pattern Alopecia*

The sole presence of androgenic alopecia as an indicator of hyperandrogenism has been less well studied. The majority of women with a primary complaint of alopecia suffer from polycystic ovaries. In a study of mixed ethnic origin women, with androgenic alopecia as primary complaint, the incidence of polycystic ovaries was 67%, while polycystic ovaries were present in only .27% of the control group. Among women with androgenic alopecia, 21% were also hirsute, compared with 4% of the control group. Interestingly, the women with alopecia had higher testosterone, androstenedione and free androgen index than controls but few had frankly abnormal androgen levels [10]. However, alopecia is a relatively poor marker of androgen excess, unless present in the oligo-ovulatory patient. The loss of scalp terminal hair is usually progressive and therefore probably under diagnosed in women with PCOS [11]. The presence of alopecia requires a familial predisposition to baldness and an associated increase in circulating androgens, consequently not all women with an excess of circulating androgens will suffer from androgenic alopecia.

8.3 Laboratory Evaluation of Hyperandrogenism

Hyperandrogenism is established by elevated circulating levels of serum total or unbound testosterone, and an increased free testosterone and/or free androgen index (FAI). Increased serum androstenedione levels are also frequently detected in PCOS women.

Testosterone in women varies not only with the menstrual cycle but also with age, race, and body mass index. Measuring total testosterone in serum has several limitations. RIAs and chemiluminescence immunoassays are the most widely used methods. Most assays are performed directly on serum or plasma ("direct" assays); however for more accurate determinations, steroids need to be extracted from plasma or serum and separated chromatographically before subjected to immunoassay. Assays after extraction and chromatography, followed by immunoassay, are more accurate and sensitive than direct assays but still require proper validation. Each laboratory should create its own reference intervals taking in consideration variables such as age, race, stage of puberty, etc.

An appropriate assay for total testosterone is necessary but not sufficient for the measurement of free testosterone (FT). FT is measured directly by RIA or much better by an equilibrium dialysis (ED) assay. The equilibrium dialysis assay is considered the gold-standard method for measuring FT.

The free androgen index (FAI) is often used to estimate FT. Because Sex Hormone Binding Globulin (SHBG) is present in excess in women, FT concentrations are driven mainly by SHBG abundance. The FAI depends on accurate measurements for testosterone and SHBG. Having measured both testosterone and SHBG, FT should be calculated, which is easily done using a fixed formula. Calculated FT, using high-quality testosterone and SHBG assays, is the most useful and a sensitive marker of hyperandrogenemia in women [12].

The access of androgens to target tissues is regulated by SHBG. Serum SHBG levels are usually decreased in women with hyperandrogenism, especially in association with PCOS. The reason for this decrease is unclear. Both high androgens and high insulin have been known to lower SHBG [13]. Obesity is also known to be associated with decreased serum SHBG levels, but SHBG values may also be genetically determined. An association of the functional (TAAAA)n polymorphism in the promoter of the SHBG gene with PCOS has been reported, with PCOS women having a significantly greater frequency of longer (TAAAA)n alleles (more than eight repeats) than normal women [14].

8.4 Biochemical Features of Hyperandrogenism

8.4.1 Ovarian Hyperandrogenism

The ovary and adrenal cortex share the bulk of the steroid biosynthesis pathways. They make equal contributions to the circulating concentrations of androstenedione and testosterone in a normal premenopausal woman.

Androgen is produced in the ovary by the theca interna layer of the ovarian follicle, whereas the zona fasciculata of the adrenal cortex synthesises adrenal androgens. The enzymes utilised in the formation of androstenedione from the initial substrate, cholesterol, are similar in both glands and are under the endocrine control of LH in the ovary and adrenocorticotrophic hormone (ACTH) in the adrenal glands. The ovary is considered the main source of excess androgens in women with PCOS, although excess adrenal androgen production may also occur. Ovarian theca cells produce androgen under the influence of LH, and it can be modulated by a number of local growth factors, hormones and cytokines. Theca cells display alterations in steroidogenic activities, including increased expression and differential regulation of genes required for steroidogenesis.

A certain amount of intraovarian androgen is essential for normal follicular growth and for the synthesis of oestradiol. Nonetheless, when the synthesis of androgens is not co-ordinated with the needs of a developing follicle, and is in excess, poor follicle maturation and increased follicular atresia results. In the normal ovary, LH acts on the theca–interstitial–stromal cells, whereas FSH acts on granulosa cells. According to the 'two-gonadotrophin, two-cell theory' of oestrogen biosynthesis, the thecal compartment secretes androgens in response to LH, and the produced androstenedione is converted in the granulosa cell to oestrogens by the action of aromatase, which in turn is under the influence of FSH. In PCOS, the ovarian theca cells are increased in number, and they have increased steroidogenic capacity caused by increased transcription and mRNA stability of steroidogenic enzymes [3].

Autocrine, paracrine and hormonal factors modulate the co-ordination of thecal and granulosa cell function, in terms of androgen synthesis. Androgens and estrogens are negative modulators of LH effects, whereas IGFs play a positive modulator role. Insulin also augments LH-stimulated androgen production, either via its own receptors or via IGF-1 receptors. Inhibin promotes androgen synthesis, whereas activin opposes the effects of inhibin. Granulosa cell development, and thereby the increase of aromatase activity, also determines androgen production. A healthy follicle >8 mm in diameter converts androstenedione to estradiol efficiently. Conversely, atretic and/or cystic follicles have a high androstenedione to estradiol ratio. The granulosa cells of the polycystic ovaries fail to increase the expression of aromatase leading to decreased oestrogens secretion and also prematurely express LH receptors and the cholesterol side-chain cleavage enzymatic activity leading to an over responsiveness to LH [3].

The action of FSH on granulosa cells determines the growth of healthy follicles that are .2–5 mm in diameter, partly mediated by the IGF system and insulin, all of which stimulate the production of estradiol. IGF-binding proteins inhibit FSH bioactivity and are markedly expressed in atretic follicles.

Nearly a half of the circulating testosterone in normal adult women is derived from the peripheral conversion of androstenedione; the remainder is derived from the ovary and adrenal cortex. The important tissues in which this conversion takes place are the lung, the liver, the adipose tissue and the skin. Adipose tissue also forms estrone from androstenedione, which explains the mild estrogen excess of obesity. Plasma dihydrotestosterone is produced virtually entirely by 5a-reductase activity in the periphery, with plasma androstenedione being its major precursor [15].

8.4.2 Adrenal Hyperandrogenism

Among PCOS women, a significant percentage ranging between 20% and 30% demonstrates adrenal androgen excess which is detectable by increased serum levels of DHEAS and androstenedione, and adrenal hyperresponsivity to ACTH stimulation test [3]. Measurements of serum DHEAS have been generally used for the assessment of adrenal androgen excess because DHEAS is secreted by 97–99% in the adrenals. DHEAS secretion declines with increasing age and is also partly influenced by a genetic component. The incidence of increased DHEAS serum levels in PCOS women range between 20 and 33% among black and white women, while in approximately 10% of PCOS patients, it may be the sole abnormality in circulating androgens [16].

Androstenedione is a weak androgen which is secreted by both the ovary and the adrenals. Although it has an adrenal component, its value in the estimation of adrenal androgen excess is unclear, although, it may be the sole androgen in excess in approximately 10% of PCOS women [17]. The adrenal androgen excess is not due to hypothalamic-pituitary alterations as both basal and circadian variation of ACTH levels and the response of ACTH to endogenous or exogenous corticotrophin-releasing hormone (CRH) are within normal limits in hyperandrogenic women [18, 19]. Adrenal androgen excess appears therefore to be due to adrenocortical steroidogenic abnormalities, abnormalities in the metabolism of adrenal products or to alterations in the responsivity of adrenals to ACTH as women with PCOS present a generalized hypersecretion of adrenocotrical products in response to ACTH stimulation [20].

Ovarian factors might also contribute to the elevation of adrenal androgens observed in women with PCOS. A 20–25% decrease in DHEAS serum levels was noted following long-acting GnRH analogue suppression in women with PCOS and elevated DHEAS levels [21]. Hyperinsulinemia plays also a critical role in enhancing adrenal androgen production.

8.5 The Molecular Basis of Hyperandrogenism

Many studies have been conducted trying to elucidate the genetic basis of functional hyperandrogenism. The familial aggregation of PCOS suggested a genetic origin at least to a subgroup of PCOS patients. Taking in consideration hyperandrogenism and chronic anovulation, an autosomal dominant mode of inheritance with variable penetrance has been suggested [22]. Different modes of inheritance like X-linked or polygenic have been suggested also. Familial aggregation of hyperandrogenism and PCOS does not exclude that clustering of PCOS within families might also result from nongenetic inheritance related to certain environmental factors.

Many genes have been considered as candidates in order to elucidate the genetic origin of PCOS mostly genes related to androgen biosynthesis and action and genes related to different aspects of insulin resistance and chronic inflammation. All genes involved in androgen biosynthesis have been used as candidates, including the CYP17 which encodes the enzyme P450c17, the CYP11A which encodes the cholesterol side-chain

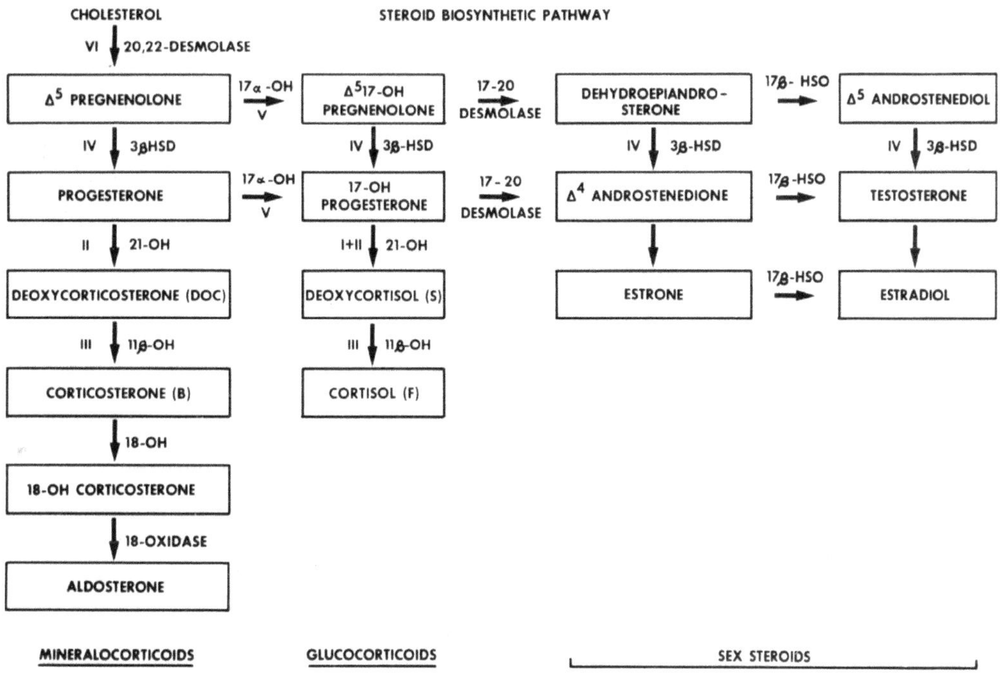

Fig. 8.1 Steroid biosynthetic pathway

cleavage enzyme, the CYP 21 which encodes the 21-hydroxylase enzyme catalyzing the conversion of 17-hydroxyprogesterone into 11-deoxycortisol, the 3β-hydroxysteroid dehydrogenase (HSD3B) which encodes the enzyme that catalyzes the conversion of Δ^5 steroids into Δ^4 steroids, the 17β hydroxysteroid dehydrogenase (17βHSD type III) which encodes the enzyme that catalyzes the conversion of androstenedione into testosterone, and the CYP 19 (the aromatase gene) which encodes the enzyme of aromatase that catalyses the conversion of androgens to estrogens (Fig. 8.1) [23, 24].

Other gene polymorphisms reported to be implicated in PCOS include those for gonadotropins, dopamine receptor, androgen receptor, aldosterone synthetase (CYP11B2), paraoxonase (PON1), follistatin, tumour necrosis factor α (TNFα), type II TNF receptor (TNFR2), interleucin 6 (IL-6) and its receptor [23, 24]

The influence of proinflamatory genotypes on PCOS and hyperandrogenism might be influenced by the interaction between different predisposing and protective genetic variants. Concerning genes related to insulin action that all reported associations in women with PCOS are mainly related to insulin resistance and obesity and not to androgen excess.

In conclusion, all candidate genes reported so far have a marginal role in the pathogenesis of hyperandrogenism. To date, no gene has been identified that directly causes or substantially contributes to the development of a PCOS phenotype [23, 24].

References

1. Azziz R, Wonds KS, Reyna R, et al. The prevalence and features of the polycystic ovary syndrome in an unselected population. J Clin Endocrinol Metab 2004; 89:2745–2749.
2. Diamanti-Kandarakis E, Kouli CR, Bergiele AT, et al. A survey of the polycystic ovary syndrome in the Greek island of Lesbos: hormonal and metabolic profile. J Clin Endocrinol Metab 1990; 51:779–786.
3. Azziz R, Nestler HE, Dewailly D. Androgen excess disorders in Women. Polycystic Ovary Syndrome and Other Disorders. Humana Press, Totowa, New Jersey, USA, second edition, 2006.
4. Ferriman D, Gallwey J. Clinical assessment of body hair growth in women. J Clin Endocrinol Metab 1961; 21:1440–1447.

5. Hassa H, Tanir H, Yildirim A, Senses T, Eskalen M, Mutlu FS. The hirsutism scoring system should be population specific. Fertil Steril 2005; 84:778–780.
6. Nikolaou D, Gilling-Smith C. Hirsutism. Current Obstertrics and Gynecology 2005; 15:174–182.
7. Carmina E, Rosato F, Jannı A`, Rizzo M, Longo RA. Relative Prevalence of Different Androgen Excess Disorders in 950 Women Referred because of Clinical Hyperandrogenism. J Clin Endocrinol Metab 2006;91:2–6
8. Slayden SM, Moran C, Sams Jr WM, et al. Hyperandrogenemia in patients presenting with acne. Fertil Steril 2001; 75: 889–892.
9. Falsetti L, Gambera A, Andrico S, Sartori E. Acne and hirsutism in polycystic ovary syndrome: clinical, endocrine-metabolic and ultrasonographic differences. Gynecological Endocrinology 2002; 16:275–284.
10. Carmina E, Lobo RA. Evidence for Increased Androsterone Metabolism in Some Normoandrogenic Women with Acne. J Clin Endocrinol Metab 1993; 76:1111–1114.
11. Cela E, Robertson C, Rush K, et al. Prevalence of polycystic ovaries in women with androgenic alopecia. Europ J Endocrinol 2003; 149:439–442.
12. Rosner W, Auchus RJ, Azziz R, Sluss PM, Raff H. Position statement: utility, limitations, and pitfalls in measuring testosterone: an endocrine society position statement. J Clin Endocrinol Metab 2007; 92:405–413.
13. Nestler JE, Powers LP, Matt DW, Steingold KA, Plymate SR, Rittmaster RS, Clore JN, Blackard WG. A direct effect of hyperinsulinaemia on serum sex-hormone-binding globulin levels in obese women with the polycystic ovary syndrome. J Clin Endocrinol Metab 1991; 72:83–89.
14. Xita N, Tsatsoulis A, Chatzikyriakidou A, Georgiou I. Association of the (TAAAA)n repeat polymorphism in the sex hormone-binding globulin (SHBG) gene with polycystic ovary syndrome and relation to SHBG serum levels. J Clin Endocrinol Metab 2003; 88(12):5976–5980.
15. Balen A. The pathophysiology of polycystic ovary syndrome: trying to understand PCOS and its endocrinology. Best Pract Res Clin Obstet Gynaecol 2004; 18(5):685–706.
16. Kumar A, Woods KS, Bartolucci AA, Azziz R. Prevalence of adrenal androgen excess in patients with the polycystic ovary syndrome (PCOS). Clin Endocrinol (Oxf) 2005; 62(6):644–649.
17. Knochenhauer ES, Key TJ, Kahsar-Miller M, Waggoner W, Boots LR, Azziz R. Prevalence of the polycystic ovary syndrome in unselected black and white women of the southeastern United States: a prospective study. J Clin Endocrinol Metab 1998; 83:3078–3082.
18. Azziz R, Black V, Hines GA, Fox LM, Boots LR. Adrenal androgen excess in the polycystic ovary syndrome: sensitivity and responsivity of the hypothalamic-pituitary-adrenal axis. J Clin Endocrinol Metab 1998; 83(7):2317–23.
19. Carmina E, Lobo RA. Pituitary-adrenal responses to ovine corticotropin-releasing factor in polycystic ovary syndrome and in other hyperandrogenic patients. Gynecol Endocrinol 1990; 4(4):225–32.
20. Moran C, Reyna R, Boots LS, Azziz R. Adrenocortical hyperresponsiveness to corticotropin in polycystic ovary syndrome patients with adrenal androgen excess. Fertil Steril 2004; 81(1):126–31.
21. Hines GA, Smith ER, Azziz R. Influence of insulin and testosterone on adrenocortical steroidogenesis in vitro: preliminary studies. Fertil Steril 2001; 76(4):730–735
22. Govind A, Obhrai MS, Clayton RN. Polycystic ovaries are inherited as an autosomal dominant trait: analysis of 29 polycystic ovary syndrome and 10 control families. J Clin Endocrinol Metabol 1999; 84(1):38–43
23. Diamanti-Kandarakis E, Kandarakis H, Legro RS. The role of genes and environment in the etiology of PCOS. Endocrine 2006. 30(1):19–26.
24. Escobar-Morreale HF, Luque-Ramírez M, San Millán JL. The molecular-genetic basis of functional hyperandrogenism and the polycystic ovary syndrome. Endocr Rev 2005; 26(2):251–82.

Chapter 9
The Risk of Diabetes and Metabolic Syndrome in PCOS

Thomas M. Barber

9.1 Adverse Metabolic Features and Cardiovascular Risk in PCOS

Polycystic ovary syndrome (PCOS) is the commonest female endocrinopathy and affects between 6 and 10% of pre-menopausal women [1]. PCOS is a highly heritable condition (heritability 0.71 [2]), the expression of which is modulated by obesity, which in turn is influenced by both genetic and environmental (principally dietary) factors [3]. Although PCOS usually presents with reproductive and hyperandrogenic features, many women with the condition (compared with the general female population and following appropriate adjustment for BMI) also have adverse metabolic features, including increased prevalence of Type 2 diabetes (T2D), hypertension, hypercholesterolaemia, hypertriglyceridaemia and increased waist circumference [4]. In a retrospective cohort study of women from the UK, involving >300 women with PCOS and >1000 age-matched control women, it was shown that the proportion of women with confirmed T2D in each group was 6.9 and 3.0% respectively ($P = 0.002$) [4]. Following adjustment for BMI and in comparison with control women, the odds ratio for T2D in the women with PCOS was 2.2 (95% CI: 0.9–5.2) [4]. Furthermore, it has been shown that impaired glucose tolerance or T2D affects between 30 and 50% of young (age <30 years) and obese women with PCOS [5].

There is a frequent concurrence of obesity with PCOS [3]: between 38 and 88% of women with PCOS are either overweight or obese [6, 7]. Obesity influences both the biochemical and clinical expression of PCOS through complex interactions that include modulation of insulin resistance and hyperinsulinaemia, discussed in more detail later in this chapter [3]. Even modest weight loss of just 5% body weight in women with PCOS results in significant improvements in fertility, hyperandrogenic and menstrual features [8, 9]. On the basis of current evidence, it is likely that the adverse metabolic profile associated with PCOS, including T2D and metabolic syndrome, is influenced by both factors inherent to the condition itself (including genetic effects) and obesity-related factors [3].

The association of PCOS with adverse metabolic features is incontrovertible [3]. However, the translation of cardiovascular *risk factors* into consequent cardiovascular *disease* and *outcomes* in women with PCOS is less clear due to a current lack of prospective and long-term studies in these women. In a retrospective study that compared middle-aged women previously diagnosed with PCOS with age-matched control women, it was demonstrated that although women with PCOS had higher rates of cardiovascular risk factors than the general female population, all-cause and cardiovascular mortality were similar between the two cohorts [4]. However, this study was limited by the relatively young age of the subjects involved. In a prospective cohort study of >82,000 female nurses, it was shown that among women with severe oligomenorrhoea (most of whom probably have PCOS), the risk of fatal myocardial infarction was twice as high than in eumenorrhoeic women [10].

Although the prevalence of T2D among women with PCOS is fairly well established [4], the actual prevalence of metabolic syndrome in women with PCOS is more controversial and influenced by a number of factors that are discussed in the next section.

T.M. Barber (✉)
Research Fellow and Specialist Registrar, Department of Endocrinology, Oxford Centre for Diabetes, Endocrinology and Metabolism, University of Oxford, Oxford, UK
e-mail: tom.barber@drl.ox.ac.uk

N.R. Farid, E. Diamanti-Kandarakis (eds.), *Diagnosis and Management of Polycystic Ovary Syndrome*,
DOI 10.1007/978-0-387-09718-3_9, © Springer Science+Business Media, LLC 2009

9.2 Prevalence of Metabolic Syndrome in PCOS

Both metabolic syndrome and PCOS are defined by more than one set of diagnostic criteria that are used commonly for both clinical and research purposes. Studies on the prevalence of metabolic syndrome in PCOS have been influenced by the particular diagnostic criteria employed and by the distribution of BMI and age among subjects within each study, as discussed in more detail below.

9.2.1 Diagnostic Criteria for Metabolic Syndrome

In 1988, Reaven coined the term, 'Syndrome X' for a constellation of disorders related to insulin resistance. Syndrome X has since become known as metabolic syndrome [11]. The precise definition and composition of metabolic syndrome has been controversial, and various diagnostic criteria have been proposed (Table 9.1). These include criteria proscribed by the National Cholesterol Education Program Adult Treatment Panel III (NCEP ATP III) [12, 13], and more recently by the International Diabetes Federation (IDF) [14]. The IDF definition of metabolic syndrome includes central obesity (waist circumference ≥80 cm in European women) as a necessary prerequisite criterion [14].

Metabolic syndrome affects between 34 and 46% of women with PCOS [15–18]. In a comparison of 129 women with PCOS versus 177 female controls, metabolic syndrome was shown to affect 34.9% (47.3% adjusted for age) versus 6.8% (4.3% adjusted for age) respectively ($P<0.001$) [16]. In further separate studies of 138 and 106 women with PCOS, metabolic syndrome was shown to affect 46% [17] and 43% [18] respectively. These figures compare with a prevalence of metabolic syndrome of just 6% (ages 20–29 years) and 15% (ages 30–39 years) among the general US female population (third National Health and Nutrition Examination Survey, NHANES III data) [18]. A limitation of these studies is that most are restricted to white US women, and most

Table 9.1 Diagnostic criteria for metabolic syndrome in women

Organisation	Diagnostic criteria for metabolic syndrome
IDF (2005) [14]	Requires the presence of central obesity (waist circumference ≥80 cm in Europid women). In addition, at least two of the following criteria are required: 1. Elevated triglycerides (≥1.7 mmol/l) 2. Reduced HDL cholesterol (<1.29 mmol/l in women) 3. Specific treatment for lipid abnormalities 4. Elevated blood pressure (systolic BP ≥130 mmHg or diastolic BP ≥85 mmHg) 5. Specific treatment of previously diagnosed hypertension 6. IFG (fasting plasma glucose ≥5.6 mmol/l) 7. Previously diagnosed T2D
NCEP ATP III [12, 13]	Three or more of the following criteria are required: 1. Abdominal obesity: waist circumference >88 cm in women 2. Elevated triglycerides (≥1.7 mmol/l) 3. Reduced HDL cholesterol (<1.3 mmol/l in women) 4. Elevated blood pressure (≥130/85 mmHg) 5. Elevated fasting glucose concentration (≥6.1 mmol/l)
WHO [19]	Requires the presence of diabetes, IFG, IGT or insulin resistance (on the basis of HOMA IR level). In addition, at least two of the following criteria are required: 1. Waist: hip ratio>0.85 in women 2. Elevated triglycerides (≥1.7 mmol/l) 3. Reduced HDL cholesterol (<1.0 mmol/l in women) 4. Urinary albumin excretion rate >20 μg/min 5. Elevated blood pressure (≥140/90 mmHg)

HOMA IR = Homeostasis model assessment of insulin resistance; IDF = International Diabetes Federation; IFG = impaired fasting glucose; IGT = impaired glucose tolerance; NCEP ATPIII = National Cholesterol Education Program Adult Treatment Panel III; WHO = World Health Organisation.

employed just one set of diagnostic criteria (NCEP ATP III [12, 13]) for metabolic syndrome [15–18]. It is likely that application of an alternative set of diagnostic criteria for metabolic syndrome would change prevalence estimates, as evidenced by a study of 43 women with PCOS in which prevalence of metabolic syndrome was just 2.3% using NCEP ATP III diagnostic criteria [12, 13] compared with 11.6% (a 5-fold increase) using WHO [19] diagnostic criteria [20, 21]. Although higher than in the general female population, the actual prevalence of metabolic syndrome in women with PCOS is influenced at least partly by the particular diagnostic criteria used to define metabolic syndrome.

9.2.2 Diagnostic Criteria for PCOS

Diagnostic criteria for PCOS are covered in a separate chapter. Application of the Rotterdam PCOS diagnostic criteria [22, 23] has led to the formation of four distinct PCOS phenotypic subgroups, including two new phenotypic subgroups that previously did not exist on the basis of the NIH diagnostic criteria [24]. These two new phenotypic subgroups define women with polycystic ovarian (PCO) morphology, hyperandrogenism but normal menstrual cyclicity ("PH" subgroup), and PCO morphology, oligo-amenorrhoea but normoandrogenaemia ("PO" subgroup). Several studies have shown significant metabolic heterogeneity between each Rotterdam-defined [22, 23] PCOS phenotypic subgroup: women in the new "PO" and "PH" subgroups have much less extreme departures from metabolic normality than women in the "PHO" subgroup (with a full-complement of PCO morphology, hyperandrogenism and oligo-amenorrhoea), in whom insulin resistance and other dysmetabolic features are confined [25–29]. In one study, it was shown that the prevalence of metabolic syndrome (defined by the IDF criteria [14]) also shows marked heterogeneity between the PCOS phenotypic subgroups: a significantly greater prevalence of metabolic syndrome was confined to the "PHO" subgroup compared with female controls (29.3% versus 3.9% respectively), whereas the "PH" (6.6%) and "PO" (7.1%) subgroups each had prevalence rates of metabolic syndrome that were statistically indistinguishable from that in the control group of women [28]. Similarly, the prevalence of metabolic syndrome using NCEP ATP III [12, 13] criteria in "PH" and "PO" PCOS subgroups in a further study was shown to be comparable to that in subjects from NHANES III, regardless of BMI [27].

The risk of metabolic dysfunction and metabolic syndrome in PCOS is confined to that subgroup with *both* hyperandrogenism *and* oligo-amenorrhoea ("PHO" subgroup). Women in each of the two new phenotypic subgroups ("PH" and "PO") that are unique to the Rotterdam diagnostic criteria [22, 23] appear to be metabolically normal. A limitation of the studies described above is that they used cross-sectional data. Therefore, the effects of possible intra-individual variability of PCOS phenotypic subgroup over time on metabolic profile and cardiovascular risk (which would require long-term prospective studies) could not be inferred. Despite this limitation, it is clear that the particular set of diagnostic criteria employed for defining PCOS is likely to influence prevalence estimates of metabolic syndrome. Compared with the NIH diagnostic criteria [24], application of the broader-based Rotterdam diagnostic criteria for PCOS [22, 23] would be expected to increase the *absolute* number of women with PCOS who also have metabolic syndrome. However, the inclusion of additional metabolically normal phenotypic subgroups ("PH" and "PO") is likely to have a 'diluting' effect on the overall *proportion* of women with PCOS who also have metabolic syndrome.

9.2.3 Distribution of BMI and Age

The prevalence of metabolic syndrome is influenced by the distribution of BMI and age within the particular group assessed. As an illustration, in a study of 394 US women with PCOS, none of the subgroup with a BMI less than or equal to 27.0 kgm^{-2} had metabolic syndrome, compared with a 40% prevalence of metabolic syndrome in the subgroup with a BMI greater than 27 kgm^{-2} [15]. As in the general population, obesity modulates the expression of metabolic syndrome in women with PCOS. However, factors related to PCOS *per se* and independent of obesity-related effects also influence metabolic dysfunction in these women [4, 28].

The prevalence of metabolic syndrome tends to increase with age in the general population [21]. Similarly, the prevalence of metabolic syndrome among older women with PCOS appears to be higher than that in their younger counterparts. In one study, the prevalence of metabolic syndrome among women with PCOS as a whole compared with that in the subgroup who were aged less than 30 years was shown to be 35% versus 24% respectively [16]. However, in the same study, it was also shown that *compared with female controls*, the younger subgroup of women with PCOS with age less than 30 years (and those with a BMI greater than 27 kgm^{-2}) were at a particularly high risk of metabolic syndrome [15, 16]. Therefore, estimates of the prevalence of metabolic syndrome in women with PCOS should take account of the BMI and age distributions among the populations studied, and appropriate matching or adjustment for these factors should be employed when comparisons are made with female controls.

9.3 Aetiology of Metabolic Dysfunction in PCOS

The aetiology of PCOS is complex and incompletely understood. It is clear from twin studies that there is a significant genetic aspect (heritability ~0.7) [2], and it is likely that PCOS is an oligogenic condition [30]. Environmental (principally dietary) factors are also likely to be involved in the modulation of the phenotypic expression of PCOS through effects on obesity [3]. The frequent concurrence of PCOS with T2D and metabolic syndrome, the heritability of metabolic traits in PCOS [31, 32] and the important role of obesity in the development of each of these conditions, raises the possibility of common pathogenic factors, the most likely being those related to obesity. These are discussed further in the rest of this section.

9.3.1 Insulin Resistance

Insulin resistance is an important factor in the development of both metabolic syndrome and PCOS [3, 33]. In PCOS, the proportion of women who also have metabolic syndrome increases significantly in relation to fasting insulin concentration [15]. Most women with PCOS (50-90%) have insulin resistance to a greater extent than in age and BMI-matched control women, this disparity being more marked in obese women [34–36]. It is clear that although worsened by obesity, insulin resistance is also a feature that is inherent to PCOS and occurs, at least partly, independently of obesity [3, 37].

Therapeutic interventions that improve insulin sensitivity and thereby hyperinsulinaemia (such as weight loss or initiation of insulin-sensitising drugs) significantly improve PCOS-related features such as hyperandrogenism, ovulatory function, menstrual cyclicity and fertility [8, 9, 38, 39]. These improved clinical features are likely to result from reduced *steroidogenic* effects of insulin. These include reduced co-gonadotrophic and stimulatory effects of insulin on P450c17α enzyme activity (with reduced biosynthesis of androgens) within ovarian theca cells [40–42] and the adrenal gland [43], reduced enhancement of pituitary LH pulse amplitude [35, 44] and reduced suppression of hepatic synthesis of sex hormone binding globulin (SHBG) [45, 46] thereby reducing free androgen index. Improved ovulatory function and menstrual cyclicity may result from reduced inhibitory effects of insulin on ovarian follicle development [29, 47].

The steroidogenic/cell growth and metabolic effects of insulin are mediated via two separate post-receptor pathways: the mitogen-activated protein kinase (MAP kinase) and phosphatidylinositol 3-kinase (PI3-kinase) pathways respectively. These pathways display tissue-specific differences in insulin sensitivity. In women with PCOS (as has been demonstrated in T2D subjects), impairment of insulin sensitivity is specific to the PI3-kinase pathway and therefore relates to the *metabolic* effects of insulin (including glucose disposal into skeletal muscle), and thus contributes towards the metabolic dysfunction characteristic of PCOS [3]. As in subjects with T2D, it is likely that in women with PCOS, signalling through the alternative MAP kinase pathway is preserved [48], which would explain how the adverse steroidogenic effects of hyperinsulinaemia can co-exist with 'metabolic' insulin resistance in women with PCOS [49].

9.3.2 Abnormal Abdominal Adiposity

Although insulin resistance is associated with abdominal/android adiposity (fat deposition in abdominal subcutaneous and visceral depots) [9, 34, 35, 50, 51], there is some controversy regarding fat distribution in PCOS, and its role in insulin resistance in this condition. There is some evidence that following prolonged exposure to *supra-physiological* doses of testosterone, non-obese female to male transsexuals [52] and postmenopausal women [53] may develop android fat distribution. Furthermore, pre-natally androgenised female Rhesus monkeys may develop a propensity towards central adiposity during adulthood [54].

Although suggestive of android fat distribution, some previous cross-sectional studies on fat distribution in women with PCOS were limited by use of techniques such as lipometer, ultrasound (operator-dependent) and dual-energy X-ray absorptiometry (DEXA, limited by its inability to delineate visceral and abdominal subcutaneous fat depots) [55, 56]. A further cross-sectional study in 50 PCOS cases versus 28 control women including a subgroup analysis of BMI/fat mass-matched pairs employed magnetic resonance imaging (MRI) to derive abdominal (visceral and subcutaneous) and gluteo-femoral (subcutaneous) fat depot cross-sectional area measurements from axial images taken at anatomically pre-defined levels [37]. In this study, fat distribution (including visceral fat) was shown to be indistinguishable between women with PCOS and female controls [37] despite significant differences in insulin resistance between the paired PCOS cases and controls, with the implication that fat distribution may be less closely linked to PCOS-related insulin resistance than has previously been thought, and that alternative mechanisms (such as abnormal ectopic fat distribution) may be involved [37].

9.3.3 Abnormal β-Cell Function

The relationship between insulin sensitivity and insulin secretion from the β-cell in women with PCOS is complex. It has been suggested that in some women with PCOS, a primary abnormality may occur within the β-cell that influences a tendency towards insulin over-secretion and consequent hyperinsulinaemia [9, 50]. Given the important role of abnormal β-cell function in the aetiology of T2D [57], it is imperative to consider whether abnormal β-cell function also features in PCOS pathogenesis.

Variants within *TCF7L2* (the gene encoding transcription factor 7-like 2) [58–60] and the E23K variant of *KCNJ11* (encoding the inwardly rectifying potassium channel Kir6.2, an essential component of the β-cell ATP-sensitive potassium [K_{ATP}] channel) [61] have been reproducibly shown to display powerful genetic associations with T2D in a number of studies. Most current evidence favours impaired β-cell insulin secretion as the mechanism by which variants within *TCF7L2* and *KCNJ11* influence T2D-susceptibility [59, 62]. Using these two genes as candidates for PCOS-susceptibility, it has been demonstrated through genetic association studies on >360 PCOS cases and >2000 controls from the UK that there are no associations between *TCF7L2* [63] and *KCNJ11* [64] variants and PCOS. These studies provide the strongest evidence yet, that despite apparent epidemiological and pathophysiological overlap, the genetic architecture of the related conditions T2D and PCOS is qualitatively distinct. These data support the notion that although abnormal β-cell function is important in defining individual risk of T2D, such a mechanism is unlikely to predominate in the aetiology of PCOS.

To summarise, based on current evidence it is likely that insulin resistance represents a key pathogenic factor that plays an important role in the development of the reproductive, hyperandrogenic and metabolic features of PCOS and which may also be implicated in the frequent concurrence of PCOS with metabolic syndrome. Insulin resistance also plays a key role in the development of T2D. Although genetically determined impairment of the *β-cell response* to insulin resistance also undoubtedly influences T2D-susceptibility, it has been hypothesised that conversely, factors involved in the *ovarian response* to insulin resistance are likely to influence PCOS susceptibility [63]. The precise tissue-specific *response* to insulin resistance (and hyperinsulinaemia) in women may therefore influence phenotypic expression within the PCOS-related spectrum of clinical features that include hyperandrogenism, menstrual disturbance, infertility, metabolic dysfunction and T2D.

9.4 Screening and Management of T2D and Dysglycaemia in PCOS

One important implication of the association of PCOS with metabolic dysfunction and presumed long-term increased risk of cardiovascular adverse events is that appropriate management of PCOS should incorporate a thorough assessment of adverse metabolic features. A simple fasting glucose level lacks the sensitivity to detect the presence of impaired glucose tolerance (IGT) [65]. Given that women with PCOS of all ages and weights are at greater risk of glucose intolerance than control women, in a position statement the Androgen Excess Society advocates that all women with PCOS (regardless of BMI and additional risk factors) should be screened for glucose intolerance through use of a standard oral glucose tolerance test (OGTT) at initial presentation [65]. Due to the high annual conversion rate from normal glucose tolerance (NGT) to IGT in women with PCOS (16–19%), it was also recommended that the subgroup of women with PCOS who have NGT should have an OGTT repeated at least every 2 years following baseline, and earlier if additional cardiovascular risk factors have been identified [65]. Due to the high rate of progression from IGT to T2D in women with PCOS, the subgroup of women with PCOS who have IGT should have an OGTT repeated annually to detect the development of T2D.

In women with PCOS who have IGT, intensive lifestyle modification (including at least 30 minutes of moderate activity on 5 days per week and a hypocaloric diet) remains the mainstay of treatment [65]. A minimum of 5–7% weight loss should be aimed for in overweight and obese women with PCOS. The addition of metformin should be considered in women with PCOS and IGT in whom weight loss is unsuccessful or impossible [65]. For those women with PCOS who also have T2D which is not effectively controlled with a maximum effective dose of metformin (2 g per day), an additional oral hypoglycaemic agent should be considered in the first instance, as per current guidance for patients with T2D. However, well-designed clinical trials of oral hypoglycaemic agents (including glitazones) for the management of T2D in women with PCOS are currently lacking.

9.5 Practice Points

- PCOS is associated with adverse metabolic features and a significantly greater prevalence of T2D and metabolic syndrome compared with control women;
- The risk of metabolic dysfunction and metabolic syndrome in PCOS is confined to that subgroup of women with both hyperandrogenism *and* oligo-amenorrhoea. Assignment of phenotypic subgroup is an important clinical assessment in women with PCOS;
- The prevalence of metabolic syndrome in women with PCOS is particularly high in the subgroup who are young (less than 30 years) and overweight or obese (BMI>27 kgm^{-2});
- The prevalence of metabolic syndrome among women with PCOS is partly dependent upon the diagnostic criteria employed to define both metabolic syndrome and PCOS, and the distribution of BMI and age among the population of women studied;
- PCOS, T2D and metabolic syndrome are likely to share common, obesity-related pathogenic factors, including insulin resistance;
- A primary β-cell defect is unlikely to influence PCOS development, although the tissue-specific *response* to insulin resistance (and hyperinsulinaemia) may influence phenotypic expression within the PCOS-related spectrum of clinical features (hyperandrogenism, menstrual disturbance, infertility, metabolic dysfunction and T2D);
- Appropriate management of PCOS should incorporate a thorough assessment of adverse metabolic features (including oral glucose tolerance test) and aggressive treatment of cardiovascular risk factors.

References

1. Asuncion M, Calvo RM, San Millan JL, et al. A prospective study of the prevalence of the polycystic ovary syndrome in unselected Caucasian women from Spain. J Clin Endocrinol Metab 2000; 85(7):2434–8.
2. Vink JM, Sadrzadeh S, Lambalk CB, et al. Heritability of polycystic ovary syndrome in a Dutch twin-family study. J Clin Endocrinol Metab 2006; 91(6):2100–4.

3. Barber TM, McCarthy MI, Wass JA, et al. Obesity and polycystic ovary syndrome. Clin Endocrinol (Oxf) 2006; 65(2): 137–45.
4. Wild S, Pierpoint T, McKeigue P, et al. Cardiovascular disease in women with polycystic ovary syndrome at long-term follow-up: a retrospective cohort study. Clin Endocrinol (Oxf) 2000; 52(5):595–600.
5. Legro RS, Kunselman AR, Dodson WC, et al. Prevalence and predictors of risk for type 2 diabetes mellitus and impaired glucose tolerance in polycystic ovary syndrome: a prospective, controlled study in 254 affected women. J Clin Endocrinol Metab 1999; 84(1):165–9.
6. Legro RS. The genetics of obesity. Lessons for polycystic ovary syndrome. Ann N Y Acad Sci 2000; 900:193–202.
7. Balen AH, Conway GS, Kaltsas G, et al. Polycystic ovary syndrome: the spectrum of the disorder in 1741 patients. Hum Reprod 1995; 10(8):2107–11.
8. Kiddy DS, Hamilton-Fairley D, Bush A, et al. Improvement in endocrine and ovarian function during dietary treatment of obese women with polycystic ovary syndrome. Clin Endocrinol (Oxf) 1992; 36(1):105–11.
9. Holte J, Bergh T, Berne C, et al. Restored insulin sensitivity but persistently increased early insulin secretion after weight loss in obese women with polycystic ovary syndrome. J Clin Endocrinol Metab 1995; 80(9):2586–93.
10. Solomon CG, Hu FB, Dunaif A, et al. Menstrual cycle irregularity and risk for future cardiovascular disease. J Clin Endocrinol Metab 2002; 87(5):2013–7.
11. Reaven GM. Role of insulin resistance in human disease. Diabetes 1988; 37:1595–607.
12. Executive Summary of The Third Report of The National Cholesterol Education Program (NCEP) Expert Panel on Detection, Evaluation, And Treatment of High Blood Cholesterol In Adults (Adult Treatment Panel III). Jama 2001; 285(19): 2486–97.
13. Third Report of the National Cholesterol Education Program (NCEP) Expert Panel on Detection, Evaluation, and Treatment of High Blood Cholesterol in Adults (Adult Treatment Panel III) final report. Circulation 2002; 106(25):3143–421.
14. Alberti KG, Zimmet P, Shaw J. Metabolic syndrome – a new world-wide definition. A Consensus Statement from the International Diabetes Federation. Diabet Med 2006; 23(5):469–80.
15. Ehrmann DA, Liljenquist DR, Kasza K, et al. Prevalence and predictors of the metabolic syndrome in women with polycystic ovary syndrome. J Clin Endocrinol Metab 2006; 91(1):48–53.
16. Dokras A, Bochner M, Hollinrake E, et al. Screening women with polycystic ovary syndrome for metabolic syndrome. Obstet Gynecol 2005; 106(1):131–7.
17. Glueck CJ, Papanna R, Wang P, et al. Incidence and treatment of metabolic syndrome in newly referred women with confirmed polycystic ovarian syndrome. Metabolism 2003; 52(7):908–15.
18. Apridonidze T, Essah PA, Iuorno MJ, et al. Prevalence and characteristics of the metabolic syndrome in women with polycystic ovary syndrome. J Clin Endocrinol Metab 2005; 90(4):1929–35.
19. Bloomgarden ZT. Definitions of the insulin resistance syndrome: the 1st World Congress on the Insulin Resistance Syndrome. Diabetes Care 2004; 27(3):824–30.
20. Vural B, Caliskan E, Turkoz E, et al. Evaluation of metabolic syndrome frequency and premature carotid atherosclerosis in young women with polycystic ovary syndrome. Hum Reprod 2005; 20(9):2409–13.
21. Azziz R. How prevalent is metabolic syndrome in women with polycystic ovary syndrome? Nat Clin Pract Endocrinol Metab 2006; 2(3):132–3.
22. Revised 2003 consensus on diagnostic criteria and long-term health risks related to polycystic ovary syndrome (PCOS). Hum Reprod 2004; 19(1):41–7.
23. Revised 2003 consensus on diagnostic criteria and long-term health risks related to polycystic ovary syndrome. Fertil Steril 2004; 81(1):19–25.
24. Zawadzki J, Dunaif A. Diagnostic criteria for polycystic ovary syndrome: towards a rational approach. In: Dunaif A GJ, Haseltine FP, Merriam GR, ed. Polycystic ovary syndrome. Boston: Blackwell Scientific, 1992; 377–84.
25. Dewailly D, Catteau-Jonard S, Reyss AC, et al. Oligo-anovulation with Polycystic Ovaries (PCO) but not overt hyperandrogenism. J Clin Endocrinol Metab 2006; 91(10):3922–7.
26. Broekmans FJ, Knauff EA, Valkenburg O, et al. PCOS according to the Rotterdam consensus criteria: change in prevalence among WHO-II anovulation and association with metabolic factors. Bjog 2006; 113(10):1210–7.
27. Welt CK, Gudmundsson JA, Arason G, et al. Characterizing Discrete Subsets of Polycystic Ovary Syndrome as Defined by the Rotterdam Criteria: The Impact of Weight on Phenotype and Metabolic Features. J Clin Endocrinol Metab 2006; 91(12): 4842–8.
28. Barber TM, Wass JA, McCarthy MI, et al. Metabolic characteristics of women with polycystic ovaries and oligo-amenorrhoea but normal androgen levels: implications for the management of polycystic ovary syndrome. Clin Endocrinol (Oxf) 2007; 66(4):513–7.
29. Robinson S, Kiddy D, Gelding SV, et al. The relationship of insulin insensitivity to menstrual pattern in women with hyperandrogenism and polycystic ovaries. Clin Endocrinol (Oxf) 1993; 39(3):351–5.
30. Franks S, Gharani N, Waterworth D, et al. The genetic basis of polycystic ovary syndrome. Hum Reprod 1997; 12(12): 2641–8.
31. Sam S, Legro RS, Bentley-Lewis R, et al. Dyslipidemia and metabolic syndrome in the sisters of women with polycystic ovary syndrome. J Clin Endocrinol Metab 2005; 90(8):4797–802.
32. Sam S, Legro RS, Essah PA, et al. Evidence for metabolic and reproductive phenotypes in mothers of women with polycystic ovary syndrome. Proc Natl Acad Sci USA 2006; 103(18):7030–5.

33. Reaven GM. The metabolic syndrome: requiescat in pace. Clin Chem 2005; 51(6):931–8.
34. Dunaif A, Segal KR, Futterweit W, et al. Profound peripheral insulin resistance, independent of obesity, in polycystic ovary syndrome. Diabetes 1989; 38(9):1165–74.
35. Dunaif A. Insulin resistance and the polycystic ovary syndrome: mechanism and implications for pathogenesis. Endocr Rev 1997; 18(6):774–800.
36. Venkatesan AM, Dunaif A, Corbould A. Insulin resistance in polycystic ovary syndrome: progress and paradoxes. Recent Prog Horm Res 2001; 56:295–308.
37. Barber TM, Golding SJ, Alvey C, et al. Global adiposity rather than abnormal regional fat distribution characterises women with polycystic ovary syndrome. J Clin Endocrinol Metab 2008; 93(3):999–1004.
38. Pasquali R, Antenucci D, Casimirri F, et al. Clinical and hormonal characteristics of obese amenorrheic hyperandrogenic women before and after weight loss. J Clin Endocrinol Metab 1989; 68(1):173–9.
39. Azziz R, Ehrmann D, Legro RS, et al. Troglitazone improves ovulation and hirsutism in the polycystic ovary syndrome: a multicenter, double blind, placebo-controlled trial. J Clin Endocrinol Metab 2001; 86(4):1626–32.
40. Nestler JE, Strauss JF 3rd. Insulin as an effector of human ovarian and adrenal steroid metabolism. Endocrinol Metab Clin North Am 1991; 20(4):807–23.
41. Franks S, Mason H, White, D, et al. Mechanisms of anovulation in polycystic ovary syndrome. Amsterdam: Elsevier, 1996.
42. White D, Leigh A, Wilson C, et al. Gonadotrophin and gonadal steroid response to a single dose of a long-acting agonist of gonadotrophin-releasing hormone in ovulatory and anovulatory women with polycystic ovary syndrome. Clin Endocrinol (Oxf) 1995; 42(5):475–81.
43. Morin-Papunen LC, Vauhkonen I, Koivunen RM, et al. Insulin sensitivity, insulin secretion, and metabolic and hormonal parameters in healthy women and women with polycystic ovarian syndrome. Hum Reprod 2000; 15(6):1266–74.
44. Adashi EY, Hsueh AJ, Yen SS. Insulin enhancement of luteinizing hormone and follicle-stimulating hormone release by cultured pituitary cells. Endocrinology 1981; 108(4):1441–9.
45. Nestler JE, Powers LP, Matt DW, et al. A direct effect of hyperinsulinemia on serum sex hormone-binding globulin levels in obese women with the polycystic ovary syndrome. J Clin Endocrinol Metab 1991; 72(1):83–9.
46. Yki-Jarvinen H, Makimattila S, Utriainen T, et al. Portal insulin concentrations rather than insulin sensitivity regulate serum sex hormone-binding globulin and insulin-like growth factor binding protein 1 in vivo. J Clin Endocrinol Metab 1995; 80(11):3227–32.
47. Willis DS, Watson H, Mason HD, et al. Premature response to luteinizing hormone of granulosa cells from anovulatory women with polycystic ovary syndrome: relevance to mechanism of anovulation. J Clin Endocrinol Metab 1998; 83(11): 3984–91.
48. Cusi K, Maezono K, Osman A, et al. Insulin resistance differentially affects the PI 3-kinase- and MAP kinase-mediated signaling in human muscle. J Clin Invest 2000; 105(3):311–20.
49. Rice S, Christoforidis N, Gadd C, et al. Impaired insulin-dependent glucose metabolism in granulosa-lutein cells from anovulatory women with polycystic ovaries. Hum Reprod 2005; 20(2):373–81.
50. Holte J, Bergh T, Berne C, et al. Enhanced early insulin response to glucose in relation to insulin resistance in women with polycystic ovary syndrome and normal glucose tolerance. J Clin Endocrinol Metab 1994; 78(5):1052–8.
51. Goodarzi MO, Erickson S, Port SC, et al. beta-Cell function: a key pathological determinant in polycystic ovary syndrome. J Clin Endocrinol Metab 2005; 90(1):310–5.
52. Elbers JM, Asscheman H, Seidell JC, et al. Long-term testosterone administration increases visceral fat in female to male transsexuals. J Clin Endocrinol Metab 1997; 82(7):2044–7.
53. Lovejoy JC, Bray GA, Bourgeois MO, et al. Exogenous androgens influence body composition and regional body fat distribution in obese postmenopausal women – a clinical research center study. J Clin Endocrinol Metab 1996; 81(6):2198–203.
54. Abbott DH, Dumesic DA, Franks S. Developmental origin of polycystic ovary syndrome - a hypothesis. J Endocrinol 2002; 174(1):1–5.
55. Kirchengast S, Huber J. Body composition characteristics and body fat distribution in lean women with polycystic ovary syndrome. Hum Reprod 2001; 16(6):1255–60.
56. Horejsi R, Moller R, Rackl S, et al. Android subcutaneous adipose tissue topography in lean and obese women suffering from PCOS: comparison with type 2 diabetic women. Am J Phys Anthropol 2004; 124(3):275–81.
57. Owen KR, McCarthy MI. Genetics of type 2 diabetes. Curr Opin Genet Dev 2007; 17(3):239–44.
58. Grant SF, Thorleifsson G, Reynisdottir I, et al. Variant of transcription factor 7-like 2 (TCF7L2) gene confers risk of type 2 diabetes. Nat Genet 2006; 38(3):320–3.
59. Zeggini E, McCarthy MI. TCF7L2: the biggest story in diabetes genetics since HLA? Diabetologia 2007; 50(1):1–4.
60. Groves CJ, Zeggini E, Minton J, et al. Association analysis of 6,736 U.K. subjects provides replication and confirms TCF7L2 as a type 2 diabetes susceptibility gene with a substantial effect on individual risk. Diabetes 2006; 55(9):2640–4.
61. Florez J, Burtt N, de Bakker P, et al. Haplotype structure and genotype-phenotype correlations of the sulfonylurea receptor and the islet ATP-sensitive potassium channel gene region. Diabetes 2004; 53(5):1360–8.
62. Freathy RM, Weedon MN, Bennett A, et al. Type 2 diabetes TCF7L2 risk genotypes alter birth weight: a study of 24,053 individuals. Am J Hum Genet 2007; 80(6):1150–61.

63. Barber TM, Bennett AJ, Groves CJ, et al. Disparate genetic influences on polycystic ovary syndrome (PCOS) and type 2 diabetes revealed by a lack of association between common variants within the TCF7L2 gene and PCOS. Diabetologia 2007; 50(11):2318–22.
64. Barber TM, Bennett AJ, Gloyn AL, et al. Relationship between E23K (an established type II diabetes-susceptibility variant within KCNJ11), polycystic ovary syndrome and androgen levels. Eur J Hum Genet 2007; 15(6):679–84.
65. Salley KE, Wickham EP, Cheang KI, et al. Glucose intolerance in polycystic ovary syndrome – a position statement of the Androgen Excess Society. J Clin Endocrinol Metab 2007; 92(12):4546–56.

Chapter 10
The Risks of Cardiovascular Disease and Diabetes in the Polycystic Ovary Syndrome

Susmeeta T. Sharma and John E. Nestler

10.1 Overview

Polycystic ovary syndrome (PCOS) is the most common cause of female infertility due to anovulation in developed countries, affecting about 5–10% of women of reproductive age [1, 2]. It is characterized by the presence of two or more of the following features: chronic oligo- or anovulation, androgen excess (either biochemically or clinically as hirsutism, acne, or male pattern alopecia), and polycystic ovarian morphology visualized on ultrasonography [3]. Although the syndrome was described more than half a century ago, much remains unknown regarding the pathophysiology of PCOS. However, recent studies have helped us to better understand the disorder and formulate more effective strategies for long-term management.

Until recently, our main concern in women with PCOS was infertility, menstrual irregularity, hirsutism, and prevention of endometrial cancer. However, we now know that insulin resistance plays an integral role in the pathophysiology of PCOS, and that women with PCOS are at a higher risk for developing type 2 diabetes and heart disease than the general population. Oral contraceptives, the traditional therapy for PCOS, have been shown in clinical trials to increase the incidence of arterial cardiovascular events, and there is some data that they may actually induce glucose intolerance in women with PCOS. In light of the above findings, although treatment of infertility and hirsutism remain important concerns both for patients and physicians, they can no longer be the sole focus, and the goals of treatment in PCOS need to be reevaluated.

PCOS, therefore, is no longer simply a reproductive disorder, but is a metabolic disorder that places affected young women at significantly higher risk of developing diabetes and heart disease. The aim of this chapter is to review the current data regarding the risks of diabetes and cardiovascular disease in women with PCOS, and to increase awareness among patients and physicians for a comprehensive evaluation and treatment of metabolic derangements in this high-risk population.

10.2 Insulin Resistance and PCOS

The association between bilateral polycystic ovaries and the clinical features of amenorrhea, hirsutism, and obesity was first recognized by Stein and Leventhal between the years 1925 and 1935. Eventually these features were grouped together under the diagnosis of *Stein–Leventhal syndrome* [4, 5]. Over the ensuing decades, multiple biochemical and clinical features have been added to form what is now known as the *polycystic ovary syndrome* or *PCOS*.

Recent evidence has shown that insulin resistance and compensatory hyperinsulinemia play a central role in the pathogenesis of the syndrome [6–12]. About 40% of PCOS women are not overweight, and studies are increasingly showing that even lean PCOS women have a form of insulin resistance that is poorly understood and

---

J.E. Nestler (✉)
Division of Endocrinology and Metabolism, Virginia Commonwealth University, Richmond, VA 23298-0111, USA
e-mail: nestler@hsc.vcu.edu

N.R. Farid, E. Diamanti-Kandarakis (eds.), *Diagnosis and Management of Polycystic Ovary Syndrome*,
DOI 10.1007/978-0-387-09718-3_10,

is intrinsic to the syndrome [6–8]. One such study conducted by Dunaif et al. in 1989 evaluated insulin sensitivity using the hyperinsulinemic-euglycemic clamp technique in lean and obese women with and without PCOS. They found that women with PCOS were more insulin resistant than their normal counterparts independent of obesity, and that the insulin resistance of obese women with PCOS was comparable to that of type 2 diabetic patients [6].

Insulin resistance or a subnormal response to a given concentration of endogenous insulin has been linked with an increased risk of several disorders and abnormalities, including diabetes mellitus type 2, hypertension, dyslipidemia, elevated plasminogen activator inhibitor type I (PAI-I), elevated endothelin-1, endothelial dysfunction, and cardiovascular disease. This constellation of aberrations associated with insulin resistance has been termed Syndrome X, insulin resistance syndrome (IRS), or dysmetabolic syndrome [13–14]. Recently, this syndrome has been recognized as a major cardiac risk factor and has been assigned a separate ICD-9 code (277.7) by the National Cholesterol Education Project's Adult Treatment Panel III [15]. In light of the association of insulin resistance with PCOS, the syndrome is no longer regarded as simply a fertility or cosmetic problem, but it is considered a part of the dysmetabolic syndrome in women. This is evidenced by the fact that the prevalence of the metabolic syndrome (MBS) is two to three times higher among women with PCOS compared to age- and BMI-matched controls, and about 20% of women with PCOS who are younger than 20 years have metabolic syndrome [16]. Given that approximately 5–6 million women of reproductive age in the United States may have PCOS, it is probably one of the most prevalent general health problems of young women.

10.3 Risk for Impaired Glucose Tolerance and Type 2 Diabetes Mellitus in PCOS

Insulin resistance is a recognized risk factor for type 2 diabetes and is probably the earliest detectable abnormality in individuals who progress to diabetes. Prospective clinical studies conducted in the United States have demonstrated a 31–35% prevalence of impaired glucose tolerance (IGT) and a 7.5–10.0% prevalence of type 2 diabetes mellitus in women with PCOS [17–18]. This is an extremely high prevalence rate compared with the 1.6% prevalence of IGT and 2.2% prevalence of type 2 diabetes in age-matched women in the United States, using data from the Third National Health and Nutrition Survey [19]. These metabolic abnormalities are not restricted to the United States. High prevalence of impaired glucose tolerance has also been documented in studies conducted in Indian, Chinese, and Thai women with PCOS [20–22]. Studies have also shown that the rate of conversion from impaired glucose tolerance to frank diabetes mellitus is increased by 5- to 10-fold in women with PCOS [17, 23]. This was recently corroborated in a controlled study conducted by Legro and colleagues, who assessed changes in glucose tolerance over an average follow-up period of 3 years in 71 women with PCOS and 23 control women with normal glucose tolerance (NGT) at baseline. The annual conversion rate from NGT to IGT was 16% in women with PCOS, and the annual conversion rate from IGT to type 2 diabetes was 2% [24].

Polycystic ovary syndrome has also been associated with an increased risk for developing gestational diabetes. In a recent meta-analysis, PCOS women were found to be 2.94 times (confidence interval for odds ratio: 1.70–5.08) more likely to develop gestational diabetes than control women [25]. These findings were confirmed by a large database study using data from the Northern California Kaiser Permanente program [26]. Studies have also looked at this from the opposite vantage point and have found that polycystic ovarian morphology is a frequent finding among women with a history of gestational diabetes [27]

Women with oligomenorrhea, defined as eight or fewer menstrual cycles per year, have been associated with an 80% chance of having PCOS; thus oligomenorrhea is a good surrogate marker of PCOS. Oligomenorrhea has also been shown to predict a 2- to 2.5-fold increase in risk for type 2 diabetes mellitus. The Nurses' Health Study, where 101,073 women in the age group of 25–42 years were followed over an eight-year period, demonstrated that the rate of conversion to type 2 diabetes was approximately 2-fold greater in women with a history of oligomenorrhea compared with women who had regular menses [28]. This risk was independent of obesity, indicating that oligomenorrhea was an independent predictor of type 2 diabetes. Although a physician-based diagnosis of PCOS was not made in the study, since most of the women with oligomenorrhea would be expected to have PCOS, this data indirectly suggests that PCOS is a strong risk factor for diabetes.

The association of PCOS and diabetes has been further substantiated by studies looking at this from the opposite perspective; i.e., is there a higher prevalence of PCOS among premenopausal women with type 2 diabetes? A retrospective study at an academic diabetes clinic in Virginia revealed that 27% of premenopausal women with type 2 diabetes had PCOS [29]. Another study conducted in a diabetes clinic in the United Kingdom reported an 82% prevalence of anatomically polycystic ovaries on transvaginal ultrasonography in premenopausal women with type 2 diabetes [30].

Collectively, the above findings indicate that women with PCOS constitute one of the groups at highest risk for the development of diabetes, and that PCOS is almost a prediabetic condition. The Diabetes Prevention Program study has shown that early identification of impaired glucose tolerance and intervention in the form of lifestyle modification and/or pharmacological agents can retard or prevent the progression to frank diabetes mellitus [31]. In view of these findings, the American Association of Clinical Endocrinologists, American College of Endocrinology, and the Androgen Excess Society have all recommended screening for diabetes, preferably with an oral glucose tolerance test, by the age of 30 years in all patients with PCOS [32–33].

10.4 Risk for Cardiovascular Disease in PCOS

Women with PCOS have an increased prevalence of several cardiovascular risk factors including hypertension [34–35] and dyslipidemia [36–39]. PCOS has also been associated with an increase in subclinical atherosclerotic disease and endothelial dysfunction [40–46]. These findings point toward an increased risk for early-onset cardiovascular disease in this population. In view of the high prevalence of PCOS in the female population, the syndrome may potentially account for a significant proportion of atherosclerotic heart disease diagnosed in women.

Probably the most common metabolic abnormality seen in women with PCOS is dyslipidemia with a 70% prevalence of an abnormal LDL level by National Cholesterol Education Program guidelines [47]. Low HDL cholesterol and high triglyceride levels are frequently found in both obese and lean women with PCOS [48–49, 16]. Small, dense LDL particles have been linked with a 3- to 7-fold increased relative risk of CAD [50]. Many studies have demonstrated a high prevalence of these atherogenic LDL particles in women with PCOS in comparison with those in control subjects [51]. Studies have also shown that with increasing age, women with PCOS have a higher incidence of hypertension than age-matched control subjects, and this increased blood pressure persisted even after adjustment for BMI, insulin sensitivity, and body fat distribution [52, 53]. Given the young age of this population, these findings of early and prolonged exposure to dyslipidemia and hypertension confer significant cardiovascular risk.

Several studies have revealed the presence of impaired endothelial function in PCOS secondary to altered insulin regulation of endothelial nitric oxide synthesis, which in turn leads to impaired nitric oxide dependent vasodilatation [43–45]. Women with PCOS have also been found to have increased levels of newly recognized surrogate markers for early atherosclerosis, including increased PAI-1 [40], endothelin-1 [41], C-reactive protein concentrations [42], and asymmetrical dimethylarginine [54].

Current data show that two major anatomic markers for subclinical cardiovascular disease in PCOS are coronary calcifications, identified by electron beam tomography, and carotid intima-media thickness, determined by ultrasonography. A Mayo Clinic study by Christian and colleagues revealed a 3-fold higher level of coronary artery calcification in nondiabetic women with PCOS than in population control subjects [55]. Obese women with PCOS, compared with BMI-matched control subjects, had a 2-fold increase in coronary artery calcification. These findings of increased prevalence of coronary artery and aortic calcifications in PCOS have been confirmed by several other studies [56, 57]. Carotid intima-media thickening, another surrogate marker for early atherogenic process, has also been found to be increased in women with PCOS compared with age-matched normal women [58]. Metabolic syndrome, a known risk factor for cardiovascular disease, is also more prevalent in women with PCOS, as noted earlier [16]. All these findings place women with PCOS at a significantly increased risk for adverse cardiovascular outcomes and mortality.

Multiple studies have reported an increased prevalence of coronary artery disease in PCOS or in women with the finding of polycystic ovarian morphology on ultrasound [59–61]. Birdsall et al. studied 143 women 60 years of age or younger who underwent coronary angiography for chest pain or valvular disease. Forty-two percent of these women were noted to have polycystic ovaries on pelvic ultrasonography – double the frequency in general population [59]. In another study, Dahlgren et al., via a risk factor model, found that compared with age-matched referents, women with PCOS had an increased risk (relative risk of 7.4) for developing myocardial infarction [61].

In contrast, a study conducted in the United Kingdom that reviewed death certificates of 786 women who were diagnosed with PCOS at an average age of 26.4 years and followed for an average duration of 30 years failed to show a statistically significant increase in cardiovascular mortality compared to expected numbers from actuarial tables [62]. Although not statistically significant, the ratio of observed to expected deaths from ischemic heart disease did increase by 1.4-fold. It is also important to note that the study had some drawbacks including the young age of women at follow-up and the limited number of subjects, decreasing the predictive power of the study.

Although outcome data specifically for women with PCOS are lacking, there is strong indirect evidence from the Nurses' Health Study looking at women with oligomenorrhea. In this study, 82,439 women were followed for 14 years. Women with highly irregular menses were found to have significantly increased relative risks of 1.5 for coronary heart disease and 1.9 for fatal myocardial infarction compared with eumenorrhic women [63]. As stated earlier, oligomenorrhic women are thought to have an 80% chance of having PCOS, and thus this study provides indirect confirmation of increased adverse cardiovascular outcomes in women with PCOS.

Most recently, cardiovascular outcomes data specifically for women with PCOS have been reported. Results from the NHLBI-sponsored Women's Ischemia Syndrome Evaluation (WISE) study revealed that post-menopausal women with clinical features of PCOS, defined by a premenopausal history of irregular menses and current biochemical evidence of hyperandrogenemia, had a higher prevalence of angiographically demonstrated coronary artery disease and a 2-fold higher incidence of cardiac events than women without PCOS [64].

Overall, current evidence supports a strong recommendation that women with PCOS should undergo comprehensive evaluation for recognized cardiovascular risk factors and receive appropriate treatment as indicated [65–66].

10.5 Clinical Significance of Insulin Resistance in PCOS

The close association of PCOS with insulin resistance, coupled with the increased risk for developing type 2 diabetes and cardiovascular disease, has established PCOS as a general health problem in women. Therefore, diagnosis and management of the co-morbidities of dysmetabolic syndrome are an essential part of the broad treatment plan in women with PCOS.

Therefore, physicians should include assessments of blood pressure, glucose tolerance (via an oral glucose tolerance test), lipids, and possibly other reversible cardiovascular risk factors such as homocysteine when evaluating women with PCOS. Detailed history taking, specifically regarding family history of diabetes, advanced age, increased BMI, and history of gestational diabetes, is particularly important as studies have shown that these are associated with an increased risk for development of type 2 diabetes and cardiovascular disease in PCOS women [18, 67–68].

Both the World Health Organization (WHO) and the American Diabetes Association (ADA) recommend using fasting plasma glucose as the initial screening test for diabetes given its convenience, low cost, and reproducibility. However, several studies have shown that the 2-hour oral glucose tolerance test (OGTT) is a more sensitive measure for the diagnosis of diabetes in women with PCOS, as many of these women have normal fasting serum glucose levels despite the presence of impaired glucose tolerance or type 2 diabetes on the OGTT [69–71]. Therefore, measurement of fasting serum glucose is not an effective tool to rule out impaired glucose tolerance and diabetes in women with PCOS. Given this fact and the high risk for diabetes in PCOS, the Androgen Excess Society recently issued a recommendation that an oral glucose tolerance test should be performed in all women with PCOS [33], regardless of weight, at the initial visit and every two years thereafter. It is important to take a detailed dietary history prior to the test, especially in this era of extreme diets, as low carbohydrate intake can result in a false positive test result [72–73].

10.5.1 Oral Contraceptives for Chronic Treatment of PCOS

In the past, oral contraceptives (OCs) have been the mainstay of treatment in PCOS. However, several studies suggest that, specifically in women with PCOS, OCs may aggravate insulin resistance and decrease glucose tolerance, and, in the female population-at-large, enhances cardiovascular risk [74–79]. A recent meta-analysis of all the relevant studies estimating the risk of cardiac or vascular arterial events associated with the current use of low dose, combined OCs in the population-at-large described a 1.85- fold increased risk for myocardial infarction and a 2.12- fold increased risk for ischemic stroke [80]. As the risk of cardiovascular outcomes is minimal in healthy women, this doubled risk with the current use of OCs continues to be minimal and is outweighed by the benefits of contraception. Moreover, OCs are used only for limited periods of time in the general population. However, in contrast to the population at large, women with PCOS at baseline are at higher risk for adverse cardiovascular outcomes and tend to be exposed to oral contraceptives for prolonged periods. These factors specific to PCOS may increase the risk for adverse vascular outcomes in this population and thus use of oral contraceptives as first-line agents in women with PCOS not desiring contraception may warrant reconsideration.

10.5.2 Insulin-Sensitizing Drugs for Chronic Treatment of PCOS

In contrast to the traditional treatment is the recent innovative use of insulin-sensitizing drugs for chronic treatment of PCOS. These drugs have been shown to improve insulin sensitivity in nondiabetic women with PCOS and to convert impaired glucose tolerance to normal glucose tolerance. Studies have also reported beneficial effects of these agents on multiple cardiovascular risk factors in PCOS, including a decrease in serum triglycerides, decrease in PAI-1 concentrations, decrease in asymmetrical dimethylarginine (ADMA) levels [54], and decrease in blood pressure [81, 82]. Studies from the diabetes literature, such as the United Kingdom Prospective Diabetes Study (UKPDS) study [83], present indirect evidence that insulin-sensitizing drugs may decrease the risk of cardiovascular events in insulin-resistant individuals.

Specific prospective randomized controlled trials addressing the prevention and treatment of IGT and diabetes in women with PCOS are lacking. However, various outcome studies in different ethnic populations have shown that interventions to improve insulin sensitivity can prevent or delay the development of diabetes in high-risk individuals at large [31, 84, 85]. A study conducted in Finland reported that improved insulin sensitivity, achieved through a combination of diet and exercise, reduced progression to type 2 diabetes by 58% over 4 years in obese men with impaired glucose tolerance [84]. More recently, the Diabetes Prevention Program Research Group conducted a study where they followed 3,234 nondiabetic high-risk individuals for an average period of 2.8 years. The study revealed that lifestyle interventions reduced the incidence of diabetes by 58%, and treatment with metformin led to a risk reduction of 31% [31]. These findings strongly suggest that improving insulin sensitivity, with lifestyle modifications or insulin-sensitizing drugs, reduces the risk for developing diabetes. Given that women with PCOS are at markedly increased risk for type 2 diabetes, it appears reasonable to presume that the demonstrated efficacy of lifestyle interventions and insulin-sensitizing drugs in individuals with impaired glucose tolerance or a history of gestational diabetes can be extrapolated to women with PCOS as well.

10.6 Insulin-Sensitizing Drugs

Lifestyle interventions, including diet and exercise to reduce weight, are the recommended first-line therapy for all obese women with PCOS. However, this may be difficult to achieve and maintain and is not an option for about 10–40% of women with PCOS who are lean. For these reasons, while not approved by the Federal Drug Administration (FDA) for the treatment of PCOS, insulin-sensitizing drugs have come to play an important role in the chronic therapy of PCOS. Prior to further discussion, we must first emphasize that whenever insulin-sensitizing drugs are used for the long-term treatment of PCOS, it is important to confirm and document the presence of regular ovulation every 2–3 months in order to obviate the risk for endometrial hyperplasia or cancer. There are two classes of commercially available insulin-sensitizing drugs: biguanides (metformin) and thiazolidinediones (mainly rosiglitazone and pioglitazone).

10.6.1 Metformin

Metformin is a biguanide first developed in 1957 and is probably the most widely prescribed oral agent for treatment of type 2 diabetes. Its primary mechanism of action is the reduction of hepatic gluconeogenesis, which is found to be pathologically increased in insulin resistant states, leading to fasting hyperinsulinemia [86]. It may also increase peripheral insulin sensitivity in other body tissues as supported by evidence that metformin lowers insulin requirements in type 1 diabetic patients [87, 88]. In addition, at least two studies suggest that metformin, when given to nondiabetic women with PCOS, specifically improves peripheral insulin sensitivity, as demonstrated by euglycemic insulin clamps [81, 82]. Because of its salutary effects in PCOS, metformin is now commonly used in the chronic treatment of PCOS [89].

The most common side effects of treatment with metformin, affecting about 10–25% of patients, are gastrointestinal (nausea and diarrhea) and can usually be minimized by starting at a low dose and gradually titrating up to the optimal dose. Malabsorption of vitamin B12 has also been reported in some patients on long-term therapy [90]. A more serious, though rare, adverse effect of metformin is lactic acidosis but this has been reported almost exclusively in high-risk populations due to renal insufficiency, liver disease, or congestive heart failure. Metformin is a category B drug and no teratogenic effects have been found in animal models.

In 1994, Velaquez et al. published the first study on the use of metformin to treat PCOS [91]. This was an uncontrolled study in which 26 obese women with PCOS were treated with metformin (1500 mg/day) for a total of 8 weeks. Metformin use significantly decreased serum insulin concentrations, lowered serum-free testosterone, and led to three spontaneous pregnancies among the 26 women treated. Subsequently, in 1996, Nestler et al. published a randomized, blinded, and placebo-controlled study using metformin (1500 mg/day) for 4–8 weeks in 24 obese women with PCOS [92]. They observed that in women treated with metformin (in the absence of any weight change), there was a decrease in circulating insulin levels, decreases in GnRH-stimulated LH release, and ovarian androgen production, a 44% decrease in serum-free testosterone levels, and a rise in serum sex-hormone binding globulin.

Ever since these initial studies, there has been mounting evidence with more than 20 placebo-controlled trials demonstrating the effect of metformin in improving ovulation and reducing insulin levels and androgen levels in women with PCOS [81, 82, 93–97]. Most of these studies have been in obese women with PCOS. However, there is some evidence for the beneficial effect of metformin in lean women with PCOS as well. In 1997, Nestler et al. reported that metformin decreased fasting and glucose-stimulated insulin levels, decreased free and total testosterone, decreased basal and GnRH-stimulated LH release, and increased SHBG specifically in lean and normal weight (BMI, 18–24 kg/m^2) women with PCOS [98]. These findings emphasize the key pathogenic role of insulin resistance in lean women with PCOS as well.

As discussed earlier, major randomized clinical trials including the Diabetes Prevention Program (DPP) and the Indian Diabetes Prevention Programme (IDDP-1) have shown that use of metformin decreases the relative risk for progression to type 2 diabetes (by 31% and 26% respectively) among patients with impaired glucose tolerance at baseline [31, 85]. It is controversial whether this was truly a decrease in progression to type 2 diabetes or simply masking of progression by decreasing the blood glucose levels. However, it should be noted that after discontinuation of metformin in the DPP study, diabetes developed in fewer subjects than would be expected if this had been solely a masking effect [99]. There has been no randomized controlled trial evaluating the effect of metformin on progression to type 2 diabetes specifically in women with PCOS. Recently however, an uncontrolled, retrospective study conducted at an academic center assessed 50 women with PCOS on metformin treatment for an average of 43 months and demonstrated that the annual conversion rate from normal glucose tolerance to impaired glucose tolerance was only 1.4% [100] compared to the 16–19% rate reported in previous studies for women not on any insulin-sensitizing therapy [24, 17]. Moreover, none of the women progressed to type 2 diabetes even though 11 of them (22%) had impaired glucose tolerance at baseline. Future prospective randomized controlled trials are needed to further establish the role of metformin in preventing progression to diabetes in this specific population.

Several studies conducted in insulin-resistant populations, including PCOS, impaired glucose tolerance, and diabetes, have reported a beneficial effect of metformin on the cardiovascular risk profile. These effects include a decrease in total cholesterol and serum triglycerides, decrease in serum PAI-1 concentrations, decrease in C-reactive protein levels and ADMA levels, and a decrease in blood pressure [54, 82, 91, 101]. The United Kingdom Prospective Diabetes Study (UKPDS) also reported a reduced incidence of myocardial infarction in obese type 2 diabetic patients who were initially treated with metformin monotherapy [83]. Although the effects of metformin on cardiovascular risk factors have been variable from study to study, no aggravation of cardiovascular risk factors has ever been reported. Therefore, in contrast to treatment of PCOS with OCs, metformin does not appear to be harmful from the cardiovascular risk perspective, and may actually be beneficial.

Some studies have found no beneficial effect of metformin in PCOS [102–104]. Of these, one study suggested that metformin did not offer additional benefit over weight loss alone in obese women with PCOS [102]. Another study used low, probably subclinical, doses of metformin (total of 1000 mg/day) [104]. One study failed to show any effect of metformin in women with PCOS who were morbidly obese (BMI as high as 50 kg/m^2) which suggests that women with extreme obesity and overwhelming insulin resistance might not respond to metformin therapy [103]. However, overall, there is overwhelming evidence in support of the use of metformin for long-term treatment in PCOS.

10.6.2 Thiazolidinediones

Thiazolidinediones (TZD) are a class of insulin-sensitizing drugs that enhance insulin-stimulated glucose uptake in adipose and muscle tissues. Their primary mechanism of action is via the activation of gamma-peroxisome proliferation activator receptors (PPAR-γ receptors). Binding of thiazolidinediones to these nuclear receptors induces gene transcription and activates genes that encode for insulin action. The first thiazolidinedione to become available in the United States was troglitazone. However, troglitazone was withdrawn by the FDA in 1999 due to numerous reports of fatal liver toxicity linked to the drug during the postmarketing phase [105]. Notably, the two thiazolidinediones (TZDs) currently available, rosiglitazone and pioglitazone, have not demonstrated similar hepatotoxicity.

Although no longer commercially available, reviewing the troglitazone literature lends insight into likely effects of this class of drug in PCOS. There are currently eight published trials that have assessed the effects of troglitazone in PCOS. All these studies reported that troglitazone decreases circulating insulin, decreases LH, reduces hyperandrogenemia, and increases the ovulation rate in women with PCOS, with variable effects on the lipid profile [106–110]. None of the trials attempted a direct comparison of metformin and troglitazone.

There is limited but growing data on use of rosiglitazone and pioglitazone in the treatment of PCOS. Multiple studies have now shown that both these medications are associated with an improvement in ovulation rates, menstrual cyclicity, insulin sensitivity, endothelial dysfunction, and androgen concentrations in PCOS women [111–118].

In 2004, Baillargeon et al. conducted a randomized, placebo-controlled trial in a group of 100 nonobese women with PCOS with no clinical or biochemical evidence of insulin resistance and studied the effects of metformin, rosiglitazone, and a combination of these drugs in these women [113]. They observed that treatment with either insulin-sensitizing drug led to an increase in the ovulation rate compared to placebo, which was significantly greater with metformin than rosiglitazone; combination therapy was not found to be more potent than metformin alone. There was a similar decrease in serum testosterone levels in all treatment groups. Measures of insulin sensitivity improved significantly after treatment with metformin and combination therapy, but not with rosiglitazone alone. These findings suggest that insulin-sensitizing drugs are useful in the treatment of nonobese women with PCOS even when they do not have any overt evidence of insulin resistance, with metformin having a greater beneficial effect than rosiglitazone.

However, it should be emphasized that this study was performed in a relatively rare subset of PCOS women (i.e., lean women with normal indices of insulin sensitivity). Since then, an increasing number of head-to-head trials of metformin versus a TZD in typical obese women with PCOS have been published. A study conducted recently in Mexico comparing the effects of pioglitazone and metformin in obese women with PCOS found that pioglitazone was as effective as metformin in improving insulin sensitivity and hyperandrogenism in this population [117]. However, pioglitazone was associated with a simultaneous increase in weight and BMI, while metformin was found to promote weight loss. In another study comparing metformin and rosiglitazone in 30 women with PCOS, metformin treatment led to a greater decrease in hyperandrogenemia while rosiglitazone treatment led to a more pronounced decrease in hyperinsulinemia [118].

Although there is increasing evidence of the beneficial effects of thiazolidinediones in women with PCOS, the majority of the reported studies are with metformin. Hence, the weight of scientific evidence is greatest for this drug. Moreover, metformin has been available worldwide for several decades, and its adverse effects and toxicities are well delineated. In addition, of all the commercially available insulin-sensitizing drugs, only metformin has a reassuring safety profile in pregnant women (Class B) [119] and is associated with facilitation of weight loss. Thiazolidinediones, on the other hand, have recently been associated with an increased risk of heart failure, bony fractures, and adverse cardiovascular outcomes [120], and it is also contraindicated in pregnancy (Class C). Therefore, metformin is currently the preferred insulin-sensitizing drug for chronic treatment of PCOS [121].

10.7 Areas of Future Research

Although recent advances afford us a better understanding of the pathophysiology of PCOS and help to form more effective strategies of management, several aspects of the disorder remain that need further investigation. OCs are now known to be associated with an increased incidence of adverse cardiovascular outcomes, and there is some evidence that they may aggravate insulin resistance and/or induce glucose intolerance specifically in women with PCOS. However, prospective, long-term studies are required to better define the effects of OCs on the metabolic and cardiovascular risk profile in this population. Prospective, randomized, controlled trials must also be conducted to assess whether treatment with insulin-sensitizing drugs prevents the development of diabetes and cardiovascular disease in women with PCOS. Head-to-head trials of various insulin-sensitizing drugs and studies looking at the combination of insulin-sensitizing drugs with OCs can further help us to form an optimal treatment strategy for PCOS. The adverse effects profile of thiazolidinediones requires further investigation and definition.

10.8 Recommendations

PCOS, a prevalent disorder in young women, has conventionally been regarded as an infertility or cosmetic problem. In the past, the aims of therapy in PCOS consisted mainly of ovulation induction, treatment of acne and hirsutism, and prevention of endometrial cancer. However, with the recognition of the prominent role of insulin resistance in the pathophysiology of the syndrome, PCOS is now considered a general health disorder associated with metabolic abnormalities, which lead to an increased risk for developing diabetes and cardiovascular disease. Moreover, oral contraceptives – the traditional therapy for PCOS – are now known to increase the risk for adverse cardiovascular outcomes and may aggravate insulin resistance and induce glucose intolerance. In light of these findings, infertility and signs of androgen excess can no longer be the sole considerations when choosing long-term pharmacological therapy for PCOS. The selection of drugs to treat PCOS needs to include consideration of the effects of the drugs on the development of diabetes and cardiovascular disease.

We recommend that when evaluating women with PCOS, physicians should consider the following:

(1) Early detection of the syndrome to reduce the incidence and severity of potential sequela associated with the disorder, keeping in mind that most women with oligomenorrhea will have PCOS.
(2) Screening for impaired glucose tolerance and diabetes with an oral glucose tolerance test, regardless of the woman's weight, and particularly in obese women with PCOS and those with a family history of type 2 diabetes.
(3) Comprehensive evaluation for recognized cardiovascular risk factors including dyslipidemia, hypertension and metabolic syndrome, and appropriate treatment as necessary.
(4) Assessment of cardiovascular risk factors and performance of an oral glucose tolerance test prior to and 3–4 months after initiation of OCs to monitor for possible detrimental effects of OCs on these parameters.
(5) Lifestyle modification with diet and exercise remain the first-line therapy for obese women with PCOS.
(6) While not approved by the FDA for this indication, consideration of insulin-sensitizing drugs as the initial therapy in women with PCOS, especially those who are overweight or are at a particularly high risk for developing diabetes. Metformin is the currently preferred insulin-sensitizing drug for chronic treatment of PCOS. When using metformin for long-term therapy, ovulation occurring every 2–3 months should be confirmed.

References

1. Knochenhauer ES, Key TJ, Kahsar-Miller M, et al. Prevalence of the polycystic ovary syndrome in unselected black and white women of the Southeastern United States: a prospective study. *J Clin Endocrinol Metab* 1998; 83(9):3078–3082.
2. Asuncion M, Calvo RM, San Millan JL, et al. A prospective study of the prevalence of the polycystic ovary syndrome in unselected Caucasian women from Spain. *J Clin Endocrinol Metab* 2000; 85(7):2434–2438.
3. The Rotterdam ESHRE/ASRM-Sponsored PCOS Consensus Workshop Group. Revised 2003 consensus on diagnostic criteria and long-term health risks related to polycystic ovary syndrome. *Hum Reprod* 2004; 19:41–7.
4. Stein IF, Leventhal ML. Amenorrhea associated with bilateral polycystic ovaries. *Am J Obstet Gynecol* 1935; 29:181–191.
5. Stein IF. Bilateral Polycystic ovaries: significance in fertility. *Am J Obstet Gynecol* 1945; 30:385–398.
6. Chang RJ, Nakamura RM, Judd HL, et al. Insulin resistance in nonobese patients with polycystic ovarian disease. *J Clin Endocrinol Metab* 1983; 57:356–359.
7. Dunaif A, Graf M, Mandeli J, et al. Characterization of groups of hyperandrogenemic women with acanthosis nigricans, impaired glucose tolerance, and/or hyperinsulinemia. *J Clin Endocrinol Metab* 1987; 65:499–507.
8. Dunaif A, Segal KR, Futterweit W, et al. Profound peripheral resistance, independent of obesity, in polycystic ovary syndrome. *Diabetes* 1989; 38:1165–1174.
9. Dunaif A, Segal KR, Shelley DR, et al. Evidence for distinctive and intrinsic defects in insulin action in polycystic ovary syndrome. *Diabetes* 1992; 41:1257–1266.
10. Ciaraldi TP, el Roeiy A, Madar Z, et al. Cellular mechanisms of insulin resistance in polycystic ovarian syndrome. *J Clin Endocrinol Metab* 1992; 75:577–583.
11. Dunaif A, Xia J, Book CB, et al. Excessive insulin receptor serine phosphorylation in cultured fibroblasts and in skeletal muscle: a potential mechanism for insulin resistance in the polycystic ovary syndrome. *J Clin Invest* 1995; 96:801–810.
12. Campbell PJ, Gerich JE. Impact of obesity on insulin action in volunteers with normal glucose tolerance: demonstration of a threshold for the adverse effect of obesity. *J Clin Endocrinol Metab* 1990; 70:1114–1118.
13. Reaven GM. Banting lecture 1988. Role of insulin resistance in human disease. *Diabetes* 1988; 37:1595–1607.
14. Reaven GM. Insulin resistance, hyperinsulinemia, hypertriglyceridemia, and hypertension. Parallels between human disease and rodent models. *Diabetes Care* 1991; 14:195–202.
15. Executive Summary of The Third Report of The National Cholesterol Education Program (NCEP) Expert Panel on Detection, Evaluation, And Treatment of High Blood Cholesterol In Adults (Adult Treatment Panel III). *JAMA* 2001; 285(19): 2486–2497.
16. Apridonidze T, Essah PA, Iuorno MJ, Nestler JE. Prevalence and characteristics of the metabolic syndrome in women with polycystic ovary syndrome. *J Clin Endocrinol Metab* 2005; 90(4):1929–1935.

17. Ehrmann DA, Barnes RB, Rosenfield RL, et al. Prevalence of impaired glucose tolerance and diabetes in women with polycystic ovary syndrome. *Diabetes Care* 1999; 22(1):141–146.
18. Legro RS, Kunselman AR, Dodson WC, Dunaif A. Prevalence and predictors of risk for type 2 diabetes mellitus and impaired glucose tolerance in polycystic ovary syndrome: a prospective, controlled study in 254 affected women. *J Clin Endocrinol Metab* 1999; 84(1):165–169.
19. Centers for Disease Control and Prevention (CDC). Prevalence of diabetes and impaired fasting glucose in adults- United States, 1999–2000. *MMWR Morb Mortal Wkly Rep* 2003; 52:833–37.
20. Norman RJ, Mahabeer S, Masters S. Ethnic differences in insulin and glucose response to glucose between White and Indian women with Polycystic Ovary Syndrome. *Fertil Steril* 1995; 63:58–62.
21. Chen X, Yang D, Li L et al. Abnormal glucose tolerance in Chinese women with polycystic ovary syndrome. *Hum Reprod* 2006; 21:2027–2032.
22. Weerakiet S, Srisombut C, Bunnag P et al. Prevalence of type 2 diabetes mellitus and impaired glucose tolerance in Asian women with polycystic ovary syndrome. *Int J Gynaecol Obstet* 2001; 75:177–84.
23. Norman RJ, Masters L, Milner CR, et al. Relative risk of conversion from normoglycemia to impaired glucose tolerance or non-insulin dependent diabetes mellitus in polycystic ovarian syndrome. *Hum Reprod* 2001; 16(9):1995–1998.
24. Legro RS, Gnatuk CL, Kunselman AR, Dunaif A. Changes in glucose tolerance over time in women with polycystic ovary syndrome: a controlled study. *J Clin Endocrinol Metab* 2005; 90(6):3236–3242.
25. Boomsma CM, Eijkemans MJ, Hughes EG, et al. A meta-analysis of pregnancy outcomes in women with polycystic ovary syndrome. *Hum Reprod Update* 2006; 12:673–83.
26. Lo JC, Feigenbaum SL, Escobar GJ, et al. Increased prevalence of gestational diabetes mellitus among women with diagnosed polycystic ovary syndrome: a population based study. *Diabetes Care* 2006; 29:1915–17.
27. Holte J, Gennarelli G, Wide L, et al. High prevalence of polycystic ovaries and associated clinical, endocrine, and metabolic features in women with previous gestational diabetes mellitus. *J Clin Endocrinol Metab* 1998; 83:1143–50.
28. Solomon CG, Hu FB, Dunaif A, et al. Long or highly irregular menstrual cycles as a marker for risk of type 2 diabetes mellitus. *JAMA* 2001; 286(19):2421–2426.
29. Peppard HR, Marfori J, Iuorno MJ, Nestler JE. Prevalence of polycystic ovary syndrome among premenopausal women with type 2 diabetes. *Diabetes Care* 2001; 24(6):1050–1052.
30. Conn JJ, Jacobs HS, Conway GS. The prevalence of polycystic ovaries in women with type 2 diabetes mellitus. *Clin Endocrinol (Oxf)* 2000; 52(1):81–86.
31. Knowler WC, Barrett-Conner E, Fowler SE, et al. (Diabetes Prevention Program Research Group). Reduction in incidence of type 2 diabetes with lifestyle intervention or metformin. *N Engl J Med* 2002; 346:393–403.
32. American Association of Clinical Endocrinologists Position Statement on Metabolic and Cardiovascular Consequences of Polycystic Ovary Syndrome. *Endocr Pract* 2005; 11(No. 2):125–134.
33. Salley KES, Wickham EP, Cheang KI, et al. Position Statement: Glucose intolerance in Polycystic Ovary Syndrome-a position statement of the Androgen Excess Society. *J Clin Endocrinol Metab* 2007; 92:4546–56.
34. Bjorntorp P. The android woman–a risky condition. *J Intern Med* 1996; 239:105–110.
35. Holte J, Gennarelli G, Wide L, et al. High prevalence of polycystic ovaries and associated clinical, endocrine, and metabolic features in women with previous gestational diabetes mellitus. *J Clin Endocrinol Metab* 1998; 83:1143–1150.
36. Talbott E, Guzick D, Clerici A, et al. Coronary heart disease risk factors in women with polycystic ovary syndrome. *Arterioscler Thromb Vasc Biol* 1995; 15:821–826.
37. Talbott E, Clerici A, Berga SL, et al. Adverse lipid and coronary heart disease risk profiles in young women with polycystic ovary syndrome: results of a case-control study. *J Clin Epidemiol (England)* 1998; 51:415–422.
38. Wild RA, Alaupovic P, Parker IJ. Lipid and apolipoprotein abnormalities in hirsute women: The association with insulin resistance. *Am J Obstet Gynecol* 1992; 166:1191–1196.
39. Wild RA. Obesity, lipids, cardiovascular risk, and androgen excess. *Am J Med* 1995; 98:27S–32S.
40. Ehrmann DA, Schneider DJ, Sobel BE, et al. Troglitazone improves defects in insulin action, insulin secretion, ovarian steroidogenesis, and fibrinolysis in women with polycystic ovary syndrome. *J Clin Endocrinol Metab* 1997; 82(7): 2108–2116.
41. Velaquez EM, Mendoza SG, Wang P, Glueck CJ. Metformin therapy is associated with a decrease in plasma plasminogen activator inhibitor-1, lipoprotein(a), and immunoreactive insulin levels in patients with the polycystic ovary syndrome. *Metabolism* 1997; 46(4):454–457.
42. Diamanti-Kandarakis E, Spina G, Kouli C, Migdalis I. Increased endothelin-1 levels in women with polycystic ovary syndrome and the beneficial effect of metformin therapy. *J Clin Endocrinol Metab* 2001; 86(10):4666–4673.
43. Kelly CC, Lyall H, Petrie JR, et al. Low grade chronic inflammation in women with polycystic ovary syndrome. *J Clin Endocrinol Metab* 2001; 86(6):2453–2455.
44. Paradisi G, Steinberg HO, Hempfling A, et al. Polycystic ovary syndrome is associated with endothelial dysfunction. *Circulation* 2001; 103(10):1410–1415.
45. Lakhani K, Constantinovici N, Purcell WM, et al. Internal carotid-artery response to 5% carbon dioxide in women with polycystic ovaries. *Lancet* 2000; 356(9236):1166–1167.
46. Kelly CJ, Speirs A, Gould GW, et al. Altered vascular function in young women with polycystic ovary syndrome. *J Clin Endocrinol Metab* 2002; 87(2):742–746.

47. Legro RS, Kunselman AR, Dunaif A. Prevalence and predictors of dyslipidemia in women with polycystic ovary syndrome. *Am J Med* 2001; 111:607–613.
48. Wild RA, Painter PC, Coulson PB, et al. Lipoprotein lipid concentration and cardiovascular risk in women with polycystic ovary syndrome. *J Clin Endocrinol Metab* 1985; 61:946–951.
49. Mather KJ, Kwan F, Corenblum B. Hyperinsulinemia in polycystic ovary syndrome correlates with increased cardiovascular risk independent of obesity. *Fertil Steril* 2000; 73:150–156.
50. Gardner CD, Fortmann SP, Krauss RM. Association of small low-density lipoprotein particles with the incidence of coronary artery disease in men and women. *JAMA* 1996; 276:875–881.
51. Dejager S, Pichard C, Giral P, et al. Smaller LDL particle size in women with polycystic ovary syndrome compared to controls. *Clin Endocrinol (Oxf)* 2001; 54:455–462.
52. Dahlgren E, Johansson S, Lindstedt G, et al. Women with polycystic ovary syndrome wedge resected in 1956 to 1965: a long-term follow-up focusing on natural history and circulating hormones. *Fertil Steril* 1992; 57:505–513.
53. Holte J, Gennarelli G, Berne C, et al. Elevated ambulatory day-time blood pressure in women with polycystic ovary syndrome: a sign of a pre-hypertensive state? *Hum Reprod* 1996; 11:23–28.
54. Heutling D, Schulz H, Nickel I, et al. Asymmetrical dimethylarginine, inflammatory and metabolic parameters in women with polycystic ovary syndrome before and after metformin treatment. *J Clin Endocrinol Metab* 2008; 93:82–90.
55. Christian RC, Dumesic DA, Behrenbeck T, et al. Prevalence and predictors of coronary artery calcification in women with polycystic ovary syndrome. *J Clin Endocrinol Metab* 2003; 88:2562–2568.
56. Talbott E, Zborowski JV, McHugh-Pemu K, et al. Metabolic cardiovascular syndrome and its relationship to coronary calcification in women with polycystic ovarian syndrome. Presented at: *3rd International Workshop on Insulin Resistance*, February 17–19, 2003, New Orleans, LA.
57. Talbott EO, Zborowski JV, Rager JR, et al. Evidence for an association between metabolic cardiovascular syndrome and coronary and aortic calcification among women with polycystic ovary syndrome. *J Clin Endocrinol Metab* 2004; 89: 5454–5461.
58. Talbott EO, Guzick DS, Sutton-Tyrrell K, et al. Evidence for association between polycystic ovary syndrome and premature carotid atherosclerosis in middle-aged women. *Arterioscler Thromb Vasc Biol* 2000; 20(11):2414–2421.
59. Birdsall MA, Farquhar CM, White HD. Association between polycystic ovaries and extent of coronary artery disease in women having cardiac catheterization. *Ann Intern Med* 1997; 126:32–35.
60. Elting MW, Korsen TJ, Bezemer PD, Schoemaker J. Prevalence of diabetes mellitus, hypertension and cardiac complaints in a follow-up study of a Dutch PCOS population. *Hum Reprod* 2001; 16:556–560.
61. Dahlgren E, Janson PO, Johansson S, et al. Polycystic ovary syndrome and risk for myocardial infarction: evaluated from a risk factor model based on a prospective population study of women. *Acta Obstet Gynecol Scand* 1992; 71:599–604.
62. Pierpoint T, McKeigue PM, Isaacs AJ, et al. Mortality of women with polycystic ovary syndrome at long-term follow-up. *J Clin Epidemiol* 1998; 51(7):581–586.
63. Solomon CG, Hu FB, Dunaif A, et al. Menstrual cycle irregularity and risk for future cardiovascular disease. *J Clin Endocrinol Metab* 2002; 87(5):2013–2017.
64. Shaw LJ, Bairey Merz CM, Azziz R, et al. Postmenopausal women with a history of irregular menses and elevated androgen measurements at high risk for worsening cardiovascular event-free survival: Results from the National Institutes of Health—National Heart, Lung, and Blood Institute sponsored Women's Ischemia Syndrome Evaluation. *J Clin Endocrinol Metab* 2008; 93(4):1276–84.
65. Legro RS. Polycystic ovary syndrome and cardiovascular disease: a premature association? *Endocr Rev* 2003; 24(3):302–312.
66. Nestler JE. Polycystic ovarian syndrome: metabolic and cardiovascular complications. In: Kreisberg RA, program director. Clinical Endocrinology Update 2003 Syllabus. Chevy Chase, MD: *The Endocrine Society Press*, 2003; 299–303.
67. Ehrmann DA, Kasza K, Azziz R, et al. Effects of race and family history of type 2 diabetes on metabolic status of women with polycystic ovary syndrome. *J Clin Endocrinol Metab* 2000; 90:66–71.
68. Trolle B, Lauszus FF. Risk factors for glucose intolerance in Danish women with polycystic ovary syndrome. *Acta Obstet Gynecol Scand* 2005; 84:1192–96.
69. Palmert MR, Gordon CM, Kartashov AI, et al. Screening for abnormal glucose tolerance in adolescents with polycystic ovary syndrome. *J Clin Endocrinol Metab* 2002; 87(3):1017–1023.
70. Gomez-Perez FJ, Aguilar-Salinas CA, Lopez-Alvarenga JC, et al. Lack of agreement between the World Health Organization Category of impaired glucose tolerance and the American Diabetes Association category of impaired fasting glucose. *Diabetes Care* 1998; 21(11):1886–1888.
71. de Vegt F, Dekker JM, Stehouwer CDA, et al. The 1997 American Diabetes Association criteria versus the 1985 World Health Organization criteria for the diagnosis of abnormal glucose tolerance: poor agreement in the Hoorn Study. *Diabetes Care* 1998; 21(10):1686–90.
72. Kaneko T, Wang PY, Tawata M, et al. A low carbohydrate intake before oral glucose-tolerance tests. Lancet 1998; 352:289.
73. Nestler JE, Sharma ST. Misleading effects of a low-carbohydrate diet on glucose tolerance testing in women with PCOS: a case report. Program of the 88th Annual Meeting of the Endocrine Society, Boston, MA, 2006, p. 857 (Abstract P3-844).
74. Korytkowski MT, Mokan M, Horwitz MJ, Berga SL. Metabolic effects of oral contraceptives in women with polycystic ovary syndrome. *J Clin Endocrinol Metab* 1995; 80:3327–3334.

75. Dahlgren E, Landin K, Krotkiewski M, et al. Effects of two anti-androgen treatments on hirsutism and insulin sensitivity in women with polycystic ovary syndrome. *Hum Reprod* 1998; 13:2706–2711.
76. Morin-Papunen LC, Vauhkonen I, Koivunen RM, et al. Endocrine and metabolic effects of metformin versus ethinyl estradiol-cyproterone acetate in obese women with polycystic ovary syndrome: a randomized study. *J Clin Endocrinol Metab* 2000; 85:3161–3168.
77. Elter K, Imir G, Durmusoglu F. Clinical, endocrine, and metabolic effects of metformin added to ethinyl estradiol-cyproterone acetate in non-obese women with polycystic ovarian syndrome: a randomized controlled study. *Hum Reprod* 2002; 17: 1729–1737.
78. Morin-Papunen L, Vauhkonen I, Koivunen R, et al. Metformin versus ethinyl estradiol-cyproterone acetate in the treatment of nonobese women with polycystic ovary syndrome: a randomized study. *J Clin Endocrinol Metab* 2003; 88(1):148–56.
79. Diamanti-Kandarakis E, Baillargeon JP, Iuorno MJ, et al. A modern medical quandary: polycystic ovary syndrome, insulin resistance, and oral contraceptive pills. *J Clin Endocrinol Metab* 2003; 88(5):1927–1932.
80. Baillargeon JP, McClish DK, Essah PA, Nestler JE. Association between the current use of low-dose oral contraceptives and cardiovascular arterial disease: a meta-analysis. *J Clin Endocrinol Metab* 2005 Jul; 90(7):3863–3870.
81. Diamanti-Kandarakis E, Kouli C, Tsianateli T, Bergiele A. Therapeutic effects of metformin on insulin resistance and hyperandrogenism in polycystic ovary syndrome. *Eur J Endocrinol* 1998; 138:269–274.
82. Moghetti P, Castello R, Negri C, et al. Metformin effects on clinical features, endocrine and metabolic profiles, and insulin sensitivity in polycystic ovary syndrome: a randomized, double-blind, placebo-controlled 6-month trial, followed by open, long-term clinical evaluation. *J Clin Endocrinol Metab* 2000 Jan; 85(1):139–146.
83. UK Prospective Diabetes Study (UKPDS) Group. Effect of intensive blood glucose control with metformin on complications in overweight patients with type 2 diabetes (UKPDS 34). *Lancet* 1998; 352(9131):854–865.
84. Tuomilehto J, Lindstrom J, Eriksson JG, et al. Finnish Diabetes Prevention Study Group. Prevention of type 2 diabetes mellitus by changes in lifestyle among subjects with impaired glucose tolerance. *N Engl J Med* 2001; 344(18):1343–1350.
85. Ramachandran A, Snehlatha C, Mary C, et al. The Indian Diabetes Prevention Programme shows that lifestyle modification and metformin prevent type 2 diabetes in Asian Indian subjects with impaired glucose tolerance (IDPP-1). *Diabetologia* 2006; 49:289–97.
86. Haechel R, Haechel H. Inhibition of gluconeogenesis from lactate by phenethylbiguanide in the perfused guinea pig liver. *Diabetologia* 1982; 7:117–124.
87. Gin H, Messerchnitt C, Brottier E. Metformin improves insulin resistance in type 1, insulin dependent, diabetic patients. *Metabolism* 1985; 34:923–925.
88. Pagano G, Tagliaferro V, Carta Q. Metformin reduces insulin requirement in type 1 diabetics. *Diabetologia* 1998; 24: 351–354.
89. Nestler JE. Metformin for the treatment of the Polycystic Ovary Syndrome. *N Eng J Med* 2008; 358:47–54.
90. Ting RZ, Szeto CC, Chan MH, et al. Risk factors of vitamin B12 deficiency in patients receiving metformin. *Arch Intern Med* 2006; 166:1975–9.
91. Velazquez EM, Mendoza S, Hamer T, et al. Metformin therapy in polycystic ovary syndrome reduces hyperinsulinemia, insulin resistance, hyperandrogenemia, and systolic blood pressure, while facilitating normal menses and pregnancy. *Metabolism*1994; 43(5):647–54.
92. Nestler JE, Jakubowicz DJ. Decreases in ovarian cytochrome P450c17α activity and serum free testosterone after reduction in insulin secretion in women with polycystic ovary syndrome. *N Eng J Med* 1996; 335:617–623.
93. De Leo V, la Marca A, Ditto A, et al. Effects of metformin on gonadotropin-induced ovulation in women with polycystic ovary syndrome. *Fertil Steril* 1999; 72(2):282–285.
94. Nestler JE, Jakubowicz DJ, Evans WS, Pasquali R. Effects of metformin on spontaneous and clomiphene-induced ovulation in the polycystic ovary syndrome. *N Engl J Med* 1998; 338(26):1876–80.
95. Chou KH, von Eye Corleta H, Capp E, Spritzer PM. Clinical, metabolic and endocrine parameters in response to metformin in obese women with polycystic ovary syndrome: a randomized, double-blind and placebo-controlled trial. *Horm Metab Res* 2003; 35(2):86–91.
96. Glueck CJ, Wang P, Fontaine R, et al. Metformin-induced resumption of normal menses in 39 of 43 (91%) previously amenorrheic women with the polycystic ovary syndrome. *Metabolism* 1999; 48(4):511–519.
97. Morin-Papunen L, Vauhkonen I, Koivunen R, et al. Metformin therapy improves the menstrual pattern with minimal endocrine and metabolic effects in women with polycystic ovary syndrome. *Fertil Steril* 1998; 69(4):691–696.
98. Nestler JE, Jakubowicz DJ. Lean women with polycystic ovary syndrome respond to insulin reduction with decreases in ovarian P450c17 activity and serum androgens. *J Clin Endocrinol Metab* 1997; 82:4075–4079.
99. *Idem.* Effects of withdrawal from metformin on the development of diabetes in the Diabetes Prevention Program. *Diabetes Care* 2003; 26:977–80.
100. Sharma ST, Wickham EP III, Nestler JE. Changes in glucose tolerance with metformin treatment in polycystic ovary syndrome: a retrospective analysis. *Endocr Pract* 2007; 88:4116–23.
101. Morin-Papunen L, Rautio K, Ruokonen A, et al. Metformin reduces C-reactive protein levels in women with polycystic ovary syndrome. *J Clin Endocrinol Metab* 2003; 88(10):4649–4654.
102. Crave JC, Fimbel S, Lejeune H et al. Effects of diet and metformin administration on sex hormone binding globulin, androgens, and insulin in hirsute and obese women. *J Clin Endocrinol Metab* 1995; 80:2057–2062.

103. Ehrmann DA, Cavaghan MK, Imperial J, et al. Effects of metformin on insulin secretion, insulin action, and ovarian steroidogenesis in women with polycystic ovary syndrome. *J Clin Endocrinol Metab* 1997; 82:524–530.
104. Unluhizarci K, Kelestimur F, Bayram F, et al. The effects of metformin on insulin resistance and ovarian steroidogenesis in women with polycystic ovary syndrome. *Clin Endocrinol (Oxf)* 1999; 51:231–236.
105. Misbin RI. Troglitazone-associated hepatic failure. *Ann Intern Med* 1999; 130(7 Pt 1):130.
106. Dunaif A, Scott D, Finegood D, et al. The insulin-sensitizing agent troglitazone improves metabolic and reproductive abnormalities in the polycystic ovary syndrome. *J Clin Endocrinol Metab* 1996; 81(9):3299–3306.
107. Hasegawa I, Murakawa H, Suzuki M, et al. Effect of troglitazone on endocrine and ovulatory performance in women with insulin resistance-related polycystic ovary syndrome. *Fertil Steril* 1999; 71(2):323–327.
108. Azziz R, Ehrmann D, Legro RS, et al. Troglitazone Study Group. Troglitazone improves ovulation and hirsutism in the polycystic ovary syndrome: a multicenter, double blind, placebo-controlled trial. *J Clin Endocrinol Metab* 2001; 86(4): 1626–1632.
109. Paradisi G, Steinberg HO, Shepard MK, et al. Troglitazone therapy improves endothelial function to near normal levels in women with polycystic ovary syndrome. *J Clin Endocrinol Metab* 2003; 88(2):576–580.
110. Legro RS, Azziz R, Ehrmann D, et al. Minimal response of circulating lipids in women with polycystic ovary syndrome to improvement in insulin sensitivity with troglitazone. *J Clin Endocrinol Metab* 2003; 88(11):5137–5144.
111. Zheng Z, Li M, Lin Y, Ma Y. Effect of rosiglitazone on insulin resistance and hyperandrogenism in polycystic ovary syndrome. *Zhonghua Fu Chan Ke Za Zhi* 2002; 37(5):271–273. Chinese.
112. Ghazeeri G, Kutten WH, Bryer-Ash M, et al. Effect of rosiglitazone on spontaneous and clomiphene citrate-induced ovulation in women with polycystic ovary syndrome. *Fertil Steril* 2003; 79(3):562–566.
113. Baillargeon JP, Jakubowicz DJ, Iuorno MJ et al. Effects of metformin and rosiglitazone, alone and in combination, in nonobese women with polycystic ovary syndrome and normal indices of insulin sensitivity. *Fertil Steril* 2004; 82(4): 893–902.
114. Tarkun I, Cetinarslan B, Tureman E, et al. Effect of rosiglitazone on insulin resistance, C-reactive protein and endothelial function in non-obese young women with polycystic ovary syndrome. *Eur J Endocrinol* 2005 Jul; 153(1):115–121.
115. Romualdi D, Guido M, Ciampelli M, et al. Selective effects of pioglitazone on insulin and androgen abnormalities in normo- and hyperinsulinaemic obese patients with polycystic ovary syndrome. *Hum Reprod* 2003; 18(6):1210–1218.
116. Brettenthaler N, De Gaytor C, Huber PR, Keller U. Effect of the insulin sensitizer pioglitazone on insulin resistance, hyperandrogenism, and ovulatory dysfunction in women with polycystic ovary syndrome. *J Clin Endocrinol Metab* 2004; 89(8):3835–3840.
117. Ortega-Gonzalez C, Luna S, Hernandez L, et al. Responses of serum androgen and insulin resistance to metformin and pioglitazone in obese, insulin-resistant women with polycystic ovary syndrome. *J Clin Endocrinol Metab* 2005 Mar; 90(3): 1360–1365.
118. Mitkov M, Pehlivanov B, Terzieva D. Metformin versus rosiglitazone in the treatment of polycystic ovary syndrome. *Eur J Obstet Gynecol Reprod Biol* 2006; 126(1):93–8.
119. Coetzee EJ, Jackson WPU. Metformin in management of pregnant insulin-dependent diabetics. *Diabetologia* 1979; 16: 241–245.
120. Nissen SE, Wolski K. Effect of rosiglitazone on the risk of myocardial infarction and death from cardiovascular causes. *N Eng J Med* 2007; 356:2457–71.
121. Sharma ST, Nestler JE. Prevention of diabetes and cardiovascular disease in women with PCOS: Treatment with insulin sensitizers. *Best Pract Res Clin Endocrinol Metab* 2006; 20(2):245–60.

Chapter 11
Pregnancy Complications in PCOS

Roy Homburg

A higher prevalence of several complications of pregnancy in women with polycystic ovary syndrome (PCOS), compared with healthy mothers with no PCOS, has been described. These include an increased prevalence of spontaneous miscarriage, gestational diabetes, pre-eclamptic toxaemia and pregnancy-induced hypertension (PIH) and the birth of small-for-gestational-age (SGA) babies.

11.1 PCOS and Miscarriage

There are three main questions regarding miscarriage in PCOS: Is there really an increased prevalence, if so, why, and what can we do in the way of possible preventative treatment?

11.2 Prevalence

Most probably, women with PCOS have an increased risk of spontaneous miscarriage. This has been difficult to establish due to several confounding factors. Treatment with ovulation-inducing agents is associated with a higher incidence of spontaneous miscarriage compared with the prevalence in the normally ovulating population, who conceive spontaneously, and the prevalence of spontaneous miscarriage for women with PCOS who conceive spontaneously is not known. In addition, obesity is often associated with PCOS, and obesity is widely reported to be an important factor associated with spontaneous miscarriage in its own right. Finally, data have been based on women attending fertility clinics who tend to receive closer scrutiny in the very early phase of a pregnancy and therefore, tend to have a higher quoted prevalence of miscarriage than those who conceive spontaneously.

The traditional first-line treatment for anovulatory PCOS is clomiphene citrate (CC) which has a quoted mean miscarriage rate of about 25% [1–3]. However, rather than an intrinsic cause associated directly to the presence of PCOS, this may well be due to a high prevalence of obesity in these patients, to the anti-oestrogenic action of CC on endometrial oestrogen receptors and suppression of pinopode formation [4] and the fact that CC also induces increased release of LH, and not just FSH, which is thought to be detrimental to the successful continuation of the pregnancy [5].

The usual second-line treatment for clomiphene failures is induction of ovulation with a low-dose FSH protocol. This also seems to produce a higher early pregnancy loss than in the spontaneously conceiving population [6]. Similarly high rates of early pregnancy loss were witnessed when using the now defunct conventional gonadotrophin ovulation induction protocols for women with PCOS [7].

R. Homburg (✉)
Professor of Reproductive Medicine, VU University Medical Centre, 1007MB Amsterdam, The Netherlands; IVF, Department of Obstetrics and Gynecology, Barzilai Medical Center, Ashkelon, Israel
e-mail: r.homburg@vumc.nl

N.R. Farid, E. Diamanti-Kandarakis (eds.), *Diagnosis and Management of Polycystic Ovary Syndrome*,
DOI 10.1007/978-0-387-09718-3_11, © Springer Science+Business Media, LLC 2009

Most of the sparse research on the subject of miscarriage in PCOS has involved a retrospective audit of patients with PCOS undergoing IVF. Here, at least, we can gain some insight into the difference in miscarriage rates between PCOS and non-PCOS patients undergoing the same treatment. Four studies indicate a clearly distinct increased prevalence of miscarriage in PCOS ranging from 25 to 37% compared with 18–25% in normal controls [7–10].

Whereas spontaneous miscarriage in non-PCOS women is highly associated with foetal chromosomal abnormalities, the aborted foetuses of women with PCOS and elevated LH levels are much more likely to have a normal karyotype [11].

Notwithstanding the constraints mentioned above, the weight of evidence points to an association between the presence of PCOS and an increased prevalence of early pregnancy loss.

11.3 Etiology

11.3.1 Fertility Treatment

The apparent increased prevalence of miscarriage in PCOS may be due to the fact that all series include women with PCOS undergoing some form of ovulation induction or ovarian stimulation, and there is no available comparison with the miscarriage rate of women with PCOS who conceive spontaneously. However, a comparison of PCOS with non-PCOS patients undergoing IVF clearly indicates that the miscarriage rate is increased in those with PCOS.

11.3.2 Obesity

Obesity is commonly associated with PCOS and has been conclusively associated with an increased prevalence of miscarriage [12]. In an attempt to define whether the increased incidence of miscarriage was due to the presence of PCOS itself or solely to the confounding factor of obesity, Wang et al. [10] analyzed 1018 women undergoing IVF, 37% of whom had PCOS. The spontaneous miscarriage rate was 28% in the women with PCOS compared with 18% in the non-PCOS group ($p<0.01$). However, this significance was lost when a multivariate analysis adjusting for obesity and treatment type was performed, the conclusion being that the higher risk of spontaneous miscarriage in PCOS was due to the higher prevalence of obesity and the type of treatment received.

11.3.3 Hyperinsulinaemia

Hyperinsulinaemia is a common feature of PCOS, particularly in the obese. It is amplified by obesity and is also strongly associated with elevated concentrations of plasminogen activator inhibitor-1 (PAI-1). Serum concentrations of PAI-1 are higher in women with PCOS compared with the general population [13]. PAI-1 is a potent inhibitor of fibrinolysis, and high serum concentrations may be a factor in the etiology of early pregnancy loss [14].

11.3.4 Hypersecretion of LH

High serum concentrations of LH (>10 IU/l) in the early to mid-follicular phase have been associated with an increased early pregnancy loss in several reports. A field study of 193 normally cycling women planning to become pregnant showed that raised mid-follicular phase serum LH concentrations were associated with a significantly higher miscarriage rate (65%), compared with those in women with normal serum LH concentrations (12%) [15].

In our own study [16] of a large group of patients with PCOS undergoing treatment with pulsatile gonadotropin hormone releasing hormone (GnRH) for induction of ovulation, follicular phase serum LH concentrations were significantly higher in those who miscarried (17.9 IU/L) compared with those who delivered successfully (9.6 IU/L). We also found that the miscarriage rate was 33% in women with PCOS compared with 10.6% in those with hypogonadotrophic hypogonadism, who were treated in a similar fashion. It was thus very clear from this first study of LH in ovulation induction that in women with PCOS, there was a significantly increased risk of miscarriage in those with an elevated follicular phase plasma LH concentration compared with those with PCOS and normal follicular phase LH levels. Furthermore, this study seemed to demonstrate that LH was the true culprit as there were no significant differences of any other hormonal parameter measured (testosterone, dihydroepiandrosterone sulphate, androstendione, FSH and prolactin) between those who delivered and who miscarried.

In 100 women with PCOS who were treated with low-dose gonadotropin therapy, the association of raised baseline and/or mid-follicular phase plasma LH concentrations with miscarriage was demonstrated [6]. Patients with an elevated LH concentration had a higher rate of miscarriage than the women with polycystic ovaries and normal LH levels. In women attending a recurrent miscarriage clinic, 82% had polycystic ovaries, as detected by ultrasound and also had abnormalities of follicular phase LH secretion [17–18].

There is also evidence that GnRH agonist, which reduces the elevated concentrations of LH found in some 50% of women with PCOS, serves to reduce the prevalence of early spontaneous miscarriage. A study from our group [7] looked at the performance of women with PCOS undergoing IVF/ET who had high mean LH concentrations, compared with a control group of normally cycling women with mechanical infertility. Pregnancy rates were similar in the two groups but whereas the GnRH agonist treatment reduced the miscarriage rate by half compared with gonadotropins alone in the PCOS group, its administration to the control group had no such effect. In a further study from our centre [19], 239 women with PCOS received hMG with or without GnRH agonist for ovulation induction or superovulation for IVF/embryo transfer. Of pregnancies achieved with GnRH agonist, 17.6% miscarried compared with 39% of those achieved with gonadotrophins alone. Cumulative live birth rates after four cycles for GnRH agonist were 64% compared with 26% for gonadotrophins only. Similarly, Balen et al. [8] analyzed the outcome of treatment in 182 women with PCO who conceived after IVF and found a highly significant reduction in the rate of miscarriage when buserelin was used to achieve pituitary desensitization followed by stimulation with hMG (15/74, 20%) compared with the use of clomiphene and hMG (51/108, 47%).

A marked decrease of serum LH concentrations is the most significant endocrine event following laparoscopic ovarian drilling for the induction of ovulation and pregnancy in women with PCOS. A report on miscarriage rates following laparoscopic ovarian diathermy involved 58 pregnancies with a miscarriage rate of 14%, much lower than that usually experienced in women with PCOS [20].

Altogether, there is compelling evidence of an etiological association between miscarriage and high LH concentrations. Further prospective controlled trials are still needed to confirm this association.

11.3.5 Endometrial Dysfunction

The association of PCOS, impaired implantation and early pregnancy loss has encouraged investigation into the state of the endometrial environment in women with PCOS. Low luteal phase serum glycodelin and insulin-like growth factor-binding protein-1 concentrations in women with PCOS, presumably induced by hyperinsulinaemia, have been demonstrated [21]. Plasma endothelin-1 levels are significantly higher in PCOS compared with controls [22]. Both these latter studies and a further study [23] have implicated hyperinsulinism in the aetiology of the inadequate endometrial blood flow that was demonstrated, affecting endometrial receptivity. These studies showed a reversal of endometrial dysfunction and, particularly, increased blood flow parameters, following treatment with metformin.

11.4 Treatment Modes

11.4.1 Metformin

Metformin, a bi-guanide, oral anti-diabetic drug, is capable of reducing insulin concentrations and consequently PAI-1 concentrations [13] without affecting normal glucose levels. In addition, it seems to be capable of enhancing uterine vascularity and blood flow [21–22], reducing plasma endothelin-1 levels [23–24], increasing luteal phase serum glycodelin concentrations [21], lowering androgen and LH concentrations and even induces weight loss in some patients [25]. These properties would suggest its theoretical clinical usefulness in the prevention of early pregnancy loss in PCOS but the two largest RCTs performed to date have not born out this promise [26–27]. In a very large trial comparing treatment with clomiphene, metformin and a combination of the two for infertile women with PCOS, the rates of first trimester pregnancy loss did not differ between these treatment groups [26]. Similarly, a large trial comparing the treatment of treatment-naïve infertile patients with PCOS with clomiphene or a combination of clomiphene and metformin found no significant differences in the rate of spontaneous abortion [27].

Two further smaller trials compared, firstly, the use of metformin versus laparoscopic ovarian diathermy of the ovaries for clomiphene resistant PCOS women who were overweight [28] and then metformin versus clomiphene in non-obese anovulatory PCOS [29]. In both series, although pregnancy rates were similar, early pregnancy loss rates with metformin were significantly decreased.

Metformin seems to be safe when continued throughout pregnancy as there has been no increase in congenital abnormalities, teratogenicity or adverse effect on infant development [30]. Preliminary data suggest that the strategy of continuing metformin throughout pregnancy can reduce the incidence of gestational diabetes, pre-eclampsia and foetal macrosomia [31]. However, as far as early pregnancy loss is concerned, any suggested effect has been said to be achieved whether metformin is discontinued when pregnancy is confirmed or continued through pregnancy [28–29].

11.4.2 Weight Loss

Overweight and frank obesity, amplifiers of insulin resistance in women with PCOS, have a profound influence on miscarriage rates [10, 32]. Loss of weight by change of life style before pregnancy is capable of reversing the deleterious effects of obesity on fertility potential. In a study examining the effect of a change in life style programme on 67 anovulatory, obese (BMI >30) women who had failed to conceive with conventional treatment for two years or more, the mean weight loss was 10.2 kg after six months [33]. Following the loss of weight, 60 of the 67 resumed ovulation and 52 achieved a pregnancy, 18 of them spontaneously. Most importantly, only 18% of these pregnancies miscarried compared with a 75% miscarriage rate in pregnancies achieved before the weight loss.

11.4.3 Reduction of LH Concentrations

GnRH agonists suppress LH concentrations before and during ovarian stimulation, avoiding premature LH surges, and this has earned them an undisputed place in IVF treatment protocols. They also neutralize any possible deleterious effect of high LH concentrations in women with PCOS. Their application during ovulation induction (not involving IVF) has not become standard treatment however, despite the fact that our experience and that of others has shown a lower miscarriage rate in women receiving combination treatment of agonist and gonadotropins when tonic LH concentrations are high. The reasons are that co-treatment with GnRH agonist and low-dose gonadotropin therapy is more cumbersome, longer, requires more gonadotropins to achieve ovulation, has a greater prevalence of multiple follicle development and consequently more OHSS and multiple pregnancies [34–35]. The combination of a GnRH agonist with low-dose gonadotropins should probably be reserved for women with high serum concentrations of LH who have repeated premature luteinization, stubbornly do not conceive on gonadotropin therapy alone or who have conceived and had early miscarriages on more than one occasion.

The use of a GnRH antagonist to suppress high LH concentrations during gonadotropin ovulation induction for PCOS could avoid several of the drawbacks of using an agonist. However, no convincing evidence has yet been forthcoming to suggest that it could be beneficial in the prevention of early pregnancy loss in these patients.

A summary of our present state of knowledge of possible therapeutic strategies to decrease early pregnancy loss in PCOS would suggest that the avoidance of overweight and obesity before pregnancy has the best potential.

11.5 Gestational Diabetes

A higher than normal finding of gestational diabetes in PCOS women would be expected considering the high prevalence of obesity and of insulin resistance among these women. This has indeed proved to be the majority opinion when examined by calculating the incidence of gestational diabetes among pregnant women with PCOS [36–40].

The prevalence of women with PCOS among those with gestational diabetes [41–44] was much higher compared with controls even when subjects and controls were weight matched [44]. The problems involved in examining this question have been the confounding factor of obesity. Indeed, some series suggested that BMI was a better predictor of gestational diabetes than PCOS [38, 45]. When PCOS women were weight matched with controls, one series with 66 women with PCOS had the same incidence of GDM as controls [46], whereas a smaller series [40] disagreed with this conclusion. The clinical conclusion from this data is that it is worthwhile screening pregnant women with PCOS for GDM especially if they are obese.

As mentioned above, the administration of metformin throughout pregnancy is a contentious issue. However, the reported reduction in the prevalence of GDM and foetal macrosomia by administering metformin [31] is logical enough to provoke further research into whether this strategy is a feasible option in our present state of knowledge.

11.6 Pregnancy-Related Hypertension

Hypertension is now well established as a possible sequela of PCOS over the age of 40, especially in those who are obese and insulin resistant. The trigger of pregnancy might be expected to produce an increased incidence of pregnancy-induced hypertension (PIH) and pre-eclamptic toxaemia (PET). Certainly, in the studies with fairly small cohorts (n = 22–47), this would seem to be true. For example, two series consisting of cohorts of 22 in each [40, 47] found that the incidence of PIH and PET respectively was increased in women with PCOS, very similar to the findings of an earlier series [48] (n = 33). Similar results [36] showed an increased incidence of PIH in women with PCOS, independent of BMI and a further report [37] demonstrated an increased incidence of PIH in PCOS but of PET only in PCOS associated with insulin resistance. A further series [49] compared blood pressure measurements throughout pregnancy in PCOS (n = 33) and controls (n = 66) and found no difference until the third trimester in which the incidence of hypertensive disorders was significantly higher in women with PCOS. In contrast, the two large series [38, 46] which examined cohorts of 66 and 99 respectively found no relation between PCOS and PIH and weight-matched controls [46], nor between PCOS and PET, despite the fact that the PCOS subjects had a higher mean BMI and an increased prevalence of nulliparity compared with controls [38].

This confusing body of evidence cannot yet convincingly point to a firm association between PCOS and hypertensive disorders of pregnancy. The only way to solve this question is to perform a prospective study employing a large cohort of women with well-defined PCOS compared with a control group matched for BMI and nulliparity.

11.7 Small-for-Gestational-Age Babies

It has been suggested, controversially, that women, later diagnosed to have PCOS, were more likely to have been born small-for-gestational-age (SGA) and that an SGA baby is more prone to develop the symptoms of PCOS later in life. While some have found a relationship between these two conditions [50–51], others found no association [52]. Less concern has been paid to the birth weight of offspring born to mothers with PCOS. Whereas the probable association of higher maternal body weight, increased weight gain during pregnancy and increased prevalence of gestational diabetes in women with PCOS would be expected to produce higher than mean birth weights, the prevalence of SGA offspring seems to be increased in women with PCOS. A comparison of the birth weights of 47 infants born from singleton pregnancies in women with PCOS with 180 infants born from singleton pregnancies in healthy controls demonstrated a significantly higher incidence of SGA infants in women with PCOS (12.8%) compared with controls (2.8%) with a similar prevalence of large-for-gestational-age infants in the two groups [53]. Insulin resistance resulting in impaired insulin-mediated growth [54] and the foetal programming hypothesis [55] are the possible explanations for this higher prevalence of SGA infants in mothers with PCOS suggested by the authors.

11.8 Summary

The prevalence of early pregnancy loss is raised in women with PCOS, particularly in those with associated obesity and hyperinsulinemia. The prevalence of gestational diabetes is increased in women with PCOS but the relation between PCOS and hypertensive disorders in pregnancy has not been clearly established. Avoiding obesity before pregnancy and screening women with PCOS for gestational diabetes and hypertension during the pregnancy, especially if they are obese, are recommended.

References

1. Kousta E, White DM, Franks S. Modern use of clomiphene citrate in induction of ovulation. Hum Reprod Update 1997; 3: 359–365.
2. Dickey RP, Taylor SN, Curole DN et al. Incidence of spontaneous abortion in clomiphene pregnancies. Hum Reprod 1996; 11: 2623–2628.
3. Macgregor AH, Johnson JE, Bunde CA. Further clinical experience with clomiphene citrate. Fertil Steril 1968; 19: 616–622.
4. Creus M, Ordi J, Fabregues F et al. The effect of different hormone therapies on integrin expression and pinopode formation in the human endometrium: a controlled study. Hum Reprod 2003; 18: 683–693.
5. Shoham Z, Borenstein R, Lunenfeld B et al. Hormonal profiles following clomiphene citrate therapy in conception and non-conception cycles. Clin Endocrinol (Oxf) 1990; 33: 271–278.
6. Hamilton-Fairley D, Kiddy D et al. Association of moderate obesity with a poor pregnancy outcome in women with polycystic ovary syndrome treated with low dose gonadotrophin. Br J Obstet Gynaecol 1992; 99: 128–131.
7. Homburg R, Levy T, Berkovitz D et al. Gonadotropin-releasing hormone agonist reduces the miscarriage rate for pregnancies achieved in women with polycystic ovary syndrome. Fertil Steril 1993; 59: 527–531.
8. Balen AH, Tan SL, MacDougall J et al. Miscarriage rates following in-vitro fertilisation are increased in women with polycystic ovaries and reduced by pituitary desensitisation with buserelin. Hum Reprod 1993; 8: 959–964.
9. Winter E, Wang J, Davies MJ et al. Early pregnancy loss following assisted reproductive technology treatment. Hum Reprod 2002; 17: 3220–3223.
10. Wang JX, Davies MJ, Norman RJ. Polycystic ovarian syndrome and the risk of spontaneous abortion following assisted reproductive technology treatment. Hum Reprod 2001; 16: 2606–2609.
11. Hasegawa I, Tanaka K, Sanada H et al. Studies on the cytogenetic and endocrinologic background of spontaneous abortion. Fertil Steril 1996; 65: 52–54.
12. Wang JX, Davies MJ, Norman RJ. Obesity increases the risk of spontaneous abortion during infertility treatment. Obes Res 2002; 10: 551–554.
13. Palomba S, Orio F Jr, Falbo A et al. Plasminogen activator inhibitor 1 and miscarriage after metformin treatment and laparoscopic ovarian drilling in patients with polycystic ovarian syndrome. Fertil Steril 2005; 84: 761–765.
14. Glueck CJ, Wang P, Fontaine RN et al. Plasmonogen inhibitor activity: an independent risk factor for the high miscarriage rate during pregnancy in women with polycystic ovary syndrome. Metabolism 1999; 48: 1589–1595.

15. Regan L, Owen EJ, Jacobs HS. Hypersecretion of luteinising hormone, infertility and miscarriage. Lancet 1990; 336: 1141–1144.
16. Homburg R, Armar NA, Eshel A, et al. Influence of serum luteinising hormone concentrations on ovulation, conception and early pregnancy loss in polycystic ovary syndrome. BMJ 1988; 297: 1024–1026.
17. Sagle M, Bishop K, Alexander FM et al. Recurrent early miscarriage and polycystic ovaries. BMJ 1988; 297: 1027–28.
18. Watson H, Hamilton-Fairley D, Kiddy D et al. Abnormalities of follicular phase luteinising hormone secretion in women with recurrent early miscarriage. J Endocrinol 1989; 123 suppl, Abstract 25.
19. Homburg R, Berkovitz D, Levy T et al. In-vitro fertilization and embryo transfer for the treatment of infertility associated with polycystic ovary syndrome. Fertil Steril 1993; 60: 858–863.
20. Armar NA, Lachelin GCL. Laparoscopic ovarian diathermy: an effective treatment for anti-oestrogen resistant anovulatory infertility in women with the polycystic ovary syndrome. Brit J Obstet Gynaecol 1993; 100: 161–164.
21. Jakubowicz DJ, Seppala M, Jakubowicz S et al. Insulin reduction with metformin increases luteal phase serum glycodelin and insulin-like growth factor-binding protein 1 concentrations and enhances uterine vacularity and blood flow in the polycystic ovary syndrome. J Clin Endocrinol Metab 2001; 86; 1126–1133.
22. alomba S, Russo T, Orio F Jr et al. Uterine effects of metformin administration in anovulatory women with polycystic ovary syndrome. Hum Reprod 2006; 21: 457–465.
23. Diamantis-Kandarakis E, Alexandraki K et al. Metformin administration improves endothelial function in women with polycystic ovary syndrome. Eur J Endocrinol 2005; 152: 749–756.
24. Orio F Jr, Palomba S, Cascella T et al. Improvement in endothelial structure and function after metformin treatment in young normal-weight women with polycystic ovary syndrome: results of a 6-month study. J Clin Endocrinol Metab 2005; 90: 6072–6076.
25. Fleming R, Hopkinson ZE, Wallace AM et al. Ovarian function and metabolic factors in women with oligomenorrhea treated with metformin in a randomized double blind placebo-controlled trial. J Clin Endocrinol Metab 2002; 87: 569–574.
26. Legro RS, Barnhart HX, Schlaff WD et al. Clomiphene, metformin, or both for infertility in the polycystic ovary syndrome. N Engl J Med 2007; 356: 551–566.
27. Moll E, Bossuyt PM, Korevaar JC et al. Effect of clomiphene citrate plus metformin and clomiphene citrate plus placebo on induction of ovulation in women with newly diagnosed polycystic ovary syndrome: randomised double blind clinical trial. BMJ 2006; 332: 1461–1462.
28. Palomba S, Orio F, Nardo LG et al. Metformin administration versus laparoscopic ovarian diathermy in clomiphene citrate resistant women with polycystic ovary syndrome: A prospective parallel randomized double-blind placebo-controlled trial. J Endocrinol Metab 2004; 89: 4801–4809.
29. Palomba S, Orio F, Falbo A et al. Prospective parallel randomized, double-blind, double-dummy controlled clinical trial comparing clomiphene citrate and metformin as first-line treatment for ovulation induction in nonobese anovulatory women with polycystic ovary syndrome. J Clin Endocrinol Metab 2005; 90: 4068–4074.
30. Glueck CJ, Goldenberg N, Pranikoff J et al. Height, weight, and motor-social development during the first 18 months of life in 126 infants born to 109 mothers with polycystic ovary syndrome who conceived on and continued metformin through pregnancy. Hum Reprod 2004; 19: 1323–1230.
31. Glueck CJ, Wang P, Kobayashi S et al. Metformin therapy throughout pregnancy reduces the development of gestational diabetes in women with polycystic ovary syndrome. Fertil Steril 2002; 77: 520–525.
32. Clark AM, Thornley B, Tomlinson L et al. Weight loss results in significant improvement in reproductive outcome for all forms of fertility treatment. Hum Reprod 1998; 13: 1502–1505.
33. Homburg R. Adverse effect of luteinizing hormone on fertility: fact or fantasy. Bailliere's Clin Obstet Gynaecol 1996; 12: 555–563.
34. Van der Meer M, Hompes PGA, Scheele F et al. The importance of endogenous feedback for monofollicular growth in low-dose step-up ovulation induction with FSH in PCOS, a randomized study. Fertil Steril 1996; 66: 571–575.
35. Homburg R, Eshel A, Kilborn J et al. Combined luteinizing hormone releasing hormone analogue and exogenous gonadotrophins for the treatment of infertility associated with polycystic ovaries. Hum Reprod 1990; 5: 32–37.
36. Urman B, Sarac E, Dogan L et al. Pregnancy in infertile PCOD patients. Complications and outcome. J Repod Med 1997; 42: 501–505.
37. Bjercke S, Dale PO, Tanbo T et al. Impact of insulin resistance on pregnancy complications and outcome in women with polycystic ovary syndrome. Gynecol Obstet Invest 2002; 54: 94–98.
38. Mikola M, Hiilesman V, Halttunen M et al. Obstetric outcome in women with polycystic ovary syndrome. Hum Reprod 2001; 16: 226–229.
39. Weerakiet S, Srisombut C, Rojanasakul A et al. Prevalence of gestational diabetes mellitus and pregnancy outcomes in Asian women with polycystic ovary syndrome. Gynecol Endocrinol 2004; 19: 134–140.
40. Radon PA, McMahon MJ, Meyer WR. Impaired glucose tolerance in pregnant women with polycystic ovary syndrome. Obstet Gynecol 1999; 94: 194–197.
41. Holte J, Gennarelli G, Wide L et al. High prevalence of polycystic ovaries and associated clinical, endocrine and metabolic features in women with previous gestational diabetes mellitus. J Clin Endocrinol Metab 1998; 83: 1143–1150.
42. Kousta E, Cela E, Lawrence N et al. The prevalence of polycystic ovaries in women with a history of gestational diabetes. Clin Endocrinol 2000; 53: 501–507.

43. Koivunen RM, Juutinen J, Vauhkonen I et al. Metabolic and steroidogenic alterations related to increased frequency of polycystic ovaries in women with a history of gestational diabetes. J Clin Endocrinol Metab 2001; 86: 2591–2599.
44. Anttila L, Karjala K, Pentilla RA et al. Polycystic ovaries in women with geatational diabetes. Obstet Gynecol 1998; 92: 13–16.
45. Turhan NO, Seckin NC, Aybar F, Inegol I. Assessment of glucose tolerance and pregnancy outcome of polycystic ovary patients. Int J Gynaecol Obstet 2003; 81: 163–168.
46. Haakova L, Cibula D, Rezabek K et al. Pregnancy outcome in women with PCOS and in controls matched by age and weight. Hum Reprod 2003; 18: 1438–1441.
47. Kashyap S, Claman P. Polycystic ovary disease and the risk of pregnancy-induced hypertension. J Reprod Med 2000; 45: 991–994.
48. Diamant YZ, Rimon E, Evron S. High incidence of preeclamptic toxemia in patients with polycystic ovarian disease. Eur J Obstet Gynecol Reprod Biol 1982; 14: 199–204.
49. Fridstrom M, Nisell H, Sjoblom P et al. Are women with polycystic ovary syndrome at an increased risk of pregnancy-induced hypertension and/or preeclampsia. Hypertens Preg 1999; 18: 73–80.
50. Ibanez L, Potau N, Francois I et al. Precocious pubarche, hyperinsulinism and ovarian hyperandrogenism in girls: relation to reduced fetal growth. J Clin Endocrinol Metab 1998; 83: 3558–3562.
51. Benitez R, Sir-Petermann T, Palomino A et al. Prevalence of metaboli c disorders among family members of patients with polycystic ovary syndrome. Rev Med Chil 2001; 129: 707–712.
52. Laitinen J, Taponen S, Martikainen H et al. Body size from birth to adulthood as a predictor of self-reported polycystic ovary syndrome symptoms. Int J Obs Relat Metab Disord 2003; 27: 710–715.
53. Sir-Petermann T, Hitchsfeld C, Maliqueo M et al. Birth weight in offspring of mothers with polycystic ovarian syndrome. Hum Reprod 2005; 20: 2122–2126.
54. Hattersley AT, Tooke JE. The fetal insulin hypothesis: an alternative explanation of the association of low birth weight with diabetes and vascular diseases. Lancet 1999; 353: 1789–1792.
55. Barker DPJ, Osmond C. Infant mortality, chidhood nutrition and ischaemic heart disease in England and Wales. Lancet 1986; i: 1077–1081.

Chapter 12
Polycystic Ovary Syndrome, Sleep Apnea, and Daytime Sleepiness and Fatigue

Alexandros N. Vgontzas and Susan Calhoun

12.1 Introduction

Although the study of sleep disorders in the general population as well as in specific groups (i.e., patients with hypothyroidism, peptic, ulcer, hypertension, and others) can be traced to the first sleep disorder clinics in the 1960s [1–3], the interest and published literature on sleep disorders and polycystic ovary syndrome (PCOS) is very recent. It was only in 2001 that the first publication on the association of sleep apnea and sleepiness with PCOS appeared in a scientific journal. The interest on sleep disorders in PCOS was triggered by the first definitive findings that sleep apnea and sleepiness are associated with insulin resistance and central obesity, the latter disorders being the primary pathogenetic mechanisms of PCOS. Thus, this chapter will begin with a summarized discussion of the findings on the association of sleep apnea with insulin resistance and central adipocity, and the role of visceral fat in sleep apnea. The chapter continues with a discussion of the association between PCOS and sleep apnea, insulin resistance, and inflammation, and concludes with the role of psychological distress and pathophysiological factors associated with excessive daytime sleepiness (EDS) in women with PCOS.

12.2 Sleep Apnea, Inflammation, Insulin Resistance, and Central Adipocity

Despite the extensive literature on the role of anatomic abnormalities in the pathogenesis of sleep apnea [4], the large majority of adult sleep apneics do not demonstrate structural abnormalities in their upper airways [5,6], whereas inversely, many patients with narrow upper airways due to clear-cut anatomic abnormalities do not have sleep apnea [7]. On physical examination, very few features have been helpful in defining the risk for sleep apnea and the response to therapy. Several reports have emphasized that a thick or large neck is an important variable [8]. However, neck size and body mass index (BMI) are highly correlated [5,9], whereas increase in waist circumference over adult life has a stronger association than neck size with sleep apnea severity [10]. Furthermore, this association has not been carefully examined outside of the apnea literature.

A number of associated features of sleep apnea suggest that this disorder is a manifestation of the metabolic syndrome. Indeed, there is a strong association of sleep apnea with obesity [5,6,11–17], male gender (android-central obesity), postmenopausal status without HT, systemic effects (e.g., hypertension and diabetes), and the natural course of symptoms [11], all of which are factors associated with the metabolic syndrome. It appears that in both sleep apnea and metabolic syndrome there is a vicious cycle of weight gain (particularly from young adulthood to middle age), snoring, development of breath cessation, daytime sleepiness, further weight gain, deterioration of breathing abnormalities, and more severe daytime sleepiness, all pointing toward a systematic

A.N. Vgontzas (✉)
Sleep Research and Treatment Center, Department of Psychiatry, Pennsylvania State University College of Medicine, Hershey, PA 17033, USA
e-mail: avgontzas@psu.edu

N.R. Farid, E. Diamanti-Kandarakis (eds.), *Diagnosis and Management of Polycystic Ovary Syndrome*,
DOI 10.1007/978-0-387-09718-3_12, © Springer Science+Business Media, LLC 2009

illness rather than a local abnormality. The high rate of failure of surgical interventions in the oropharynx and the fact that even modest weight gain or loss, respectively, result in a significant worsening or improvement of sleep apnea in middle-aged individuals [18] suggest that anatomic abnormalities are not primary in adult sleep apnea.

In 1997, we published our first report on cytokines and disorders of excessive daytime sleepiness [19]. In that controlled study, we first demonstrated that tumor necrosis factor-alpha (TNFα) was significantly elevated in sleep apneics and narcoleptics compared to that in normal controls (Fig. 12.1). Second, interleukin-6 (IL-6) concentrations were markedly and significantly elevated in sleep apneics compared to normal controls. Both

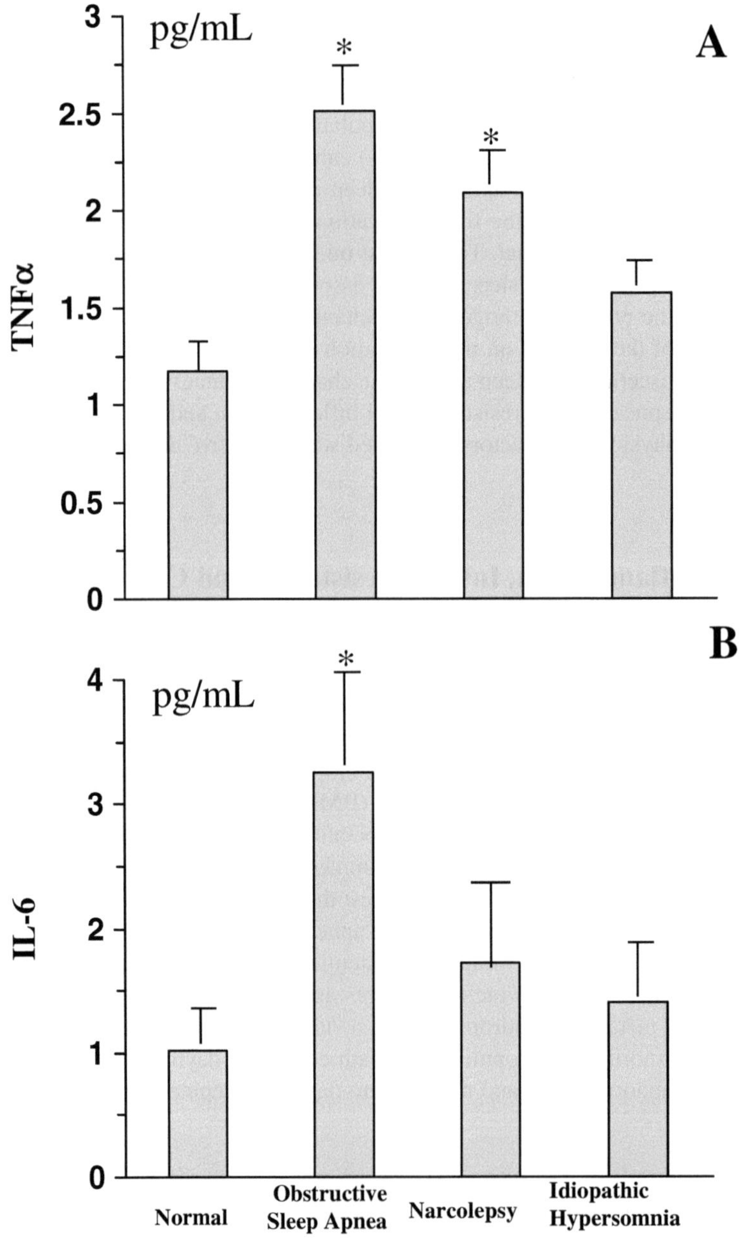

Fig. 12.1 Plasma TNFα and IL-6 levels in normal subjects and patients with EDS. (**A**) *, $P<0.001$ vs. normal. (**B**) *, $P=0.028$ vs. normal

TNFα and IL-6 plasma concentrations were positively correlated with the presence of EDS, and IL-6 plasma levels were positively correlated with BMI.

In a follow-up study, we demonstrated that in sleep apneic men, plasma concentrations of TNFα, IL-6, and leptin were elevated independently of obesity [20]. Both cytokines and leptin correlated positively with BMI, whereas leptin and IL-6 levels correlated positively with plasma insulin levels. In the last several years, many studies have confirmed the association of sleep apnea with inflammation both in adults and in children [21–23].

The data, showing that sleep apnea is associated with hypercytokinemia, in connection with (a) the emerging literature linking cytokines to obesity and insulin resistance [24–32], (b) the well-known relationships between insulin resistance and cardiovascular disease risk [33–38], and (c) the increased prevalence of cardiovascular disease in sleep apnea [19,17] have prompted us to explore whether sleep apnea is associated with insulin resistance independently of obesity.

Earlier studies reported inconsistent modest associations between sleep apnea and insulin resistance [39–43]. The weak correlations between sleep apnea and insulin levels in clinical samples and the absence of insulin resistance in otherwise asymptomatic apneics, as reported in some studies, may be due to the possibility that sleep apnea is a heterogeneous disorder in terms of its association with insulin resistance and/or that sleep apnea without symptoms has a weak association with insulin resistance.

In our study, we compared obese men with symptomatic sleep apnea and BMI- and age-matched, obese, nonapneic controls [20]. Mean fasting blood glucose levels were higher in the apneics than in obese controls. Mean plasma insulin levels were also higher in sleep apneics than in obese controls.

Similarly, two subsequent studies published in the *American Journal of Respiratory and Critical Care Medicine* in March of 2002 that employed larger samples reported an association between sleep apnea and insulin resistance independently of obesity [44,45]. Importantly, Ip and associates observed that the association between sleep apnea and insulin resistance was present even in nonobese subjects [44], while Punjabi and co-workers reported insulin resistance even in mild forms of sleep apnea [45]. Taken together, these studies supported an independent association between sleep apnea and insulin resistance [46].

At the same time, several investigational and epidemiologic studies suggested that partial sleep restriction may lead to decreased glucose tolerance and insulin sensitivity and that short sleep duration (subjectively assessed) is associated with an increased risk for obesity and diabetes [47]. It is possible that sleep apnea, through sleep loss, sleep fragmentation, and hypoxia, exacerbates the severity of metabolic disturbances.

12.3 Visceral Fat is the Predominant Fat Problem in Sleep apnea

Based on our finding that sleep apnea is associated with insulin resistance independently of obesity, we proceeded to examine whether visceral fat, which is closely associated with insulin resistance, correlates more strongly to sleep apnea than subcutaneous (SC) or total fat. We assessed body fat distribution using computed tomographic (CT) scanning. There were no significant differences between the two groups in terms of total body fat or SC fat. However, sleep apneics compared to obese controls had a significantly greater amount of visceral fat at L1. Interestingly, BMI correlated significantly with total body fat and SC fat but not with visceral fat. Importantly, visceral, but not SC fat, was significantly correlated with indices of sleep apnea (Fig. 12.2). These findings are consistent with reports that visceral fat accumulation is an important risk factor for sleep apnea in obese subjects [48], and the apnea/hypopnea index (number of apneas/hypopneas per hour of sleep) is significantly correlated with intra-abdominal fat but not with subcutaneous fat in the neck region or parapharyngeal fat [49]. Notably, our findings on the key role of visceral fat in the pathogenesis of sleep apnea were replicated in a recent study by our group that included obese apneics, obese controls, and nonobese controls [50].

Based on these results, we proposed that visceral obesity/insulin resistance is determined by both genetic/constitutional and environmental factors, which progressively lead to worsening metabolic syndrome manifestations and sleep apnea. Sleep apnea may lead to a worsening of visceral obesity and the metabolic syndrome by providing a stress stimulus and causing nocturnal elevations of hormones, such as cortisol and insulin, that promote visceral adiposity, metabolic abnormalities, and cardiovascular complications [20, 51].

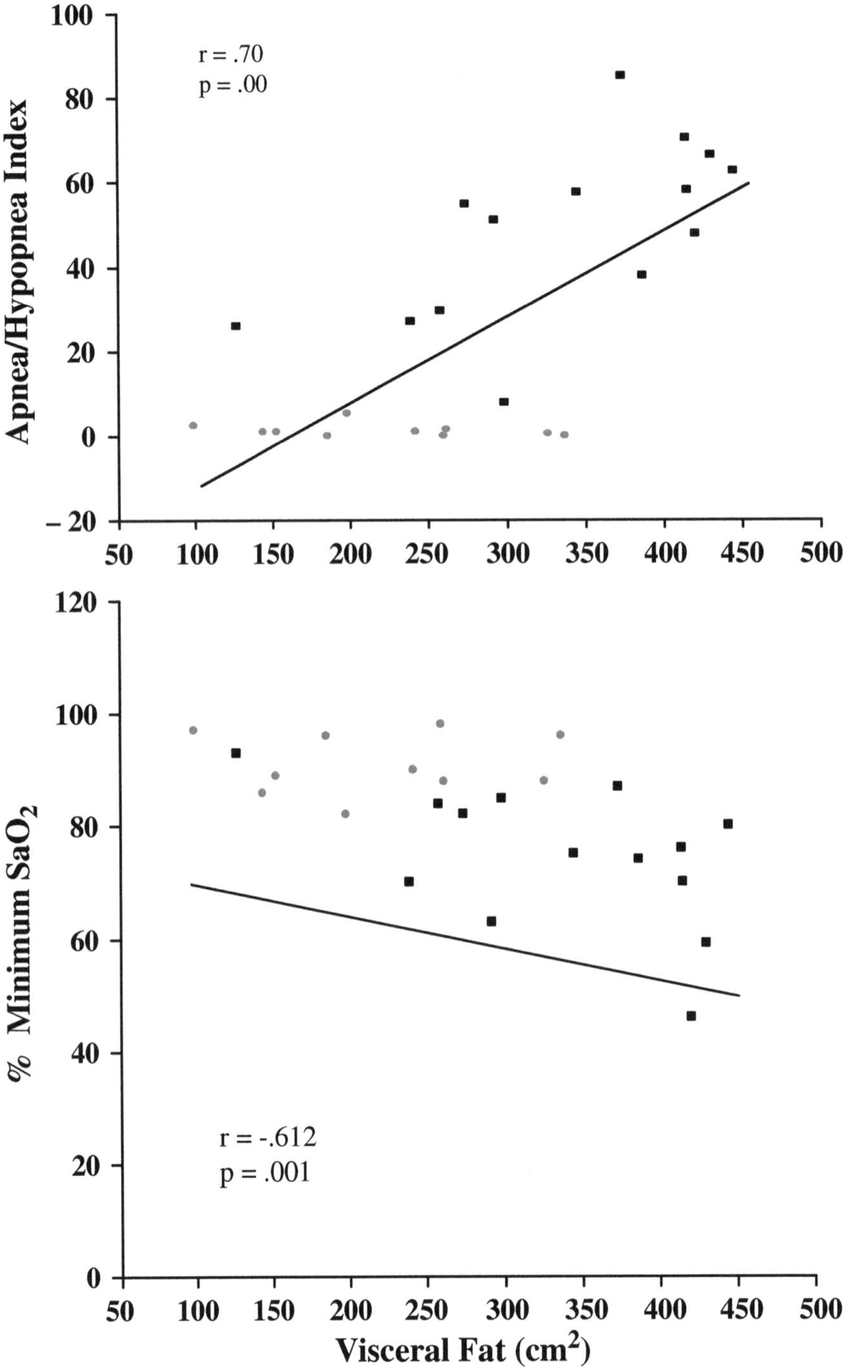

Fig. 12.2 Visceral fat significantly correlates with indices of sleep apnea. ■, sleep apneics; ○, obese controls

12.4 Sleep Apnea is Very Frequent in Women with PCOS

Our finding that sleep apnea is associated with insulin resistance independently of obesity prompted us to explore the other side of this bi-directional association. In other words, if insulin resistance is underlying sleep apnea's pathogenetic mechanisms, then the latter should be more prevalent in disorders in which insulin resistance is a primary abnormality, such as PCOS [52,53].

12.5 PCOS is Associated with Sleep Apnea and EDS Independent of Obesity

Fifty-three premenopausal women with PCOS (BMI range, 24.3–67.7) were prospectively studied in the sleep laboratory. The diagnosis of PCOS was made by the presence of chronic anovulation (six or fewer menstrual periods per year) in association with elevated circulating androgen levels [52]. Control women were 452 premenopausal women (BMI range, 16.1–59.9) selected from a general random sample [14]. Sleep apnea was diagnosed using Sleep Disorders Clinic criteria, which employed sleep laboratory (apnea/hypopnea index ≥ 10) and clinical findings [13,14].

In this study, women with PCOS were 30 times more likely to suffer from sleep apnea than controls (Fig. 12.3). Specifically, nine of the women with PCOS (17.0%) were given treatment for sleep apnea or upper airway resistance syndrome in contrast to only three (0.6%) controls (two for sleep apnea and one for upper airway resistance syndrome). The difference between the two groups remained significant even when we controlled for BMI.

Three more studies replicated the strong association between sleep apnea and PCOS. In a study by Fogel et al. [54], 18 obese PCOS women were compared to 18 age- and weight-matched controls. Women with PCOS had a higher A/HI (22.5 vs. 6.7) and were more likely to suffer from symptomatic sleep apnea syndrome (44.4% vs. 5.5%). In a subsequent study by Gopal et al. [55], 23 premenopausal women with PCOS were recorded in the sleep laboratory. Sixteen of 23 (69.6%) met criteria for sleep apnea, whereas five were treated with continuous positive airway pressure (CPAP).

In a more recent study by Tasali et al. [56], the risk for sleep apnea was assessed in two cohorts of women with PCOS. Cohort 1 included 40 non-diabetic women who completed the subjective questionnaires to assess the risk of sleep apnea. Cohort 2 included eight women who had a polysomnographic study. Thirty of the

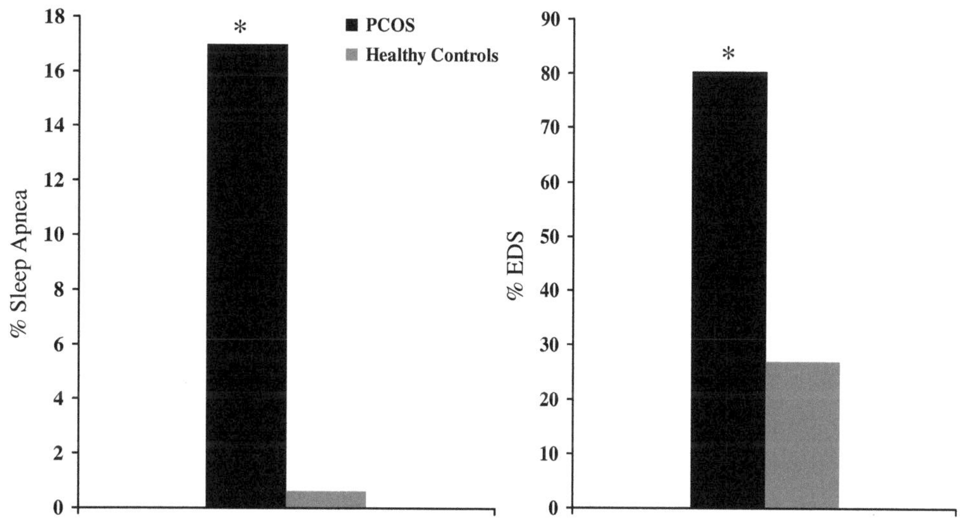

Fig. 12.3 Prevalence of obstructive sleep apnea and excessive daytime sleepiness (EDS) in women with the polycystic ovary syndrome is markedly higher than in healthy controls. *, $P<0.05$

40 women had a high risk of sleep apnea by the subjective questionnaires. Women in cohort 2 had rapid eye movement (REM)-predominant sleep apnea.

Cumulatively, these four studies suggest that sleep apnea is highly prevalent in women with PCOS.

12.6 Insulin Resistance is the Strongest Predictor of Sleep Apnea in PCOS

In order to understand further the relationship between the presence of sleep apnea in women with PCOS and potential predictive factors, i.e., age, BMI, free and total testosterone, fasting insulin levels and glucose-to-insulin ratio, were included in a logistic regression analysis. The backward conditional analysis eliminated all variables but insulin and glucose-to-insulin ratio, suggesting that insulin resistance was a stronger predictor for sleep apnea than age, BMI, or testosterone.

In the study by Fogel et al. [54], elevated serum androgen and central obesity were both significantly associated with the severity of sleep apnea. In the study by Tasali et al. [56], insulin levels and measures of glucose tolerance in PCOS were strongly correlated with the risk and severity of sleep apnea. Similar to our study, they found no significant relationship between the androgen levels and the severity of sleep apnea. In conclusion, it appears that insulin resistance is the strongest predictor of sleep apnea in PCOS.

The role of inflammation and insulin resistance in the pathogenesis of sleep apnea in women is further supported by data on the prevalence of sleep apnea in postmenopausal women. In a recent large epidemiologic study, Bixler and colleagues demonstrated that the prevalence of sleep apnea is quite low in premenopausal women (0.6%) as well as postmenopausal women on hormone therapy (HT) [14]. Further, in these women, the presence of sleep apnea appeared to be associated exclusively with obesity (BMI $\geq$ 32.3%). Postmenopausal women without HT had a prevalence of sleep apnea that was close, although still lower, to the prevalence in men. Loss of estrogen after menopause is associated with elevated IL-6, increasing obesity (primarily central), and an increase of cardiovascular disease [57]. It is possible that elevation of inflammatory cytokines, central obesity, and/or insulin resistance are risk factors for increased prevalence of sleep apnea and cardiovascular disease in postmenopausal women. In support of this speculation, a recent study from the Women's Health Initiative Hormone Trial reported that estrogen plus progestin decreased diabetes and insulin resistance in postmenopausal women, which might be a mechanism through which HT protects women from sleep apnea [58]. The adverse effect of menopause and the protective role of gonadal hormones in sleep apnea in women was confirmed in the Sleep Heart Health Study as well as in a Wisconsin cohort [59,60].

Given the association of insulin resistance with pro-inflammatory cytokines, which are proposed mediators of sleepiness and sleep apnea, we examined whether IL-6 and TNFα are elevated in PCOS. Women with PCOS exhibited higher plasma concentrations of IL-6 than obese controls, who had intermediate values, or normal-weight controls, who had the lowest values. TNFα values were higher in PCOS and obese controls compared to normal-weight controls, but the difference was not statistically significant. Furthermore, within the PCOS group, IL-6 and TNFα correlated more strongly with indices of insulin resistance than obesity. We concluded that IL-6 levels are elevated in obese women with PCOS independently of obesity or sleep apnea and may represent a pathophysiologic link to insulin resistance and daytime sleepiness in this disorder [61].

12.7 Excessive Daytime Sleepiness: Prevalence and its Association with Metabolic Disorders

EDS and fatigue (tiredness without increased sleep propensity) are the most common complaints of patients referred to a sleep disorders clinic [11,62]. In fact, approximately 70% of those evaluated in a sleep clinic report a complaint of sleepiness. In the general population, the prevalence of EDS is estimated to range from 5 to 20% based on the question asked [63–71]. From published epidemiologic studies, it is clear that there has been a significant increase of sleepiness over the last two decades. For example, Bixler et al. reported a prevalence of 4% of "hypersomnia" in Los Angeles in 1979 [63], whereas moderate to severe EDS was present in about 10%

of the general population in central Pennsylvania in 2005 [69]. It has been suggested that self-induced sleep restriction may be a major factor underlying this "epidemic" of sleepiness and fatigue [62]. However, it appears, depression, and obesity and its associated comorbid conditions might be much stronger factors underlying this "epidemic" of sleepiness and fatigue. Certainly, EDS is a major health issue, both in terms of its impact on personal suffering and as a major safety issue for the public.

It appears that obesity, a prevalent condition among women with PCOS, is associated with excessive daytime sleepiness and might be a significant factor underlying the current epidemic of fatigue and sleepiness in modern societies [11,62]. One study using objective measures for assessment of daytime sleepiness demonstrated that obese patients without sleep apnea compared with controls were sleepier during the day [72]. Three other studies showed similar findings in regard to an independent contribution of obesity in sleepiness [73–75]. These findings are consistent with a recent study in a large general, randomized sample that was evaluated in the sleep laboratory and showed that obesity was a significant risk factor for excessive daytime sleepiness independently of sleep-disordered breathing and age [69] (Fig. 12.4). Two other large cross-sectional population studies reported that a higher body mass index was associated with self-reported daytime sleepiness and fatigue [70,71]. It appears that obesity per se is a major contributor of EDS and should be considered in the differential diagnosis of patients who present with a primary complaint of daytime sleepiness.

Fatigue is a frequent complaint of patients with diabetes. The underlying mechanisms are unknown. In 1993, Feinberg alerted sleep specialists to the possibility that untreated diabetes should be considered in patients with severe sleepiness for which other causes had been ruled out [76]. He postulated that sleepiness in diabetics may be explained either by the nocturia which might have produced a chronic sleep curtailment and/or that the derangement of glucose metabolism in diabetes could interfere with the hypothesized restorative processes of sleep.

Bixler and his colleagues assessed the association of EDS with diabetes or hyperglycemia (fasting blood glucose > 126 mg/dl) in a large sample of 1,741 subjects. In the multiple logistic regression analysis, EDS was shown to have a significant association with diabetes when controlling for sleep apnea, obesity, depression, and age [69] (Fig. 12.5). The authors concluded that diabetes or impaired glucose tolerance should be considered in the differential diagnosis whenever excessive daytime sleepiness is present.

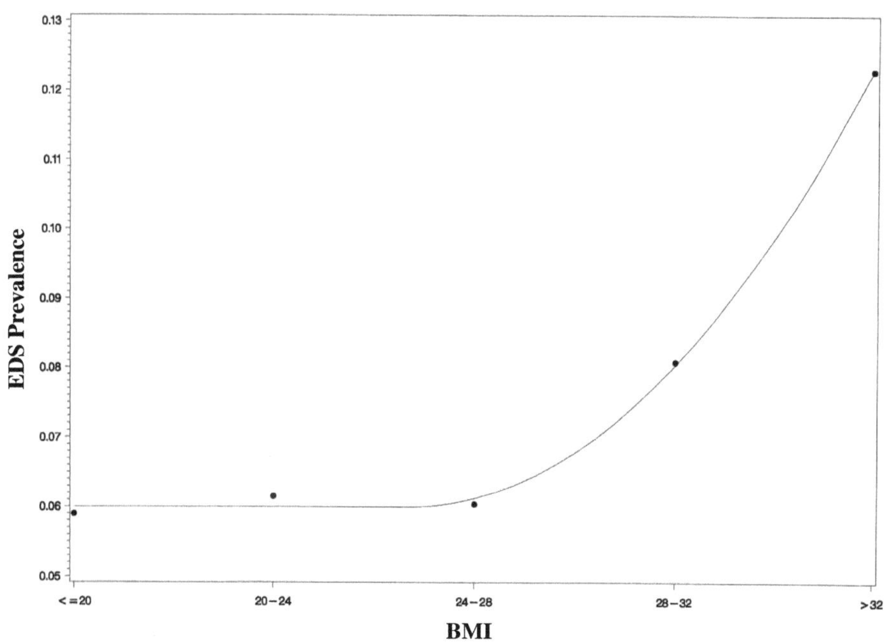

Fig. 12.4 BMI-specific prevalence of EDS

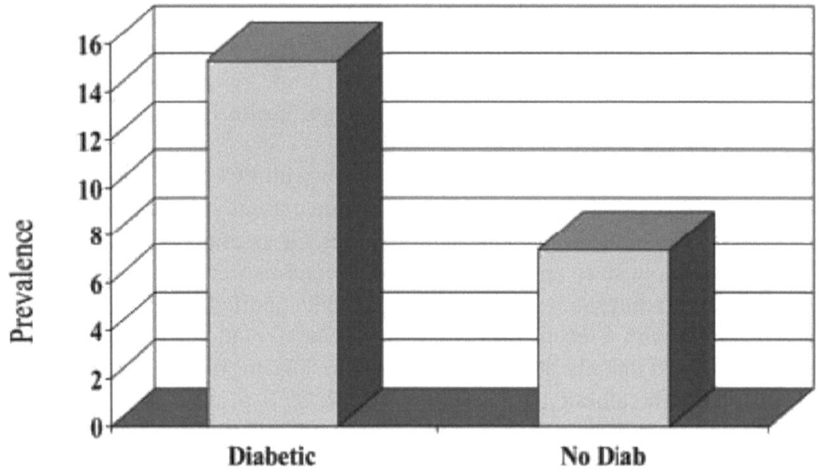

Fig. 12.5 Prevalence of EDS in subjects with known diabetes, compared with those without diabetes. OR ($\pm$ 95% CI) = 1.9 (1.6, 2.4), $P<0.001$

12.8 Daytime Sleepiness in PCOS

Daytime sleepiness is reported very frequently by women with PCOS in whom insulin resistance is a common metabolic abnormality [52,53,56]. In a sample of 53 premenopausal women with PCOS, sleep apnea was diagnosed in 17%, whereas 80% complained of EDS (Fig. 12.3). Furthermore, in the nonobese category (BMI $\leq$ 32.3), 75.0% of PCOS complained of EDS in contrast to only 22.5% of nonobese controls [53]. This suggests that in this syndrome of glucose dysregulation, EDS is present independently of sleep apnea or obesity [53–56]. This finding is consistent with another study that showed that daytime sleepiness was equally distributed among obese and nonobese women with PCOS [55], suggesting that in PCOS women, daytime sleepiness exists independently of obesity or sleep apnea [53,55].

Psychological stress and depression are the most common risk factors of EDS in general population samples [13,14]. Furthermore, it appears that the presence of EDS is even more strongly associated with depression than with sleep apnea [69]. Previous studies [77–84] have reported some level of psychological distress including depression, anxiety, and aggression among this group of women. In order to explore whether psychological stress is a major risk factor for EDS in women with PCOS, in a recent study, we examined the association between psychological stress and EDS in a sample of women with PCOS and controls [85]. Fifty-seven premenopausal women with PCOS were recorded in the sleep laboratory and completed an extensive widely used psychometric instrument (MMPI-2) as a measure of psychological distress. Controls were 68 nonobese premenopausal women and 69 obese premenopausal women selected from The Penn State Cohort, a general randomized sample of adults. Comparison between groups revealed no significant differences on the MMPI-2 clinical scales, and remained nonsignificant after considering the variance related to treatment for depression and age. The results of our study demonstrated that women with PCOS do not experience more chronic psychological distress than obese and nonobese women from the general population, whereas it is possible that they experience situational stress (i.e., secondary to infertility problems) as shown in previous studies. Furthermore, the results of this study indicate that psychological stress is only weakly associated with increased complaints of sleepiness in women with PCOS versus obese controls and thin controls even when controlling for the effects of A/HI or percent sleep time. Thus, the increased report of sleepiness cannot be simply explained by chronic psychological distress. We concluded that sleepiness in PCOS is related to pathophysiological rather than emotional factors associated with the disorder, such as obesity, insulin resistance, and hormonal imbalance, which are known risks factors for daytime sleepiness [11,14,69]. Of interest is the recent report that increased levels of IL-6 in women with PCOS, independently of obesity and sleep apnea [61], may function as mediators of the sleepiness and fatigue in PCOS. Methods to improve these pathophysiological factors (i.e., weight loss, exercise, specific antagonists to TNFα or IL-6, and insulin-sensitivity agents) may benefit the patient's sleepiness and fatigue.

12.9 Summary

PCOS is the most common endocrine disorder in premenopausal women and is associated with insulin resistance and central adipocity. Sleep apnea is strongly associated with insulin resistance and visceral obesity and there is evidence for the pathogenetic role of these metabolic disturbances. In the last several years, a number of studies have demonstrated that sleep apnea is very prevalent in women with PCOS. It appears also that the primary pathogenetic mechanism is insulin resistance and visceral adipocity. Furthermore, there is increasing evidence that PCOS is associated very frequently with excessive daytime sleepiness and fatigue, which is independent of psychological distress. The causal role of obesity, insulin resistance, and visceral adipocity in the pathogenesis of these disturbances in women with PCOS should be explored and may shed light on the overall pathogenetic mechanism of these two very prevalent sleep disorders. From a clinical standpoint, sleep apnea and daytime sleepiness are very prevalent in women with PCOS and should be considered as primary clinical manifestations of that disorder. Thus, women with PCOS should be screened systematically for these two sleep disorders.

References

1. Kales A, Kales J. Evaluation, diagnosis, and treatment of clinical conditions related to sleep. JAMA 1970; 213:2229–2235.
2. Dement W, Holman RB, Guilleminault C. Neurochemical and neuropharmacological foundations of the sleep disorders. Psychopharmacol Commun 1976; 2:77–90.
3. Lugaresi E, Coccagna G, Petrella A, Berti Ceroni G, Pazzaglia P. The disorder of sleep and respiration in the Pickwick syndrome. [Italian] Sist Nerv 1968; 20:38–50.
4. Kuna S, Remmers JE. Anatomy and physiology of upper airway obstruction. In: Kryger MH, Roth T, Dement WC, editors. Sleep medicine. Philadelphia: WB Saunders; 2000:840–858.
5. Strohl, KP, Redline S. Recognition of sleep apnea. Am J Respir Crit Care Med 1996; 154:279–289.
6. Lugaresi E, Cirignotta F, Geraldi R, Montagna P. Snoring and sleep apnea: natural history of heavy snorers disease. In: Guilleminault C, Partinen M, editors. Sleep apnea syndrome. New York: Raven Press; 1990:25–36.
7. Smith PL, Schwartz AR. Biomechanics of the upper airway during sleep. In: Pack AI, editor. Sleep apnea: pathogenesis, diagnosis, and treatment. New York: Marcel Dekker, Inc.; 2002:31–52.
8. Hoffstein V, Szalai JP. Predictive value of clinical features in diagnosing sleep apnea. Sleep 1993; 16:18–22.
9. Young T, Peppard P, Palta M, Hla M, Finn L, Morgan B, Skatrud J. Population-based study of sleep-disordered breathing as a risk factor for hypertension. Arch Intern Med 1997; 157:1746–1752.
10. Carmelli D, Swan GE, Bliwise DL. Relationship of 30-year changes in obesity to sleep-disordered breathing in the Western Collaborative Group Study. Obes Res 2000; 8:632–637.
11. Vgontzas AN, Kales A. Sleep and its disorders. Annu Rev Med 1999; 50-387-400.
12. Young T, Palta M, Dempsey J, Skatrud J, Weber S, Badr S. The occurrence of sleep-disordered breathing among middle-age adults. N Engl J Med 1993; 328-1230-5.
13. Bixler EO, Vgontzas AN, Ten Have T, Tyson K, Kales A. Effects of age on sleep apnea in men: I. Prevalence and severity. Am J Respir Crit Care Med 1998; 157:144–148.
14. Bixler EO, Vgontzas AN, Lin H-M, Ten Have T, Rein J, Vela-Bueno A, Kales A. Prevalence of sleep-disordered breathing in women. Am J Respir Crit Care Med 2001; 163:608–613.
15. Guilleminault C, van den Hoed J, Mitler MM. Clinical overview of the sleep apnea syndromes. In: Guilleminault C, Dement WC, editors. Sleep apnea syndromes. New York: Alan R. Liss, Inc.; 1978:1–12.
16. Lugaresi E, Coccagna G, Montavani M. Hypersomnia with periodic apneas. In: Weitzman E, editor. Advances in sleep research. New York: Spectrum Publications; 1978:4.
17. Lavie P. Sleep apnea in the presumably healthy working population-revisited. Sleep 2002; 25:380–386.
18. Peppard PE, Young T, Palta M. Dempsey J, Skatrud J. Longitudinal study of moderate weight change and sleep-disordered breathing. JAMA 2000; 284:3015–3021.
19. Vgontzas AN, Papanicolaou DA, Bixler EO, Kales A, Tyson K, Chrousos GP. Elevation of plasma cytokines in disorders of excessive daytime sleepiness: role of sleep disturbance and obesity. J Clin Endocrinol Metab 1997; 82:1313–1316.

20. Vgontzas AN, Papanicolaou DA, Bixler EO, Hopper K, Lotsikas A, Lin HM, Kales A, Chrousos GP. Sleep apnea and daytime sleepiness and fatigue: relation to visceral obesity, insulin resistance, and hypercytokinemia. J Clin Endocrinol Metab 2000; 85:1151–1158.
21. Ryan S, Taylor CT, McNigholas WT. Predictors of elevated nuclear factor-kappaβ-dependent genes in sleep apnea syndrome. Am J Respir Crit Care Med 2006; 174:824–830.
22. Punjabi NM, Beamer BA. C-reactive protein is associated with sleep apnea independent of adiposity. [see comment]. Sleep 2007; 30:29–34.
23. Gozal D, Crabtree VM, Sans Capdevila O, Witcher LA, Kheirandish-Gozal L. C-reactive protein, sleep apnea, and cognitive dysfunction in school-aged children. Am J Respir Crit Care Med 2007; 176:188–193.
24. Fried SK, Bunkin DA, Greenberg AS. Omental and subcutaneous adipose tissues of obese subjects release interleukin-6: depot difference and regulation by glucocorticoid. J Clin Endocrinol Metab 1998; 83:847–850.
25. Orban Z, Remaley AT, Sampson M, Trajanoski Z, Chrousos GP. The differential effect of food intake and β-adrenergic stimulation on adipose-derived hormones and cytokines in man. J Clin Endocrinol Metab 1999; 84:2126–2133.
26. Mohamed-Ali V, Goodrick S, Rawesh A, Katz DR, Miles JM, Yudkin JS, Klein S, Coppack SW. Subcutaneous adipose tissue releases interleukin-6, but not tumor necrosis factor-α, *in vivo*. J Clin Endocrinol Metab 1997; 82:4196–41200.
27. Gotamisligil GS, Shargill NS, Spiegelman BM. Adipose expression of tumor necrosis factor-α: direct role in obesity-linked insulin resistance. Science 1993; 259:87–91.
28. Flier JS. Diabetes. The missing link with obesity? Nature 2001; 409:292–293.
29. Vgontzas AN, Bixler EO, Papanicolaou DA, Chrousos GP. Chronic systemic inflammation in overweight and obese adults. JAMA 2000; 283:2235–2236.
30. Bastard JP, Jardel C, Bruckert E. Elevated levels of interleukin 6 are reduced in serum and subcutaneous adipose tissue of obese women after weight loss. J Clin Endocrinol Metab 2000; 85:3338–3342.
31. Fernandez-Real J-M, Vayreda M, Richart C, Gutierrez C, Broch M, Vendrell J, Ricart W. Circulating interleukin 6 levels, blood pressure, and insulin sensitivity in apparently healthy men and women. J Clin Endocrinol Metab 2001; 86:1154–1159.
32. Bastard JP, Maachi M, Tran Van Nheiu J, Jardel C, Bruckert E, Grimaldi A, Robert JJ, Capeau J, Hainque B. Adipose tissue IL-6 content correlates with resistance to insulin activation of glucose uptake both *in vivo* and *in vitro*. J Clin Endocrinol Metab 2002; 87:2084–2089.
33. Reaven GM. Role of insulin resistance in human disease. Diabetes 1988; 37:1595–1607.
34. Reaven GM, Lithell H, Landsberg L. Hypertension and associated metabolic abnormalities: the role of insulin resistance and the sympathoadrenal system. N Engl J Med 1996; 334:374–381.
35. Chrousos GP. The role of stress and the hypothalamic-pituitary-adrenal axis in the pathogenesis of the metabolic syndrome: neuro-endocrine and target tissue-related causes (review). Int J Obes 2000; 24:S50–S55.
36. DeFronzo R, Ferrannini E. Insulin resistance: a multifaceted syndrome responsible for NIDDM, obesity, hypertension, dyslipidemia and atherosclerotic cardiovascular disease. Diabetes Care 1991; 14:173–194.
37. Bixler EO, Vgontzas AN, Lin H-M, Ten Have T, Leiby BE, Vela-Bueno A, Kales A. Association of hypertension and sleep-disordered breathing. Arch Intern Med 2000; 161:2634–2635.
38. Peppard PE, Yount T, Palta M, Skatrud J. Prospective study of the association between sleep-disordered breathing and hypertension. N Engl J Med 2000; 342:1378–1384.
39. Strohl KP, Novak RD, Singer W, Cahan C, Boehm KD, Denko CW, Hoffstem VS. Insulin levels, blood pressure and sleep apnea. Sleep 1994; 17:614–618.
40. Tiihonen M, Partinen M, Närvänen S. The severity of obstructive sleep apnoea is associated with insulin resistance. J Sleep Res 1993; 2:56–61.
41. Brooks B, Cistulli PA, Borkman M, Ross G, McGhee S, Grunstein RR, Sullivan CE, Yue DK. Sleep apnea in obese noninsulin-dependent diabetic patients: effect of continuous positive airway pressure treatment on insulin responsiveness. J Clin Endocrinol Metab 1994; 79:1681–1685.
42. Davies RJO, Turner R, Crosby J, Stradling JR. Plasma insulin and lipid levels in untreated obstructive sleep apnoea and snoring: their comparison with matched controls and response to treatment. J Sleep Res 1994; 3:180–185.
43. Stoohs RA, Facchini F, Guilleminault C. Insulin resistance and sleep-disordered breathing in healthy humans. Am J Respir Crit Care Med 1996; 154:170–174.
44. Ip MSM, Lam B, Ng MMT, Lam WK, Tsant KWT, Lam KSL. Sleep apnea is independently associated with insulin resistance. Am J Respir Crit Care Med 2002; 165:670–676.
45. Punjabi NM, Sorkin JD, Katzel L, Goldberg A, Schwartz A, Smith PL. Sleep-disordered breathing and insulin resistance in middle aged and overweight men. Am J Respir Crit Care Med 2002; 165:677–682.
46. Tasali E, Van Cauter E. Sleep-disordered breathing and the current epidemic of obesity. Am J Crit Care Respir Care Med 2002; 165:562–563.
47. Spiegel K, Knutson K, Leproult R, Tasali E, Van Cauter E. Sleep loss: a novel risk factor for insulin resistance and Type 2 diabetes. J Appl Physiol 2005; 99:2008–2019.
48. Shinohara E, Kihara S, Yamashita S, Yamane M, Nishida M, Arai T, Kotani K, Nakamura T, Takemura K, Matsuzawa Y. Visceral fat accumulation as an important risk factor for obstructive sleep apnoea syndrome in obese subjects. J Intern Med 1997; 241:11–18.
49. Schäfer, Pauleit D, Sudhop T, Gouni-Berthold I, Ewig S, Berthold HK. Body fat distribution, serum leptin, and cardiovascular risk factors in men with sleep apnea. Chest 2002, 122:829–839.

50. Vgontzas AN Zoumakis E, Bixler EO, Lin H-M, Collins B, Basta M, Pejovic S, Chrousos GP. Selective effects of CPAP on sleep apnea-associated manifestations. Eur J Clin Invest 2008; 38:585–595.
51. Rosmond R, Dallman MF, Björntorp P. Stress-related cortisol secretion in men: relationships with abdominal obesity, endocrine, metabolic, and hemodynamic abnormalities. J Clin Endocrinol Metab 1998; 83:1853–1859.
52. Dunaif A. Insulin resistance and the polycystic ovary syndrome: mechanism and implications for pathogenesis. Endocr Rev 1997; 18:774–800.
53. Vgontzas AN, Legro RS, Bixler EO, Grayev A, Kales A, Chrousos GP. Polycystic ovary syndrome is associated with sleep apnea and daytime sleepiness: role of insulin resistance. J Clin Endocrinol Metab 2001; 86:517–520.
54. Fogel RB MA, Pillar G, Pittman SD, Dunaif A, White DP. Increased prevalence of sleep apnea syndrome in obese women with polycystic ovary syndrome. J Clin Endocrinol Metab 2001; 86:1175–1178.
55. Gopal M, Duntley S, Uhles M, Attarian H. The role of obesity in the increased prevalence of sleep apnea syndrome in patients with polycystic ovarian syndrome. Sleep Med 2002; 3:401–404.
56. Tasali E, Van Cauter E, Ehrmann DA. Relationships between sleep apnea and glucose metabolism in polycystic ovary syndrome. J Clin Endocrinol Metab 2006; 91:36–42.
57. Papanicolaou DA, Wilder RL, Manolagas SC, Chrousos GP. The pathophysiologic roles of interleukin-6 in human disease. Ann Intern Med 1998; 128:127–137.
58. Margolis KL, Bonds DE, Rodabough RJ, Tinker L, Phillips LS, Allen C, Bassford T, Burke G, Torrens J, Howard BV, Women's Health Initiative Investigators. Effect of oestrogen plus progestin on the incidence of diabetes in postmenopausal women: results from the Women's Health Initiative Hormone Trial. Diabetologia 2004; 47:1175–1187.
59. Shahar E, Redline S, Young T, Boland LL, Baldwin CM, Nieto FJ, O'Connor GT, Rapoport DM, Robbins JA. Hormone replacement therapy and sleep-disordered breathing. Am J Respir Crit Care Med 2003; 167:1186–1192.
60. Young T, Finn L, Austin D, Peterson A. Menopausal status and sleep-disordered breathing in the Wisconsin Sleep Cohort Study. Am J Respir Crit Care Med 2003; 167:1181–1185.
61. Vgontzas AN, Trakada G, Bixler EO, Lin H-M, Pejovic S, Zoumakis E, Chrousos GP, Legro RS. Plasma interleukin 6 levels are elevated in polycystic ovary syndrome independently of obesity or sleep apnea. Metabolism 2006; 55:1076–1082.
62. Roehrs T, Carskadon MA, Dement WC, Roth T. In Kryger M, Roth T, Dement W, editors. Principles and practice of sleep medicine, third edition. Philadelphia, PA: WB Saunders Company; 2000:43–52.
63. Bixler EO, Kales A, Soldatos CR, Kales JD, Healey S. Prevalence of sleep disorders in the Los Angeles metropolitan area. Am J Psychiatry 1979; 136:1257–1262.
64. Martikainen K, Hasan J, Urponen H, Vuori I, Partinen M. Daytime sleepiness: a risk factor in community life. Acta Neurol Scand 1992; 86:337–341.
65. Ohayon MM, Caulet M, Philip P, Guilleminault C, Priest RG. How sleep complaints and mental disorders are related to complaints of daytime sleepiness. Arch Intern Med 1997; 157:2645–2652.
66. Ford D, Kamerow D. Epidemiologic study of sleep disturbances and psychiatric disorders. An opportunity for prevention? JAMA 1989; 262:1479–1484.
67. Breslau N, Roth T, Rosenthal L, Andreski P. Daytime sleepiness; an epidemiological study of young adults. Am J Public Health 1997; 87:1649–1653.
68. National Sleep Foundation. Omnibus Sleep in America Poll. Washington, DC: National Sleep Foundation. 2001.
69. Bixler EO, Vgontzas AN, Lin HM, Calhoun SL, Vela-Bueno A, Kales A. Excessive daytime sleepiness in a general population sample: the role of sleep apnea, age, obesity, diabetes and depression. J Clin Endocrinol Metab 2005; 90:4510–4515.
70. Resnick HE, Carter EA, Aloia M, Phillips B. Cross-sectional relationship of reported fatigue to obesity, diet, and physical activity: results from the Third National Health and Nutrition Examination Survey. J Clin Sleep Med 2006; 2:163–169.
71. Theorell-Haglöw JE, Lindberg E, Janson C. What are the important risk factors for daytime sleepiness and fatigue in women? Sleep 2006; 29:751–757.
72. Vgontzas AN, Bixler EO, Tan TL, Kantner D, Martin LF, Kales A. Obesity without sleep apnea is associated with daytime sleepiness. Arch Intern Med 1998; 158:1333–1337.
73. Punjabi NM, O'hearn DJ, Neubauer DN, Nieto FJ, Schwartz AR, Smith PL, Bandeen-Roche K. Modeling hypersomnia in sleep-disordered breathing. Am J Respir Crit Care Med 1993; 159:1703–1709.
74. Resta O, Foschino-Barbaro MP, Legari G, Talamo S, Bonfitto P, Palumbo A, Minenna A, Giorgino R, De Pergola G. Sleep-related breathing disorders, loud snoring and excessive daytime sleepiness in obese subjects. Int J Obes Relat Metab Disord 2001; 25:669–675.
75. Resta O, Foschino Barbaro MP, Bonfitto P, Giliberti T, Depalo A, Pannacciulli N, De Pergola G. Low sleep quality and daytime sleepiness in obese patients without obstructive sleep apnoea syndrome. J Intern Med 2003; 253:536–543.
76. Feinberg I. Untreated type 2 diabetes as a cause of daytime somnolence. Sleep 1993; 16:82.
77. Himelein MJ, Thatcher SS. Depression and body image among women with polycystic ovary syndrome. J Health Psychol 2006; 11:613–625.
78. Bruce-Jones WG, White P. Polycystic ovary syndrome and psychiatric morbidity. J Psychosom Obstet Gynaecol 1993; 14: 111–116.
79. Elsenbruch S, Hahn S, Kowalsky D, Offner AH, Schedlowski M, Mann K, Janssen OE. Quality of life, psychosocial well-being and sexual satisfaction in women with polycystic ovary syndrome. J Clin Endocrinol Metab 2003; 88:5801–5807.
80. Elsenbruch S, Benson S, Hahn S, Tan S, Mann K, Pleger K, Kimmig R, Janssen OE. Determinants of emotional distress in women with polycystic ovary syndrome. Hum Reprod 2006; 21:1092–1099.

81. Rasgon NL, Rao RC, Hwang S, Altshuler LL, Elman S, Zuckerbrow-Miller J, Korenman S. Depression in women with polycystic ovary syndrome: clinical and biological correlates. J Affect Disord 2003; 74:299–304.
82. Wiener CL, Primeau M, Ehrmann DA. Androgens and mood dysfunction in women: comparison of women with polycystic ovarian syndrome to healthy controls. Psychosom Med 2004; 66:356–362.
83. Keegan A, Liao LM, Boyle M. 'Hirsutism': a psychological analysis. J Health Psychol 2003; 8:327–45.
84. Hahn S, Janssen OE, Tan S, Pleger K, Mann K, Schedlowski M, Kimmig R, Benson S, Balamitsa E, Elsenbruch S. Clinical and psychological correlates of quality-of-life in polycystic ovary syndrome. Eur J Endocrinol 2005 153:853–860.
85. Calhoun SL, Vgontzas AN, Legro R, Bixler EO. Women with polycystic ovary syndrome are situationally not chronically stressed: therapeutic implications (submitted).

Chapter 13
Polycystic Ovarian Syndrome and Gynaecological Cancer

Alexandra Lawrence and W. Peter Mason

13.1 Introduction

Polycystic ovarian syndrome(PCOS) is the most common female endocrine disturbance and is associated with an increased risk of gynaecological cancers. Endometrial adenocarcinoma has long been associated with PCOS particularly in premenopausal women. Breast cancer is more common in women with PCOS. The studies on epithelial ovarian cancer are conflicting but overall do not suggest a major increase in risk (Fig. 13.1).

Epidemiological studies are difficult to compare due to the difference between diagnostic criteria for PCOS in Europe and North America. A number of studies have also included patients with infertility or non-specific ovarian dysfunction, which causes further clouding of the evidence. In addition, several studies have not corrected for the known effects of obesity.

13.2 Endometrial Cancer

13.2.1 Epidemiology

Endometrial cancer is the second most common cancer of the female genital tract in the United Kingdom after ovarian cancer, affecting 16.8 per 100,000 women in 2004 [1]. The mortality in 2005 was 3.5 per 100,000 women.

An increased incidence of endometrial cancer has long been observed in women with PCOS. In 1957, Jackson reported 16 cases of endometrial cancer in women ranging in age from 27 to 48 years. These women had a high incidence of prolonged amenorrhoea, obesity and hypertension. Of the 15 married women, 13 were nulliparous [2]. A study on 1270 women at the Mayo clinic examined the risk of developing endometrial cancer in the presence of chronic anovulation without hypoestrogenaemia. Compared to the population-based rate, the study group had a relative risk of 3.1 (95% confidence interval 1.1–7.3) with a prevalence of 1% [3]. A large case–control study found an increased risk of endometrial cancer in women with low levels of sex hormone-binding globulin (SHBG) [4] and elevated levels of insulin [5], both of which are characteristic of women with PCOS.

Infertility confers an increased risk of endometrial cancer, in particular anovulatory infertility. A study of 2672 women with primary or secondary infertility with over 31,000 patient years of follow-up showed that these women had a 4.8 times increased risk of developing endometrial cancer as compared to the population mean. The subset of women with anovulatory infertility as opposed to male, mechanical or unclassified had a 10.3-fold increased risk of endometrial cancer [6]. These findings were supported by Escobado in 1991 who carried out a case–control study of 399 women with endometrial cancer below the age of 55 years. Women with

A. Lawrence (✉)
Subspeciality Trainee in Gynaecological Oncology, Hammersmith Hospital, Du Cane Road, London, W12 0HS, UK
e-mail: AlexandraC.Lawrence@imperial.nhs.uk

N.R. Farid, E. Diamanti-Kandarakis (eds.), *Diagnosis and Management of Polycystic Ovary Syndrome*,
DOI 10.1007/978-0-387-09718-3_13, © Springer Science+Business Media, LLC 2009

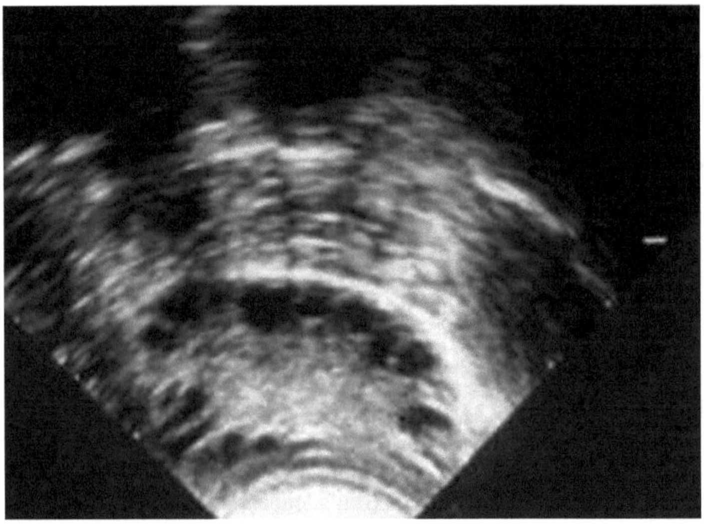

Fig. 13.1 A polycystic ovary with typical increase in ovarian stroma and peripherally distributed cysts

above 2 years of infertility had a 1.7-fold risk, whereas those with infertility due to ovarian factors had a 4.2-fold increased risk [7].

Nulliparity is associated with an increased incidence of endometrial cancer. Brinton investigated 405 women in a multicentre case–control study and found nulliparous women to have a 2.8-fold risk compared to women with a previous pregnancy [8]. Other risk factors for endometrial cancer include hypertension and diabetes with relative risks of 2.1 and 2.8, respectively [9]. Hirsutism and obesity are also factors associated with PCOS. Dahlgren studied Scandinavian women with endometrial cancer and found an increased risk of both hirsutism and obesity in premenopausal and postmenopausal women compared with controls [10]. A high-fat diet increases the likelihood of developing endometrial cancer [11] as does a sedentary lifestyle [12]. Countries with a higher rate of obesity have an increased prevalence of endometrial cancer [13].

13.2.2 Pathogenesis

Prolonged stimulation of the endometrium by oestrogen unopposed by progesterone has been known to be a precursor of endometrial hyperplasia and cancer since 1947 [14]. The chronic anovulation typical of polycystic ovarian syndrome leads to prolonged oestrogen stimulation of the endometrium. Endometrial hyperplasia is a precursor to endometrial carcinoma. Three histopathological types are recognised: simple hyperplasia, complex or adenomatous hyperplasia and complex hyperplasia with atypia. Simple hyperplasia is a common finding in women with anovulatory cycles but has a low rate of progression to endometrial carcinoma (0.4–1.1% [15,16]). Complex hyperplasia has a higher rate of progression to endometrial cancer. There is variation in the reported rate of progression in the literature from 0 to 26.7% due to inclusion of cases with coexistent atypia in earlier studies [17]. More recent studies have provided a clearer definition of the cytological findings and support a low rate of progression [15,16]. Atypical complex hyperplasia is defined by the presence of glands with nuclear atypia. It may coexist with endometrial carcinoma in up to 50% of cases. The reported risk of progression to invasive disease ranges from 22 to 88.9% [15–17] (Figs. 13.2 and 13.3).

A number of oncogenes have been implicated in the development of endometrial cancer. Kohler et al. found mutations of the p53 tumour suppressor gene in 21% of a series of 107 endometrial cancers. Gene mutation was associated with advanced stage of disease with a higher incidence of positive peritoneal cytology and metastatic disease [18]. Further work by the same group demonstrated the absence of p53 mutation in 117 women with endometrial hyperplasia, suggesting that mutation is likely to be a late event in carcinogenesis [19].

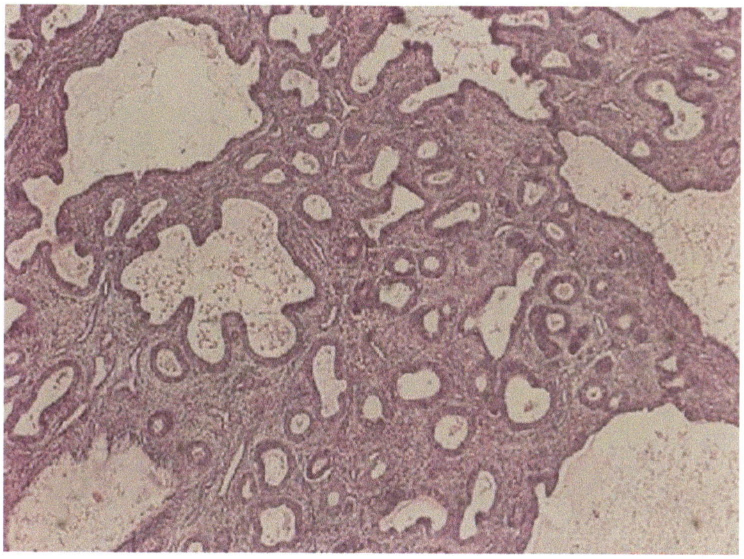

Fig. 13.2 Simple endometrial hyperplasia

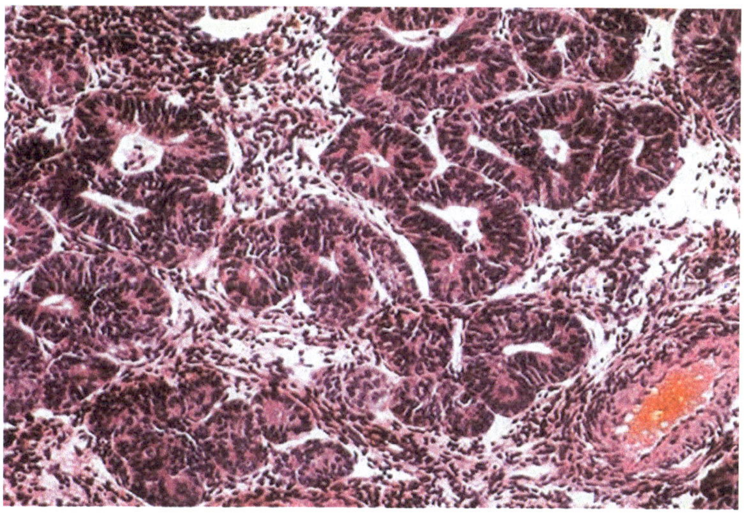

Fig. 13.3 Complex endometrial hyperplasia with atypia

Twenty percent of endometrial cancers demonstrate mutations in the Ki-ras oncogene, the majority of which are on codon 12 and 13. Ki-ras mutations are found in atypical endometrial hyperplasia and endometrial cancer although not in simple hyperplasia or complex hyperplasia without atypia. This suggests that Ki-ras mutation is a relatively early event in endometrial carcinogenesis and is implicated in the progression to atypical hyperplasia [20]. Recent research has demonstrated the overexpression of steroid cell coactivators in the endometrium of women with polycystic ovarian syndrome as compared to healthy volunteers. This increased sensitivity of the endometrium to both estrogens and androgens is a possible mechanism in the development of endometrial hyperplasia and carcinoma [21] (Fig. 13.4).

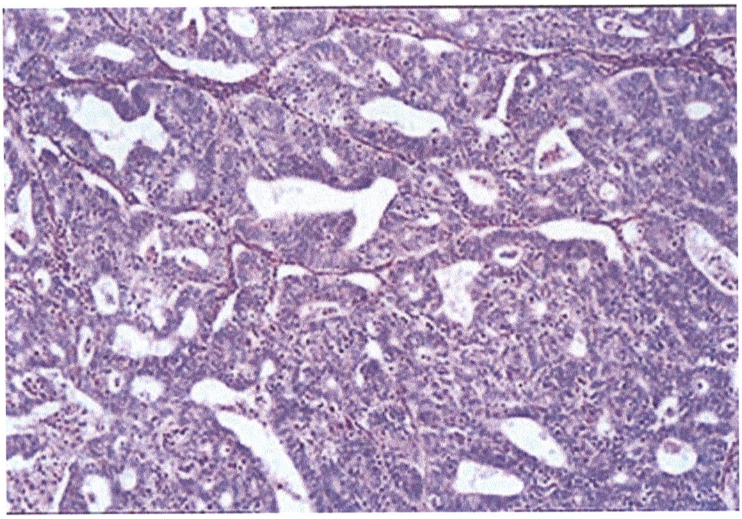

Fig. 13.4 Endometrioid endometrial adenocarcinoma

13.2.3 Screening for Endometrial Cancer

The prevalence of endometrial cancer in the premenopausal population has not been widely investigated. A study including 2586 pre and postmenopausal asymptomatic American women found a background rate of 0.8% endometrial hyperplasia and 0.7% endometrial carcinoma [22].

There is no diagnostic non-invasive screening test available currently. Based on a risk assessment, women are advised to undergo either a blind endometrial sampling or a hysteroscopically directed biopsy. Transvaginal ultrasound is a valuable screening tool for endometrial cancer in postmenopausal women. Both measurement of the endometrial thickness and assessment of the morphology of the endometrium provide high sensitivity in the diagnosis of endometrial carcinoma. A Swedish study including 394 women with postmenopausal bleeding showed a cut off level of 4 mm had 100% sensitivity with 60% specificity in the diagnosis of endometrial cancer and hyperplasia. After 10 years follow-up, no women with an endometrial thickness of less than or equal to 4 mm went on to develop endometrial cancer or hyperplasia [23]. A study of over 400 asymptomatic women on hormonal replacement therapy showed ultrasound to give a high negative predictive value in the exclusion of endometrial pathology with an endometrial thickness of less than 5 mm [24]. The positive predictive value of a measurement of greater than 5 mm was only 9% in this study due to a low prevalence of pathology (Figs. 13.5 and 13.6).

13.2.4 Prevention and Treatment of Endometrial Hyperplasia

Induction of regular withdrawal bleeds in women with oligomenorrhoea or amenorrhoea is accepted as appropriate management in the United Kingdom [25]. It is known that intervals of greater than 3 months between menstruation are associated with an increased risk of endometrial hyperplasia [26]. Most authors advocate shedding of the endometrium at least every 90 days using progestin therapy or the combined oral contraceptive pill to avoid endometrial hyperplasia. An alternative is the use of a progesterone-releasing intrauterine device (Mirena IUS®), which has the additional benefit of providing contraception. In a woman wishing to avoid hormonal manipulation, a pelvic ultrasound is recommended every 6–12 months. An endometrial thickness of greater than 10 mm in an amenorrheic woman should be treated with a withdrawal bleed. If the endometrium remains thick following the bleed, an endometrial biopsy is advised [27].

The choice and duration of progesterone or oral contraceptive treatment are largely empirical. Use of the combined pill in a population of healthy women has shown a reduction of the incidence of endometrial cancer

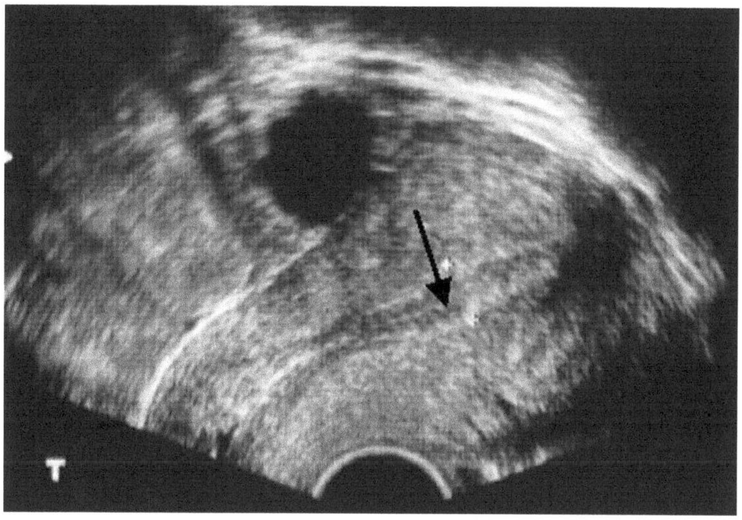

Fig. 13.5 Normal periovulatory endometrium on transvaginal scan. Note the hypoechogenic endometrium with a clear midline echo (*arrowed*)

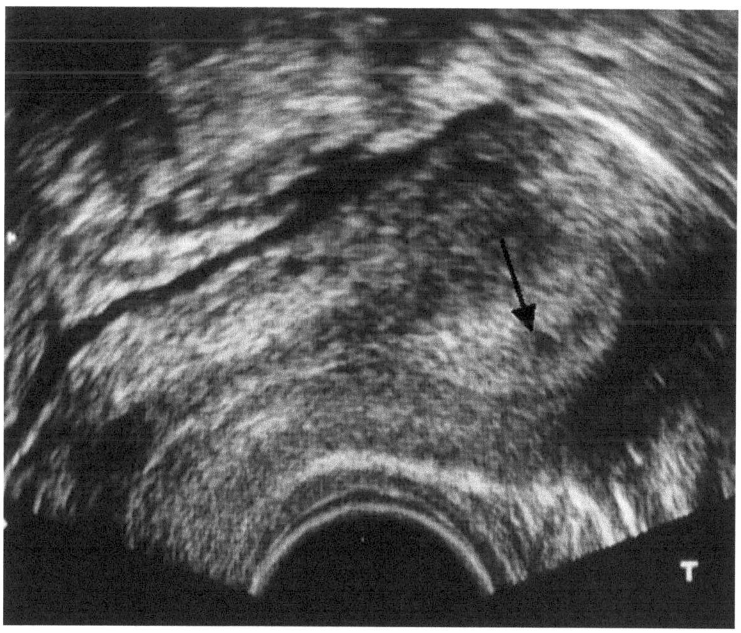

Fig. 13.6 Hyperplastic endometrium demonstrating echogenic endometrium with central hypoechogenic cystic spaces (*arrowed*)

of over 50% for at least 10 years after discontinuation [28,29]. An additional benefit of the contraceptive pill is the reduction in relative risk of epithelial ovarian cancer by 60% [29].

Hyperplasia can be treated conservatively with progestin therapy. Most authors recommend the use of megestrol acetate and follow-up hysteroscopy and endometrial biopsy every three months to ensure regression of the hyperplasia. However, careful follow up for these women is essential. Recently a case of progression of atypical complex hyperplasia after 2 years of progestin treatment has been reported. The woman developed grade 2 endometrioid adenocarcinoma with lymph node metastases at the time of diagnosis [30] (Figs. 13.7, 13.8 and 13.9).

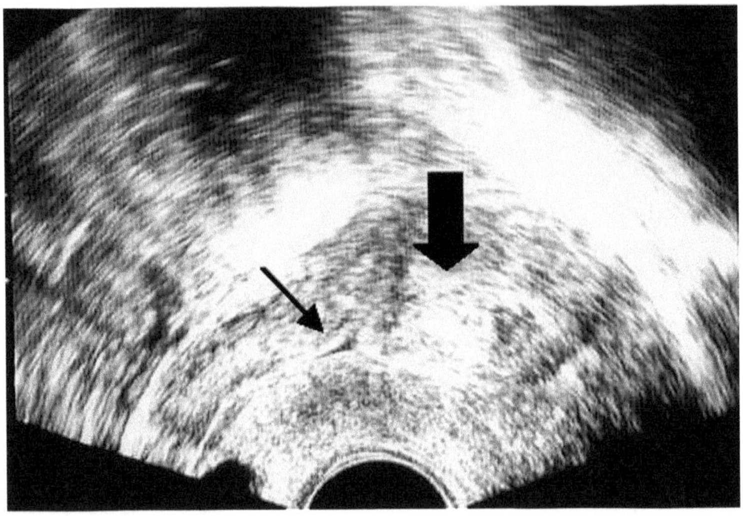

Fig. 13.7 Endometrial polyp occupying the endometrial cavity. It is echogenic with central cystic spaces but the endometrium can be seen surrounding it (*large arrow*) and there is a triangle of hypoechoic fluid below it at the internal os (*small arrow*)

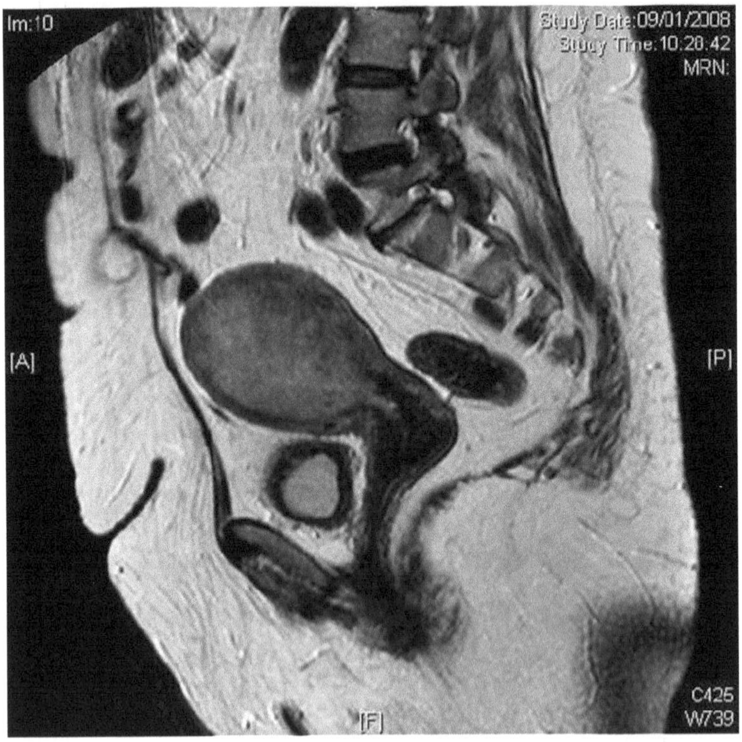

Fig. 13.8 MRI of Stage 1b endometrial cancer. Note the expansion of the endometrial cavity and the projection of the echogenic tissue in the cavity into the myometrium through the junctional zone of the myometrium

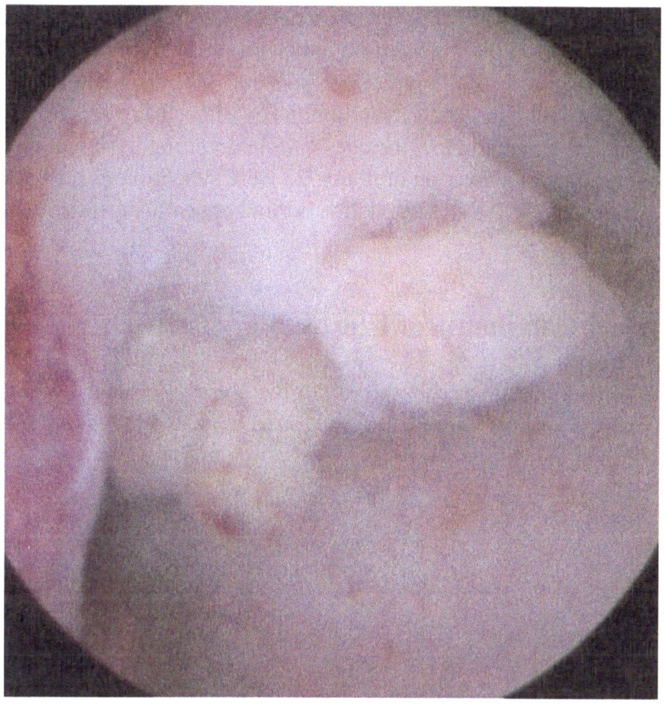

Fig. 13.9 Stage 1a endometrioid adenocarcinoma seen at saline hysteroscopy

13.2.5 Management of Endometrial Cancer

Endometrial cancer has historically been managed with hysterectomy and bilateral salpingo-oophorectomy either abdominally or laparoscopically. This allows assessment of the upper abdomen, peritoneal cavity and diagnostic washing of the peritoneum. A number of young women with PCOS and low-grade endometrioid adenocarcinoma have been managed conservatively. The rationale behind this approach is that this cancer presents early, tends to be well differentiated and is unlikely to metastasise. There is also a clear cause for the development of endometrial cancer in women with polycystic ovarian syndrome, which is amenable to therapy. They are often young women who are desirous of fertility. However, the literature on women with endometrial abnormalities and PCOS suggests that they have impaired fertility both from the factors predisposing to endometrial cancer (obesity, anovulation, impaired glucose tolerance, diabetes) and the presence of abnormal endometrium impairing implantation.

Fechner and Kaufman reported on two such women below the age of 34 years with well-differentiated carcinoma. One woman underwent a wedge resection of the ovaries and subsequently developed a regular menstrual cycle and had no evidence of recurrence 12 years later. The second was treated with clomifene citrate and a wedge resection but underwent a hysterectomy 2 years later for persistent metromenorrhagia. Her hysterectomy specimen showed a Stage 1a endometrial adenocarcinoma [31]. A second series of ten women below the age of 25 years was reported, seven of which had clinical features of PCOS and three had histologically proven polycystic ovaries. Three women were successfully managed with endometrial curettage and high-dose progestagens and one woman went on to have two successful pregnancies. The remaining seven women required a hysterectomy [32]. An Israeli group treated 13 women with progestin therapy and found a complete histological response within 3.5 months in all cases. Six women had a recurrence of cancer, which responded to a second course of progestins [33].

Two separate Japanese groups reported that the response to progestin treatment is associated with the expression of progesterone receptor. The first series treated 12 women with grade 1 disease with 600 mg medroxyprogesterone acetate (MPA) daily. Eight patients required hysterectomy for recurrent disease or no response to treatment and one woman died of metastatic disease to the liver and brain [34]. The second series treated nine women, seven of whom had a complete response to 400 mg MPA daily. Two women developed recurrent disease and both were found to have a synchronous ovarian cancer [35].

A retrospective review of 102 women below the age of 45 undergoing hysterectomy for endometrial cancer, 26 women were found to have epithelial ovarian tumours: 23 were synchronous primary tumours and three were metastases. Interestingly, four women had ovaries with a normal appearance at the time of surgery [36].

13.3 Non-Endometrioid Carcinoma of Uterus

Several anecdotal reports of endometrial adenosarcoma of the uterus in young women with PCOS exist in the literature [37,38]. A 19-year-old woman with PCOS was found to have a malignant mixed mullerian tumour of the endometrium [39]. There have been no case series suggesting an increased risk of these tumours in women with PCOS.

13.3.1 Breast Cancer

Obesity, infertility and hyperandrogenism are all risk factors for the development of breast cancer. This suggests that the incidence of breast cancer may be higher in women with PCOS.

Four large trials have reported on the subject. A retrospective cohort study of 1270 women with chronic anovulation at the Mayo clinic were followed up and compared to population incidence rates for breast cancer. The investigators found five cases of breast cancer in the postmenopausal group against 1.4 expected cases giving a relative risk of 3.6 (95% confidence interval 1.2–8.3). This study did not control for potential confounding factors such as obesity and infertility [40]. A case–control study carried out at Columbia University included 4730 women with breast cancer and 4688 controls. The self-reported rate of PCOS was 0.49 which is lower than other population-based estimates. The odds ratio of breast cancer was 0.52 (95% CI 0.32–0.87) suggesting a protective effect of PCOS [41].

The Iowa Women's Health Study was a prospective cohort study which included 41,837 women of which 1.35% reported a history of PCOS. The findings were of an increased risk of benign breast disease (RR 1.8) but not an increased risk of breast cancer (RR 1.2, 95% CI 0.7–2) after adjustment for age [42]. A UK retrospective cohort study included 786 women with histologically proven PCOS followed up over 30 years. Mortality from breast cancer was the leading cause of death with a standardised mortality ratio of 1.48 (95% CI 0.79–2.54) [43].

13.3.2 Ovarian Cancer

Ovarian cancer is the fourth most common cause of death from malignancy in women in the United Kingdom [44]. There has recently been extensive debate surrounding the incidence of ovarian cancer in infertile women and a potential link to the use of ovulation induction. The incessant ovulation theory proposed by Fathalla in 1971 suggested that ovarian neoplasia resulted from repeated trauma or mitotic activity in the ovarian epithelium following ovulation [45]. Therefore, increasing the number of ovulations using ovulation induction would be expected to increase the risk of ovarian cancer. Conversely, any factor that decreases the number of lifetime ovulations such as pregnancy, lactation, use of the oral contraceptive pill or early menopause would theoretically decrease the ovarian cancer risk. This theory provides an explanation of the observed link between nulliparous women with an early menarche and late menopause, who have multiple ovulations, and an increased risk of ovarian cancer [46]. Women with PCOS who are oligo- or anovulatory might therefore be expected to have a lower risk of ovarian cancer than the general population. However, women who had undergone superovulation might be expected to be at increased risk.

A case–control study of 2197 women with ovarian cancer suggested that infertile nulligravid women had an odds ratio of 2.1 of developing epithelial ovarian cancer. In addition, nulligravid women who had used ovulation induction had an odds ratio of 27.0. These findings were limited by the small numbers of women who had used fertility medication, the lack of detail on the cause of infertility and the type and duration of medication and also a potential recall bias [47]. A further study examining the link between type of infertility, treatment and ovarian cancer included 3837 infertile women. The risk of cancer was increased in ovulatory abnormalities and with the use of clomifene citrate for greater than 12 months (relative risk 11.1) [48].

Few studies have addressed the incidence of ovarian cancer specifically in women with PCOS. The Mayo clinic cohort study showed no increased risk of ovarian cancer in anovulatory women [40]. The Cancer and Steroid Hormone study of 476 women with ovarian cancer below the age of 55 years found an odds ratio of 2.5 (95% CI 1.1–5.9) among women with self-reported PCOS. This risk was higher in women who had never used oral contraceptives (OR 10.5, 95% CI 2.5–44.2). The study included only 31 women with PCOS and the authors acknowledged that there was a possibility of recall bias in the women who were affected by ovarian cancer [49]. The retrospective UK cohort study of women with PCOS showed the standardized mortality rate of ovarian cancer was 0.39 (95% CI 0.01–2.17) [43].

It has been suggested that these findings, although inconclusive, support the choice of the combined oral contraceptive pill to reduce the long-term risk of ovarian cancer in women with PCOS who are not desirous of fertility.

13.4 Conclusion

There is significant evidence to link PCOS with an increased risk of both endometrial hyperplasia and endometrial cancer. The standard management of endometrial cancer is surgical although there have been recent series of successful management with medical treatment. There may be an increased risk of breast cancer in this group of women. However, it is difficult to distinguish the risks attributable to obesity and diabetes from that conferred by PCOS. There is no conclusive evidence of an increased risk of ovarian cancer women with PCOS.

References

1. Office for National Statistics. Cancer statistics – registrations, England, 2004. Series MB1 no. 35. London: Office for National Statistics, 2005.
2. Jackson RL, Dockerty MB. The Stein-Leventhal Syndrome: analysis of 43 cases with special reference to association with endometrial carcinoma. American Journal of Obstetrics and Gynaecology 1957;73:161–173.
3. Coulam CB, Annergers JF, Kranz JS. Chronic anovulation syndrome and associated neoplasia. Obstetrics and Gynecology 1983;61:403–407.
4. Potischman N, Hoover RN, Brinton LA, Siiteri P. Case-control study of endogenous steroid hormones and endometrial cancer. Journal of the National Cancer Institute 1996;88:1127–1135.
5. Troisi R, Potischman N, Hoover RN, Siiteri P, Brinton LA. Insulin and endometrial cancer. American Journal of Epidemiology 1997;146:476–482.
6. Ron E, Lunenfeld B, Menczer J, Blumstein T, Katz L. Cancer incidence in a cohort of infertile women. American Journal of Epidemiology 1987;125:780–790.
7. Escobado LG, Lee NC, Peterson HB, Wingo PA. Infertility associated endometrial cancer risk may be limited to specific subgroups of infertile women. Obstetrics and Gynecology 1991; 77:124–128.
8. Brinton LA, Berman ML, Mortel, R, Twiggs LB, Barrett RJ. Reproductive, menstrual and medical risk factors for endometrial cancer: results from a case control study. American Journal of Obstetrics and Gynaecology 1992;167:1317–1325.
9. Elwood JM, Cole P Rothman KJ. Epidemiology of ovarian cancer. Journal of the National Cancer Institute 1977;59:1055–1060.
10. Dahlgren E, Friberg L-G, Johansson S, Lindstrom B. Endometrial carcinoma; ovarian dysfunction – a risk factor in young women. Journal of Obstetrics, Gynecology and Reproductive Biology 1991;41: 143–150.
11. Key TJ, Allen NE, Spencer EA, Travis RC. The effect of diet on the risk of cancer. Lancet 2002;360:861–868.

12. Levi F, LaVecchia C, Negri E, Franceschi S. Selected physical activities and the risk of endometrial cancer. British Journal of Cancer 1993;67:846–851.
13. Akhmedkhanov A, Zeleniuch-Jacquotte A, Toniolo P. Role of exogenous and endogenous hormones in endometrial cancer: review of the evidence and research perspectives. Annals of the New York Academy of Science 2001;943:296–315.
14. Gusberg SB. Precursors of corpus carcinoma. Estrogens and adenomatous hyperplasia. American Journal of Obstetrics and Gynecology 1947;53:419–423.
15. Kurman R, Kamisnski P, Norris H. The behaviour of endometrial hyperplasia, a long-term study of untreated hyperplasia in 170 patients. Cancer 1985;56:403–412.
16. Lindahl B, Willen R. Spontaneous endometrial endometrial hyperplasia. A prospective, 5 year follow up of 246 patients after abrasion only, including 380 patients followed up for 2 years. Anticancer research 1994;14:2141–2146.
17. Wentz W. Progestin therapy in endometrial hyperplasia. Gynecologic oncology 1974;2:362–367.
18. Kohler M, Berchuck A, Davidoff A. Overexpression and mutation of p53 in endometrial carcinoma. Cancer Research 1992; 52:1622–1625.
19. Kohler M, Nishii H, Humphrey P. Mutation of the p53 tumor-suppressor gene is not a feature of endometrial hyperplasias. American Journal of Obstetrics and Gynecology 1993; 169:690–695.
20. Sasaki H, Nishii H, Takahashi H. Mutation of the Ki-ras protooncogene in human endometrial hyperplasia and carcinoma. Cancer research 1993;53:1906–1911.
21. Gregory C, Wilson E, Apparao K. Steroid receptor coactivator expression throughout the menstrual cycle in normal and abnormal endometrium. Journal of Clinical Endocrinology and Metabolism 2002;85:2960–2966.
22. Koss L, Schreiber K, Oberlander S. Detection of endometrial carcinoma and hyperplasia in asymptomatic women. Obstetrics and Gynecology 1984;64:1–11.
23. Gull B, Karlsson B, Milsom I, Granberg S. Can ultrasound replace dilation and curettage? A longitudinal evaluation of postmenopausal bleeding and transvaginal sonographic measurement of the endometrium as predictors of endometrial cancer. American Journal of Obstetrics and Gynecology 2003;188:401–408.
24. Langer R, Pierce J, O'Hanlan K. Transvaginal ultrasonography compared with endometrial biopsy for the detection of endometrial disease. Postmenopausal estrogen/progestin interventions trial. New England Journal of Medicine 1997;337:1792–1798.
25. RCOG Green Top Guideline No. 33 Long Teem consequences of polycystic ovarian syndrome. May 2003. RCOG Press.
26. Cheung AP. Ultrasound and menstrual history in predicting endometrial hyperplasia in polycystic ovary syndrome. Obstetrics and Gynecology 2001;98:325–331.
27. Balen AH. Polycystic ovary syndrome and cancer. Human Reproductive Update 2001;7:522–525.
28. Hulka B, Chambless L, Kaufman D. Protection against endometrial carcinoma by combination-product oral contraceptives. Journal of the American Medical Association 1982;247:475–477
29. Vessey M, Painter R. Endometrial and ovarian cancer and oral contraceptives-findings in a large cohort study. British Journal of Cancer 1995;71:1340–1342
30. Rubatt JM, Slomovitz BM, Burke TW, Broaddus RR. Development of metastatic endometrial endometrioid adenocarcinoma while on progestin therapy for endometrial hyperplasia. Gynecolgical Oncology 2005;99:472–476.
31. Fechner R, Kaufman R. Endometrial adenocarcinoma in Stein-Leventhal syndrome. Cancer 1974;34:444–452.
32. Farhi D, Nosanchuk J, Silverberg S. Endometrial adenocarcinoma in women under 25 years of age. Obstetrics and Gynecology 1986;68:741–745.
33. Gotlieb WH, Beiner ME, Shalmon B. Outcome of fertility-sparing treatment with progestins in young patients with endometrial cancer. Obstetrics and Gynecology 2003;102:718–725.
34. Ota T, Yoshida M, Kimura M, Kinoshita K. Clinicopathologic study of uterine endometrial carcinoma in young women aged 40 years and younger. International Journal of Gynecological Cancer. 2005;15:657–662.
35. Yamazawa K, Hirai M, Fujito A. Fertility-preserving treatment with progestin, and pathological criteria to predict responses, in young women with endometrial cancer. Human Reproduction 2007;22:1953–1958.
36. Walsh C, Holschneider C, Hoang Y. Coexisting ovarian malignancy in young women with endometrial cancer. Obstetrics and Gynecology 2005;106:693–699.
37. Hallak M, Peipert JF, Heller PB, Sedlacek T, Schauer G. Mullerian adenosarcoma of the uterus with sarcomatous overgrowth. Journal of Surgical Oncology 1992;51:68–70.
38. Press M, Scully R. Endometrial sarcomas complicating ovarian thecoma, polycystic ovarian disease and estrogen therapy. Gynecological Oncology 1985;21:135–154.
39. Chumas J, Mann W, Tseng L. Malignant mixed Mullerian tumour of the endometrium in a young woman with polycystic ovaries. Cancer 1983;52:1478–1481.
40. Coulam C, Annegers J, Kranz J. Chronic anovulation syndrome and associated neoplasia. Obstetrics and Gynecology 1983;61:403–407.
41. Gammon M, Thompson W. Polycystic ovaries and the risk of breast cancer. American Journal of Epidemiology 1991;134: 818–824.
42. Anderson K, Sellers T, Chen P, Rich S, Hong C, Folsom A. Association of Stein-Leventhal syndrome with the incidence of postmenopausal breast carcinoma in a large prospective study of women in Iowa. Cancer 1997;79:494–499.
43. Pierpoint T, McKeigue P, Isaacs A. Mortality of women with polycystic ovarian syndrome at long term follow up. Journal of Clinical Epidemiology 1998;51:581–586.

44. Quinn M, Babb P, Brock A. Cancer trends in England and Wales 1950 to 1999. Studies on medical and population subjects no. 66, 2001, Her Majesty's Stationery Office, London.
45. Fathalla M. Incessant ovulation- a factor in ovarian neoplasia? Lancet 1971; 11:163.
46. McGowan L, Parent L, Lednar W. The woman at risk for developing ovarian cancer. Gynecological Oncology 1979;7:325–344.
47. Whittemore A, Harris R, Itnyre J. Characteristics relating to ovarian cancer risk: collaborative analysis of 12 US case-control studies II. Invasive epithelial cancers in white women. Collaborative ovarian cancer group. American Journal of Epidemiology 1992;136:1212–1220.
48. Rossing M, Daling J, Weiss N. Ovarian tumours in a cohort of infertile women. New England Journal of Medicine 1994;331:771–776.
49. Schildkraut J, Schwingl P, Bastos E, Evanoff A, Hughes C. Epithelial ovarian cancer risk among women with polycystic ovarian syndrome. Obstetrics and Gynecology 1996;88:554–559.

Chapter 14
PCOS, Depression, and Alzheimer's Disease

Pascale G. Stemmle, Heather A. Kenna, and Natalie L. Rasgon

14.1 Introduction

Polycystic ovary syndrome (PCOS) is an endocrine disorder characterized primarily by insulin resistance (IR), as well as hyperandrogenism and chronic anovulation [1]. PCOS is one of the most common endocrine disorders occurring in reproductive-aged women, with an estimated prevalence of between 4 and 6% [2]. Standard PCOS treatment entails insulin-sensitizing medications, such as biguanides (e.g., metformin) or peroxisome proliferator-activated receptors (PPAR) agonists (e.g., rosiglitazone, pioglitazone, and troglitazone) which generally results in improved metabolic and reproductive function in women with PCOS [3]. Depressive disorders are among the most common psychiatric diagnosis in America [4], and data indicate that women have double the lifetime risk of depression compared to men [4–7]. Mood disorders are the leading cause of disability among women aged 15–44 [8].

We were first to postulate a link between PCOS and depressive symptomatology [9], although the pathophysiology of this connection has yet to be fully elucidated. Some evidence suggests that depressive disorders in women with PCOS may be driven by the pathophysiological consequences of IR [10]. As will be discussed in this chapter, IR may be associated with depressive symptomatology via numerous reciprocal interactions in regulating systems.

Depression has been shown to be a significant risk factor for cognitive decline and Alzheimer's disease (AD) [11–17]. We were first to suggest IR as a link between depressive disorders and AD [18, 19], postulating that IR causes inadequate glucose metabolism in the brain, resulting in cognitive dysfunction. Inadequate glucose utilization resulting from IR may underlie neuronal changes in crucial brain regions observed among patients with depressive disorders [18, 19]. Further, such neuronal changes in glucose utilization, if unresolved, may result in treatment-resistant depressive disorders, cumulative cognitive impairment, and eventually, neurodegeneration and facilitation of AD onset.

Although there is no empirical evidence at this point to suggest a direct association between PCOS and AD, PCOS has been directly associated with several other comorbidities that greatly increase risk of AD. These include IR and cardiovascular disease (CVD), in addition to depressive disorders. Herein, we review the evidence linking PCOS with depression, depression with AD, and IR with AD. In addition, CVD is a common thread that may moderate the relationship between PCOS and AD. Taken together, these data indirectly suggest a link between PCOS and AD or cognitive decline.

P.G. Stemmle (✉)
Department of Psychiatry and Behavioral Sciences, Stanford University, School of Medicine, Stanford, CA, USA
e-mail: pascale@stanford.edu

N.R. Farid, E. Diamanti-Kandarakis (eds.), *Diagnosis and Management of Polycystic Ovary Syndrome*,
DOI 10.1007/978-0-387-09718-3_14,

14.2 Depressive Disorders in Women with PCOS

Research has suggested that women with PCOS have high rates of affective disturbances [20], including both depressive disorders [9, 20–22] and bipolar disorder [23]. In the only study to screen for bipolar disorder among women diagnosed with PCOS, Klipstein and Goldberg (2006) found that 24.4% of women with PCOS screened positive for bipolar disorder, using on the Mood Disorders Questionnaire, while 7.7% had a prior diagnosis of bipolar disorder [23]. Only 4% of these subjects had a prior lifetime exposure to treatment with valproate, and none were currently treated with valproate at the time of evaluation. As such, the pharmacologic effects of treatment with valproate compound were not responsible for this relationship. These results suggest that rates of bipolar disorder may be much higher among women in PCOS than in the general population. Most recently, the National Comorbidity Survey Replication estimated the lifetime prevalence of DSM-IV bipolar disorder to be 3.9% [24]. The authors surmised that the reported connection between PCOS and bipolar disorder might be due to a shared hypothalamic–pituitary–gonadal axis defect, although this hypothesis has yet to be evaluated [23].

In our 2003 study, we examined rates of depression among 32 women seeking treatment for PCOS using the Center for Epidemiological Studies Depression Rating Scale (CES-D) [25] self-report measure [9]. Sixteen of these women (50%) exhibited CES-D scores $\geq$16, which are indicative of depression. Notably, depression was significantly associated with greater insulin resistance (p=0.02) and obesity (p=0.05). Analysis of CES-D scores revealed higher rates of depression among untreated women (66%) compared to those receiving oral contraceptive treatment for PCOS (29%). Contrary to previous findings [26–28], we did not find elevated serum bioavailable testosterone in depressed patients with PCOS. Interpretation of our findings was limited by the lack of an age-matched healthy comparison group, as well as by the fact that we utilized a self-report measure without a corresponding clinician-administered diagnostic evaluation. Although the CES-D was designed for and has gained general acceptance as a useful tool for screening depressive symptomatology in primary care settings [29], some researchers have found it to have low specificity and modest positive predictive power for detecting DSM depressive disorders [30–32].

A subsequent study from Weiner and colleagues (2004) compared a BMI-matched sample of 27 women with PCOS to 27 women with normal menstruation cycles [20]. Both state and trait depression were significantly increased among women with PCOS, and these differences remained statistically significant even after controlling for the moderating effects of physical symptomatology (e.g., acne, body dissatisfaction) and other mood states (e.g., anxiety, aggression). This study reported a curvilinear relationship between negative mood and free testosterone (FT) levels. Whereas the highest negative mood-scale scores were associated with FT values just beyond the upper limits of normal, lower negative mood scores corresponded to both normal and extremely high values of FT. This curvilinear pattern was an unexpected finding and has yet to be replicated by other researchers. The authors postulated that women with the highest FT values may have suffered from a more extreme form of PCOS and may have cycled less than those with lower FT values. Alternatively, they suggested that these women may have become desensitized to the higher levels of FT, such that they no longer contributed to producing negative affect.

Elsenbruch and colleagues (2003) reported higher scores for depression, using the German version of the Symptom Checklist Revised (SCL-90), in 50 women with PCOS compared to 50 healthy controls [21]. However, the results of this study may have been affected by a selection bias, since one-third of PCOS patients in this sample were referred to the study by a gynecologist due to infertility problems. Oddens and colleagues (1999) found that women with infertility problems experienced more negative emotional feelings while trying to conceive than women who conceived spontaneously [33]. Further, as our own review of the literature suggests, a range of existing studies suggest that mood disorders and fertility are related in a complex way [34], and there is still much to be learned about the specifics of this relationship. These findings suggest that infertility may have mediating effects on the relationship between PCOS and depressive disorders.

Most recently, Hollinrake and colleagues (2007) used the Primary Care Evaluation of Mental Disorders Patient Health Questionnaire (PRIME-MD PHQ) to evaluate depressive symptoms in 103 PCOS patients and 103 control subjects [22]. They found that women with PCOS were at an increased risk for depressive disorders compared with controls (21% compared to 3%; odds ratio 5.11 [95% confidence interval (CI) 1.26–20.69]; $p<0.03$). The overall risk of depressive disorders in women with PCOS was 4.23 (95% CI 1.49–11.98; $p<0.01$), which was independent of obesity and infertility. Compared with non-depressed PCOS subjects, depressed PCOS subjects had a higher body mass index (BMI) ($p<0.01$) and elevated fasting insulin ($p<0.02$). Although several previous studies have suggested that elevated androgens in women with PCOS may influence mood [26, 28], the results of this study did not find a significant difference in ovarian or adrenal androgen levels between depressed and non-depressed PCOS subjects [22]. Of note, a large percentage of the women with PCOS in this sample (47% compared to 6% of controls, $p<0.05$) were attempting pregnancy at the time of assessment. However, among depressed women with PCOS, there was no significant difference in infertility rates compared to non-depressed women with PCOS. These results would suggest that the relationship between depression and PCOS is not necessarily related to fertility problems [22].

14.2.1 Psychosocial Aspects of PCOS: Additional Contribution to Depression

Although PCOS is a neuroendocrine disorder, its phenotype is likely to cause a significant level of emotional distress [35]. Changes in physical appearance that are associated with PCOS, particularly hirsutism, cystic acne, seborrhea, alopecia, and obesity [36] may negatively affect self-esteem. Up to 50% of women with PCOS are overweight or obese [37]. In addition, the disorder's effect on female fertility may also be a significant stressor. PCOS is associated with irregular menstrual periods (dysmenorrhea) or the absence of menstruation altogether (amenorrhea), as well as difficulty conceiving, and sometimes, changes in sexual attitudes and behaviors [38]. The impact of these disturbances on psychosocial well-being is significant, since PCOS typically manifests during a time when women may be focused on partnering and starting a family. Finally, the long-term medical sequelae associated with PCOS, including non-insulin dependent type-2 diabetes and risk of cardiovascular events, including atherosclerosis, may also negatively affect psychosocial well-being. Women with PCOS have also been found to report feeling anxiety and frustration as a result of their diagnosis of PCOS [39].

Indeed, several studies have examined health-related quality of life (QoL) in patients with PCOS. Elsenbruch et al (2003) investigated the impact of PCOS on psychological well-being [21], QoL, and sexuality in 50 women with PCOS and 50 age-matched controls. PCOS patients and healthy controls did not differ with respect to education, family status, or employment, yet they exhibited greater psychological disturbances, as measured by the SCL-90-R [40], in the obsessive-compulsive, depression, anxiety, interpersonal sensitivity, aggression, and psychoticism domains.

PCOS patients and healthy controls also completed two self-report QoL measures: the FLZ [41], which assesses satisfaction with various aspects of life, including health, work, finances, leisure activities, marriage/relationship, self, sexuality, friends/relatives, and living conditions; and the MOS SF-36 [42], which assesses health-related quality of life (HRQL). Women with PCOS reported a lower degree of life satisfaction as measured by the FLZ with respect to health, self, and sexuality. Women with PCOS also reported significantly decreased scores on the SF-36 for physical role function, bodily pain, vitality, social function, emotional role function, and mental health. Finally, although both women with PCOS and controls rated having a satisfying sex life as equally important, women with PCOS reported feeling significantly less satisfied with their sex life and less sexually attractive [21].

The authors of this study recognized the potentially confounding effects of obesity and performed additional analyses using BMI as the covariate. After adjusting for BMI, women with PCOS still reported significantly lower HRQL in the domains of physical role function, vitality, emotional role function, and mental health. Differences in life satisfaction in the areas of health, self, and sexuality also remained statistically significant after controlling for BMI. Scores on the SCL-90-R depression dimension were still significantly different for women with PCOS after controlling for BMI [21]. However, as mentioned above, the high prevalence of infertility problems in this sample is also a potential confound. In our own research, depression was highly correlated with BMI, but did not correlate with other possibly distressing physical symptoms of PCOS, such as hirsutism, irregular menses, alopecia, or acne [9].

14.3 Cardiovascular Disease and PCOS

A growing body of evidence supports a relationship between PCOS and depression. In addition, a number of recent studies have suggested that depression is a risk factor for the development of CVD [43]. Several associated features of PCOS are established risk factors for CVD. These factors, specifically obesity, insulin resistance, and immunological responses, will be briefly reviewed herein. Finally, although the precise risk of CVD in women with PCOS remains unclear, we review a growing body of evidence that points to a possible increased risk of cardiovascular events in women with menstrual abnormalities and hyperandrogenism.

14.3.1 Obesity

Obesity is a common feature of PCOS [44]. Up to 50% of women with PCOS are overweight or obese [37], compared to approximately one-third of the general population [45]. Obese PCOS patients, particularly those with an abdominal obesity phenotype, tend to be more insulin resistant and more hyperinsulinemic than their normal-weight counterparts [37, 46]. Even if they are normal weight, individuals with PCOS tend to have a higher proportion of abdominal body fat [47, 48]. Although the exact nature of the relationship between the weight gain and the development of PCOS is not clear, one possibility is that obesity may intensify the degree of insulin resistance and hyperinsulinemia in these individuals [44].

Abdominal fat accumulation is associated with an increase in low-grade chronic inflammation [49], insulin resistance [47], and metabolic dysfunction in women with PCOS [50]. Several studies have clearly demonstrated that menstrual abnormalities are more frequent in obese women with PCOS compared to normal-weight PCOS women [51]. Moreover, there is evidence that a reduced incidence of pregnancy as well as a blunted responsiveness to pharmacological treatments that induce ovulation (such as clomiphene citrate) may be more common in obese PCOS women [52]. Finally, obesity in general and abdominal fat in particular are established risk factors for the development of cardiovascular disease (CVD) [53].

14.3.2 Insulin Resistance (IR)

Insulin resistance is a primary characteristic of women with PCOS. Research has demonstrated higher rates of IR in populations of women with PCOS, with findings that up to 40% of women with PCOS exhibit this abnormality [54, 55]. IR has been found among both lean and obese women with PCOS, and rates are thought to be higher in both groups than in the general populations [56]. IR may be more severe among anovulatory women with PCOS compared to ovulatory women with polycystic ovaries [57]. As might be expected given the higher rates of IR, women with PCOS also show a higher prevalence of non-insulin dependent type-2 diabetes (NIDDM) (estimated at 7.5–10%) and impaired glucose tolerance (estimated at 31 to 35%) [58]. It has been reported that the rate of conversion from impaired glucose tolerance to type-2 diabetes increases 5 to 10-fold in PCOS populations [54, 59, 60]. In a study of 28 women who had undergone ovarian wedge resection compared to 752 controls, Cibula and colleagues found that 32% of women with PCOS had NIDDM, compared to 8% of controls ($p<0.001$) [61]. Wild and colleagues reported that PCOS women had lower HDL levels, higher LDL/HDL ratios, and higher triglyceride levels than regularly menstruating women [62], which may suggest insulin resistance [63, 64] and are also established risk factors for cardiovascular disease [65–68]. Finally, prospective research by Solomon and colleagues (2001) suggests that women with PCOS-like menstrual abnormalities may be at significantly increased risk for the development of type-2 diabetes, independent of obesity [60]. Compared to women with a typical cycle length of 26–31 days at age 18–22 years, the relative risk (RR) of type-2 diabetes among women with long menstrual cycles was 2.08 (95% confidence interval [CI], 1.62–2.66), after adjusting for BMI at age 18, family history of type-2 diabetes, physical activity level, cigarette smoking, weight change, age, race, and use of oral contraceptives. The RR for type-2 diabetes was not significantly increased among women with a short cycle length. The RR of type-2 diabetes associated with long menstrual cycles was greater in obese women, but was also increased in non-obese women [60], suggesting that this relationship may be somewhat independent of weight gain.

14.3.3 Elevated Immunological Response

Women with PCOS demonstrate other risk factors for CVD, such as elevated immunological response, which are in turn closely linked to obesity. Multiple reports have found significantly increased serum concentrations of hsCRP, IL-6, and increased numbers of leukocytes, granulocytes, and lymphocytes in women with PCOS compared to healthy controls [69, 70]. In the only study to examine the correlation between depression and immune markers in women with PCOS, Benson (2008) found that depression, assessed using the German version of the Beck Depression Inventory, was not associated with increases in the inflammatory markers hsCRP, IL-6, and leukocytes. These markers were, however, significantly increased in women with PCOS compared to healthy controls (although controls were not matched by BMI). Further, these markers were correlated with BMI and several cardiovascular risk factors, such as HDL, diastolic blood pressure, and insulin resistance. This data would suggest that the primary association between PCOS and immune activation is due to obesity, rather than other factors of the disorder [69]. In either case, these inflammatory processes can lead to the subclinical CVD and impairment of endothelial structure that have been reported in PCOS women [71–75].

14.3.4 Risk of CVD in Women with PCOS

The precise risk of CVD in women with PCOS remains unclear, due to a paucity of prospective studies examining cardiovascular events or mortality in this population. However, a few studies do call attention to a possible increased risk of cardiovascular events in women with menstrual abnormalities and hyperandrogenism.

Most recently, Shaw and colleagues (2008) evaluated the risk of cardiovascular events in 390 postmenopausal women [76]. Clinical features of PCOS were considered present if a woman had a premenopausal history of irregular menses and current biochemical evidence of hyperandrogenemia. Twenty-seven percent of the sample met this criterion (n=104). Diabetes (p=0.0001), obesity, (p= 0.005), metabolic syndrome (p=0.0001), insulin resistance (p=0.0001), and angiographic coronary artery disease (p=0.04) were significantly more likely among women with clinical features of PCOS. Almost one-third (32%) of women with PCOS-like features had coronary artery disease, compared to 25% of women without PCOS-like features. At 5-year follow-up, women with clinical features of PCOS had a significantly lower cardiovascular event-free survival rate (p=0.006) than women without clinical features of PCOS (78.9% for women with clinical features of PCOS (n=104), compared to 88.7% for women without clinical features of PCOS (n= 286)) [76].

Solomon and colleagues (2002) examined fatal and nonfatal cardiovascular events at 14-year follow-up in women with a self-reported history of irregular menses at baseline [77]. Because they did not examine clinical and biochemical indicators of PCOS –associated hyperandrogenism, per the Rotterdam criteria [78], they could not confirm a diagnosis of PCOS. However, because PCOS is frequently the reason for irregular menses, they speculated that many women in the sample did suffer from the disorder [77]. Menstrual cycle regularity was assessed by a retrospective self-report question administered to all participants at study inception. Women with a self-report of very irregular menses had a 50% higher risk of fatal and nonfatal coronary heart disease (CHD) compared to controls. This elevated risk remained statistically significant after adjusting for several known risk factors of CVD, including BMI, cigarette smoking, parity, oral contraceptive use, alcohol intake, aspirin, multivitamin use, vitamin E use, menopausal status, and postmenopausal hormone use (RR = 1.53; 95% CI = 1.24–1.90; trend for increasing irregularity, $p < 0.0001$). Increased risks were observed for both nonfatal myocardial infarction (multivariate RR = 1.38; 95% CI = 1.06–1.80) and fatal CHD (multivariate RR = 1.88; 95% CI = 1.32–2.67). The authors concluded that menstrual irregularity may be a marker of underlying metabolic dysfunction, which may predispose an individual to increased risk of CVD [77]. Increased risk of myocardial infarction [79], coronary atherosclerosis, elevated triglycerides, and low HDL-C levels [80] have also been reported among women with PCOS.

Not all studies have demonstrated an association between PCOS and CVD [79, 80]. Pierpoint et al (1998) identified 786 women who were previously diagnosed with PCOS by wedge resection of the ovaries [83] and followed them through their medical records over a 30-year period [79]. The authors reported that rates of death from ischemic heart disease or circulatory disease were not greater among women with PCOS than the national rates of death from these causes. The authors also conducted follow-up with survivors, and again failed to find increased rates of cardiovascular mortality among women with PCOS compared to controls [80]. However, women with PCOS did have higher levels of several cardiovascular risk factors: diabetes ($p = 0.002$) hypertension ($p = 0.04$), hypercholesterolemia ($p < 0.001$), hypertriglyceridemia ($p = 0.02$), and increased waist to hip ratio ($p = 0.004$). After controlling for BMI, odds ratios were 2.2 (0.9–5. 2) for diabetes, 1.4 (0.9–2.0) for hypertension, and 3.2 (1.7–6.0) for hypercholesterolemia. A history of coronary heart disease (CHD) was not significantly more common in women with PCOS (crude odds ratio [95% CI] =1.5 [0.7–2.9]) but the crude odds ratio for cerebrovascular disease was 2.8 (1.1–7.1) [80].

Although there are no prospective studies that clearly demonstrate increased risk of CVD in women with PCOS, the above studies suggest that women with PCOS may be at increased risk of fatal and nonfatal cardiovascular events, as do a number of other studies which have found that women with PCOS exhibit evidence of subclinical cardiovascular disease [81, 82].

14.4 PCOS and Alzheimer's Disease

14.4.1 Cognitive Performance in Women with PCOS

To date, there are no studies that examine whether women with PCOS are at increased risk of developing cognitive decline or dementia. However, several studies have suggested that testosterone plays a role in cognitive performance. The results of these studies suggest that higher levels of testosterone in women may enhance performance on tasks of visuospatial ability [83–88] while impairing performance on tasks of verbal fluency and verbal memory [89, 90]. However, these studies have utilized healthy women, not women with an endocrinologic disorder that causes hyperandrogenemia, such as PCOS. As such, they have administered exogenous doses of testosterone after the pre-test battery in order to measure its effect on post-test performance.

A recent study by Schattman and Sherwin investigated the possible influence of testosterone on cognitive functioning in women with PCOS [91]. They hypothesized that women with PCOS would perform better than controls on masculinized tasks (such as visuospatial tasks) and worse than controls on female-favored tasks (such as verbal fluency ad verbal memory). Twenty-nine women with PCOS and 22 age- and education-matched healthy control women completed a battery of neuropsychological tests and underwent a blood draw to measure testosterone levels. Women with PCOS had significantly higher levels of free testosterone and demonstrated significantly poorer performance on tests of verbal fluency, verbal memory, manual dexterity, and visuospatial working memory than healthy control women. However, no differences between the groups were found on tests of mental rotation, spatial visualization, spatial perception, or perceptual speed [87].

Although these findings may point to differential verbal abilities in women with PCOS compared to controls, it is difficult to state with certainty that these differences are due to the influence of higher levels of testosterone. As noted by the authors, there is another culprit that could possibly account for this difference, impaired glucose tolerance [91]. Glucose testing was not performed on this sample, so it is impossible to know whether insulin resistance was present in PCOS patients. As discussed below, IR is associated with cognitive decline in both diabetic and non-diabetic individuals. The authors hypothesize that because women with PCOS had a mean BMI of 27.5, they were unlikely to be IR. However, as described by Abbasi, IR can be present in lean, non-diabetic individuals [92].

In a follow-up study, Schattmann and Sherwin [93] examined cognitive function in 19 PCOS women, who completed a battery of neuropsychological tests before and after being randomized to 3 months of treatment with either an androgen receptor antagonist (cyproterone acetate) plus estrogen or a placebo. Hormone treatment of women with PCOS was effective in that it caused a significant reduction in free testosterone levels, but did not affect performance on tests visuospatial ability, verbal memory, manual dexterity, or perceptual speed. Women treated with hormone therapy did significantly improve on one test of verbal fluency compared to their own pre-treatment scores ($p<0.01$), but not on a second test of verbal fluency.

The findings reported by Schattmann and Sherwin are novel, and pose several interesting questions for future research efforts. First, the selection of 3 months treatment time is arbitrary. PCOS is a chronic condition, and there is no reason to suggest that changes in cognitive functioning could be observed during this short-time frame. A longer treatment interval may produce different results. Second, PCOS is a disorder that has an impact on many different hormones in the reproductive milieu. In addition to hyperandrogenism, PCOS is frequently characterized by low-normal levels of follicle stimulating hormone (FSH), in conjunction with increased levels of luteinizing hormone (LH) [94, 95]. These abnormalities reflect an increase in gonadotropin releasing hormone (GnRH) release, and possibly an underlying dysregulation of the hypothalamic system [96]. The specific role these hormones might play in altering cognitive performance among women with PCOS is not clear. Finally, cyproterone acetate is a medication that exerts multiple endocrinological effects [93]; it suppresses the actions of testosterone and luteinizing hormone and also functions as a weak progestational agonist. Thus, it is possible that changes in serum levels of other hormones may have been responsible for the results observed in this study.

Finally, in a large Internet-based study, Barnard et al. (2007) compared performance on computerized cognitive neuropsychological tests in right-handed women with and without PCOS. The sample was first stratified according to use of anti-androgen medications and level of depression. Performance on visuospatial tasks, including mental rotation and spatial location, did not differ between groups. However, women with PCOS demonstrated slightly impaired performance in terms of speed and accuracy on reaction time and word recognition tasks [97].

Taken together, these findings do not bear out the hypothesis that women with PCOS show masculinized performance on neuropsychological tests due to increased serum testosterone levels. However, there is some evidence to suggest that women with PCOS may show a slight impairment in verbal abilities, although it is not yet clear why this may be the case. More research is needed to characterize the cognitive deficits seen in women with PCOS, to chart these deficits prospectively, and to determine whether they can be improved with treatment.

14.4.2 Associated Conditions of PCOS may also Confer Risk of AD

There are several conditions associated with PCOS that have clear evidence of association with the development of Alzheimer's disease (AD), vascular dementia, and other disorders of cognitive decline. The finding that about half of women with PCOS also suffer from depressive disorders, as described earlier in this chapter, suggests a possible connection between PCOS and AD. Several lines of neurochemical, neuropsychological, and radiological evidence demonstrate an association between depression and Alzheimer's disease (AD), which are both characterized by significant cognitive dysfunction [98]. Increasing data show that IR, the primary feature of PCOS, is a pathological link between depression and risk of AD [18, 19]. Aside from the other deleterious effects of IR, such as stiffening of the arterial walls [99], it is thought that peripheral IR also leads to inadequate glucose metabolism in the brain, resulting in cognitive dysfunction. As we have postulated, when inadequate glucose utilization occurs in the IR patient, it leads to neuronal changes in crucial brain regions that appear to modulate mood and higher thinking in depressive disorders [18, 19]. Further, such neuronal alteration in glucose utilization, if unresolved, may result in treatment-resistant depression, cumulative cognitive impairment, and eventually, more widespread neurodegeneration and facilitation of the onset of AD.

Depression itself has been shown to be a significant risk factor in the development of AD and in more debilitating cognitive dysfunction once AD develops [11, 12, 14–17, 100]. Further, depression is often a prodromal symptom in clinical cases of AD [101–108]. Most recently, a meta-analysis by Ownby et al. found that rather than being a prodromal symptom, depression is rather a risk factor for development of AD, as demonstrated by the long interval between diagnosis of depression and AD [109]. Given that even young and middle-aged depressed patients show problems with memory and attention [110], further investigation of the relationship between depression and dementia is warranted.

Epidemiological data suggest a relationship between depression and AD, although study designs and results have been mixed (for review, see [109]). Complicating the investigation of depression as a risk factor for AD is the temporal onset of depression with respect to cognitive decline and AD. [11–17, 111–114], as the majority of studies have examined depression in late-life (60 years of age and older). However, data have shown a significantly increased prevalence of AD in patients with a history of depression, even when the depression occurred more than 25 years prior to onset of AD [111] and increasing risk with increasing number of depressive episodes [112].

A number of large population-based studies of type II diabetes IR provide evidence of a strong association with dementia, as well as cognitive deficits in non-demented older adults [115–123]. Contrary to these results, a recent post-mortem study found a negative association between type II diabetes and AD neuropathology [124]. However, these results raise the possibility that the link between type II diabetes and dementia may be specific to as yet ill-defined subgroups of dementia and patients with deficits in glucose utilization. In fact, AD has recently been proposed to be a kind of "Type 3 diabetes" because of its combination of cognitive and neuroendocrine abnormalities [125]. Furthermore, longitudinal studies report an association of hyperinsulinemia with greater risk of AD and decline in memory [126, 127].

Presence of obesity may obscure findings on potential IR links between DD and AD, given that obesity is highly correlated with degree of IR. One large longitudinal study found a positive correlation between obesity and AD development later in life [128], while two other large longitudinal studies found no association between obesity at midlife and AD prevalence in late-life [129, 130]. Research has shown that even lean individuals can have IR [131], and differences in IR within lean individuals appears to be due to the differences in postprandial skeletal muscle glycogen synthesis and net hepatic triglyceride synthesis [132].

14.5 Conclusion

A growing body of evidence suggests a relationship between PCOS and affective disorders, including both depression and bipolar disorder, although the pathophysiology of these connections has yet to be elucidated. While there is no empirical evidence at this time to support a direct association between PCOS and AD, PCOS is directly linked with several other comorbidities that greatly increase risk of AD, including IR and CVD, in addition to depression. PCOS may also be associated with differing cognitive abilities in women, specifically mild impairment in verbal abilities. More research is needed to clarify whether a direct relationship might exist between PCOS and AD, or whether risk is conferred by the obesity, IR, and depression frequently seen in women with PCOS. Nonetheless, clinicians should be mindful of a history of PCOS in patients presenting with cognitive complaints.

References

1. Dunaif A. Current concepts in the polycystic ovary syndrome. Annu Rev Med 2001;52:401–419.
2. Franks S. Polycystic ovary syndrome. N Engl J Med 1995;333(13):853–861.
3. Dunaif A. The insulin-sensitizing agent troglitazone improves metabolic and reproductive abnormalities in the polycystic ovary syndrome. J Clin Endocrinol Metab 1996;81(9):3299–3306.
4. Kessler RC, McGonagle KA, Swartz M, Blazer DG, Nelson CB. Sex and depression in the National Comorbidity Survey. I: lifetime prevalence, chronicity and recurrence. J Affect Disord 1993;29(2–3):85–96.
5. Bebbington P, Dunn G, Jenkins R, et al. The influence of age and sex on the prevalence of depressive conditions: report from the National Survey of Psychiatric Morbidity. Psychol Med 1998;28(1):9–19.
6. Nolen-Hoeksema S. Sex differences in depression. Stanford: Stanford University Press; 1990.
7. Weissman MM. Cross-national epidemiology of major depression and bipolar disorder. JAMA 1996;276(4):293–299.
8. Murray CJL, Lopez AD. Alternative visions of the future: projecting mortality and disability, 1990–2020. In: Murray CJL, Lopez AD, eds. The Global Burden of Disease: A Comprehensive Assessment of Mortality and Disability from Diseases, Injuries, and Risk Factors in 1990 and Projected to 2020. Boston: Harvard University Press; 1996:325–395.

9. Rasgon NL, Rao RC, Hwang S, et al. Depression in women with polycystic ovary syndrome: clinical and biochemical correlates. J Affect Disord 2003;74(3):299–304.
10. Rasgon NL, Carter MS, Elman S, Bauer M, Love M, Korenman SG. Common treatment of polycystic ovarian syndrome and major depressive disorder: case report and review. Curr Drug Targets Immune Endocr Metabol Disord 2002;2(1):97–102.
11. Cooper B, Holmes C. Previous psychiatric history as a risk factor for late-life dementia: a population-based case-control study. Age Ageing 1998;27:181–188.
12. French LR, Schuman LM, Mortimer JA, Hutton JT, Boatman RA, Christians B. A case-control study of dementia of the Alzheimer type. Am J Epidemiol 1985;121(3):414–421.
13. Kokmen E, Beard CM, Chandra V, Offord KP, Schoenberg BS, Ballard DJ. Clinical risk factors for Alzheimer's disease: a population-based case-control study. Neurology 1991;41(9):1393–1397.
14. Shalat SL, Seltzer B, Pidcock C, Baker EL. Risk factors for Alzheimer's disease: a case-control study. Neurology 1987;37(10):1630–1633.
15. Speck CE, Kukull WA, Brenner DE, et al. History of depression as a risk factor for Alzheimer's disease. Epidemiology 1995;6(4):366–369.
16. Steffens DC, Plassman BL, Helms MJ, Welsh-Bohmer KA, Saunders AM, Breitner JC. A twin study of late-onset depression and apolipoprotein E epsilon 4 as risk factors for Alzheimer's disease. Biol Psychiatry 1997;41(8):851–856.
17. Wetherell JL, Gatz M, Johansson B, Pedersen NL. History of depression and other psychiatric illness as risk factors for Alzheimer disease in a twin sample. Alzheimer Dis Assoc Disord 1999;13(1):47–52.
18. Rasgon N, Jarvik GP, Jarvik L. Affective disorders and Alzheimer disease: a missing-link hypothesis. Am J Geriatr Psychiatry 2001;9(4):444–445.
19. Rasgon NL, Jarvik L. Insulin resistance, affective disorders, and Alzheimer's disease: review and hypothesis. J Gerontol A Biol Sci Med Sci 2004;59(2):178–183.
20. Weiner CL, Primeau M, Ehrmann DA. Androgens and mood dysfunction in women: comparison of women with polycystic ovarian syndrome to healthy controls. Psychosom Med 2004;66(3):356–362.
21. Elsenbruch S, Hahn S, Kowalsky D, et al. Quality of life, psychosocial well-being, and sexual satisfaction in women with polycystic ovary syndrome. J Clin Endocrinol Metab 2003;88(12):5801–5807.
22. Hollinrake E, Abreu A, Maifeld M, Van Voorhis BJ, Dokras A. Increased risk of depressive disorders in women with polycystic ovary syndrome. Fertil Steril 2007;87(6):1369–1376.
23. Klipstein KG, Goldberg JF. Screening for bipolar disorder in women with polycystic ovary syndrome: a pilot study. J Affect Disord 2006;91:205–209.
24. Kessler RC, Berglund P, Demler O, Jin R, Merikangas KR, Walters EE. Lifetime prevalence and age-of-onset distributions of DSM-IV disorders in the National Comorbidity Survey Replication. Arch Gen Psychiatry 2005;62:593–602.
25. Radloff L. The CES-D Scale: a self-report depression scale for research in the general population. Appl Psych Meas 1977;1(3):385–401.
26. Baischer W, Koinig G, Hartmann B, Huber J, Langer G. Hypothalamic-pituitary-gonadal axis in depressed premenopausal women: elevated blood testosterone concentrations compared to normal controls. Psychoneuroendocrinology 1995;20(5):553–559.
27. Shulman LH, DeRogatis L, Spielvogel R, Miller JL, Rose LI. Serum androgens and depression in women with facial hirsutism. J Am Acad Dermatol 1992;27(2 Pt 1):178–181.
28. Weber B, Lewicka S, Deuschle M, Colla M, Heuser I. Testosterone, androstenedione and dihydrotestosterone concentrations are elevated in female patients with major depression. Psychoneuroendocrinology 2000;25(8):765–771.
29. Brantley PJ, Mehan DJJ, Thomas JL. The Beck Depression Inventory (BDI) and the Center for Epidemiologic Studies Depression scale (CES-D). In: Maruish MM, ed. Handbook of Psychological Assessment in Primary Care Settings. New Jersey: Lawrence Erlbaum Associates, Inc.; 1999.
30. Coyne JC, Schwenk TL. The relationship of distress to mood disturbance in primary care and psychiatric populations. J Consult Clin Psychol 1997;65(1):161–168.
31. Myers JK, Weissman MM. Use of a self-report symptom scale to detect depression in a community sample. Am J Psychiatry 1980;137(9):1081–1084.
32. Schulberg HC, Saul M, McClelland M, Ganguli M, Christy W, Frank R. Assessing depression in primary medical and psychiatric practices. Arch Gen Psychiatry 1985;42(12):1164–1170.
33. Oddens BJ, den Tonkelaar I, Nieuwenhuyse H. Psychosocial experiences in women facing fertility problems—a comparative survey. Hum Reprod 1999;14(1):255–261.
34. Williams KE, Marsh WK, Rasgon NL. Mood disorders and fertility in women: a critical review of the literature and implications for future research. Hum Reprod Update 2007;13(6):607–616.
35. Eggers S, Kirchengast S. The polycystic ovary syndrome–a medical condition but also an important psychosocial problem. Coll Antropol 2001;25(2):673–685.
36. Venkatesan AM, Dunaif A, Corbould A. Insulin resistance in polycystic ovary syndrome: progress and paradoxes. Recent Prog Horm Res 2001;56(1):295–308.
37. Pasquali R, Casimirri F. The impact of obesity on hyperandrogenism and polycystic ovary syndrome in premenopausal women. Clin Endocrinol 1993;39:1–16.

38. Kitzinger C. The thief of womanhood: women's experience of polycystic ovarian syndrome. Soc Sci Med 2002;54(3): 349–361.
39. Sills ES, Perloe M, Tucker M, Kaplan C, Genton M, Schattman G. Diagnostic and treatment characteristics of polycystic ovary syndrome: descriptive measurements of patient perception and awareness from 657 confidential self-reports. BMC Womens Health 2001;1(1):3.
40. Derogatis LR, Lipman RS, Covi L. SCL-90: an outpatient psychiatric rating scale–preliminary report. Psychopharmacol Bull 1973;9(1):13–28.
41. Henrich G. Questions on life satisfaction (FLZ M): a short questionnaire for assessing subjective quality of life. Eur J Psychol Assess 2000;16(3):150–159.
42. Ware Jr, JE, Sherbourne CD. The MOS 36-Item short-form health survey (SF-36): conceptual framework and item selection. Med Care 1992;30(6):473–483.
43. Lett HS, Blumenthal JA, Babyak MA, et al. Depression as a risk factor for coronary artery disease: evidence, mechanisms, and treatment. Psychosom Med 2004;66:305–315.
44. Gambineri A, Pelusi C, Vicennati V, Pagotto U, Pasquali R. Obesity and the polycystic ovary syndrome. Int J Obes 2002;26(7):883–896.
45. Flegal KL. Prevalence and trends in obesity among US adults, 1999–2000. JAMA 2002;288(14):1723–1727.
46. Ciaraldi TP, Morales AJ, Hickman MG, Odom-Ford R, Olefsky JM, Yen SS. Cellular insulin resistance in adipocytes from obese polycystic ovary syndrome subjects involves adenosine modulation of insulin sensitivity. J Clin Endocrinol Metab 1997;82(5):1421–1425.
47. Carmina E, Bucchieri S, Esposito A, et al. Abdominal fat quantity and distribution in women with polycystic ovary syndrome and extent of its relation to insulin resistance. J Clin Endocrinol Metab 2007;92(7):2500–2505.
48. Kirchengast S, Huber J. Body composition characteristics and body fat distribution in lean women with polycystic ovary syndrome. Hum Reprod 2001;16(6):1255–1260.
49. Puder JJ, Varga S, Kraenzlin M, De Geyter C, Keller U, Muller B. Central fat excess in polycystic ovary syndrome: relation to low-grade inflammation and insulin resistance. J Clin Endocrinol Metab 2005;90(11):6014–6021.
50. Lord J, Thomas R, Fox B, Acharya U, Wilkin T. The central issue? Visceral fat mass is a good marker of insulin resistance and metabolic disturbance in women with polycystic ovary syndrome. BJOG 2006;113(10):1203–1209.
51. Kiddy DS, Sharp PS, White DM, et al. Differences in clinical and endocrine features between obese and non-obese subjects with polycystic ovary syndrome: an analysis of 263 consecutive cases. Clin Endocrinol 1990;32(2):213–220.
52. Galtier-Dereure F, Pujol P, Dewailly D, Bringer J. Choice of stimulation in polycystic ovarian syndrome: the influence of obesity. Hum Reprod 1997;12 Suppl 1:88–96.
53. Larsson B, Bengtsson C, Bjorntorp P, et al. Is abdominal body fat distribution a major explanation for the sex difference in the incidence of myocardial infarction? the study of men born in 1913 and the study of women, Goteborg, Sweden. Am J Epidemiol 1992;135(3):266–273.
54. Ehrmann DA. Prevalence of impaired glucose tolerance and diabetes in women with polycystic ovary syndrome. Diabetes Care 1999;22(1):141–146.
55. Legro RS, Kunselman AR, Dodson WC, Dunaif A. Prevalence and predictors of risk for type II diabetes mellitus and impaired glucose tolerance in polycystic ovary syndrome: a prospective controlled study in 254 affected women. J Clin Endocrinol Metab 1999:165–169.
56. Dunaif A, Graf M, Mandeli J, Laumas V, Dobrjansky A. Characterization of groups of hyperandrogenic women with acanthosis nigricans, impaired glucose tolerance, and/or hyperinsulinemia. J Clin Endocrinol Metab 1987;65(3):499–507.
57. Sharp PS, Kiddy DS, Reed MJ, Anyaoku V, Johnston DG, Franks S. Correlation of plasma insulin and insulin-like growth factor-I with indices of androgen transport and metabolism in women with polycystic ovary syndrome. Clin Endocrinol 1991;35(3):253–257.
58. Legro RS, Kunselman AR, Dunaif A. Prevalence and predictors of dyslipidemia in women with polycystic ovary syndrome. Am J Med 2001;111(8):607–613.
59. Norman RJ, Masters L, Milner CR, Wang JX, Davies MJ. Relative risk of conversion from normoglycaemia to impaired glucose tolerance or non-insulin dependent diabetes mellitus in polycystic ovarian syndrome. Hum Reprod 2001;16(9): 1995–1998.
60. Solomon CG, Hu FB, Dunaif A, et al. Long or highly irregular menstrual cycles as a marker for risk of type 2 diabetes mellitus. JAMA 2001;286(19):2421–2426.
61. Cibula D, Cifkova R, Fanta M, Poledne R, Zivny J, Skibova J. Increased risk of non-insulin dependent diabetes mellitus, arterial hypertension and coronary artery disease in perimenopausal women with a history of polycystic ovary syndrome. Hum Reprod 2000;15(4):785–789.
62. Wild RA, Painter PC, Coulson PB, Carruth KB, Ranney GB. Lipoprotein lipid concentrations and cardiovascular risk in women with polycystic ovary syndrome. J Clin Endocrinol Metab 1985;61(5):946–951.
63. McLaughlin T, Reaven G, Abbasi F, Lamendola C, Saad M, Waters D, Simon J, Krauss RM. Is there a simple way to identify insulin-resistant individuals at increased risk of cardiovascular disease? Am J Cardiol 2005;96:399–404.
64. McLaughlin T, Abbasi F, Cheal K, Chu J, Lamendola C, Reaven G. Use of metabolic markers to identify overweight individuals who are insulin resistant. Ann Intern Med 2003;139(10):802–809.

65. Carlson L, Bottiger L, Ahfeldt P. Risk factors for myocardial infarction in the Stockholm prospective study: a 14-year follow-up focusing on the role of plasma triglycerides and cholesterol. Acta Med Scand 1979;206:351–360.
66. Castelli W, Garrison R, Wilson P, Abbott R, Kalonsdian S, Kannel W. Incidence of coronary heart disease and lipoprotein cholesterol levels: the Framingham Study. JAMA 1986;256:2385–2387.
67. Hokanson J, Austin M. Plasma triglyceride level is a risk factor for cardiovascular disease independent of high-density lipoprotein cholesterol level: a meta-analysis of population-based prospective studies. J Cardiovasc Risk 1996;3:213–219.
68. Miller G, Miller N. Plasma high-density-lipoprotein concentration and development of ischemic heart disease. Lancet 1975;1:16–19.
69. Benson S, Janssen OE, Hahn S, et al. Obesity, depression, and chronic low-grade inflammation in women with polycystic ovary syndrome. Brain Behav Immun 2008;22(2):177–184.
70. Diamanti-Kandarakis E, Paterakis T, Alexandraki K, et al. Indices of low-grade chronic inflammation in polycystic ovary syndrome and the beneficial effect of metformin. Hum Reprod 2006;21(6):1426–1431.
71. Cussons AJ, Stuckey BGA, Watts GF. Cardiovascular disease in the polycystic ovary syndrome: new insights and perspectives. Atherosclerosis 2006;185(2):227–239.
72. Orio F, Palomba S, Spinelli L, et al. The cardiovascular risk of young women with polycystic ovary syndrome: an observational, analytical, prospective case-control study. J Clin Endocrinol Metab 2004;89(8):3696–3701.
73. Paradisi G, Steinberg HO, Hempfling A, et al. Polycystic ovary syndrome is associated with endothelial dysfunction. Circulation 2001;103(10):1410–1415.
74. Tiras MB, Yalcin R, Noyan V, et al. Alterations in cardiac flow parameters in patients with polycystic ovarian syndrome. Hum Reprod 1999;14(8):1949–1952.
75. Vural B, Caliskan E, Turkoz E, Kilic T, Demirci A. Evaluation of metabolic syndrome frequency and premature carotid atherosclerosis in young women with polycystic ovary syndrome. Hum Reprod 2005;20(9):2409–2413.
76. Shaw LJ, Bairey Merz CN, Azziz R, et al. Postmenopausal women with a history of irregular menses and elevated androgen measurements at high risk for worsening cardiovascular event-free survival: results from the National Institutes of Health–National Heart, Lung, and Blood Institute sponsored women's ischemia syndrome evaluation. J Clin Endocrinol Metab 2008;93(4):1276–1284.
77. Solomon CG. Menstrual cycle irregularity and risk for future cardiovascular disease. J Clin Endocrinol Metab 2002;87(5):2013–2017.
78. Revised 2003 consensus on diagnostic criteria and long-term health risks related to polycystic ovary syndrome (PCOS). Hum Reprod 2004;19:41–47.
79. Pierpoint T, McKeigue PM, Isaacs AJ, Wild SH, Jacobs HS. Mortality of women with polycystic ovary syndrome at long-term follow-up. J Clin Epidemiol 1998;51(7):581–586.
80. Wild S, Pierpoint T, McKeigue P, Jacobs H. Cardiovascular disease in women with polycystic ovary syndrome at long-term follow-up: a retrospective cohort study. Clin Endocrinol 2000;52(5):595–600.
81. Battaglia C, Mancini F, Cianciosi A, et al. Vascular risk in young women with polycystic ovary and polycystic ovary syndrome. Obstet Gynecol 2008;111(2):385–395.
82. Meyer C, McGrath BP, Teede HJ. Overweight women with polycystic ovary syndrome have evidence of subclinical cardiovascular disease. J Clin Endocrinol Metab 2005;90(10):5711–5716.
83. Aleman A, Bronk E, Kessels RPC, Koppeschaar HPF, van Honk J. A single administration of testosterone improves visuospatial ability in young women. Psychoneuroendocrinology 2004;29(5):612–617.
84. Gouchie C, Kimura D. The relationship between testosterone levels and cognitive ability patterns. Psychoneuroendocrinology 1991;16(4):323–334.
85. Hausmann M, Slabbekoorn D, Van Goozen SH, Cohen-Kettenis PT, Gunturkun O. Sex hormones affect spatial abilities during the menstrual cycle. Behav Neurosci 2000;114(6):1245.
86. Moffat SD, Hampson E. A curvilinear relationship between testosterone and spatial cognition in humans: possible influence of hand preference. Psychoneuroendocrinology 1996;21(3):323–337.
87. Postma A, Meyer G, Tuiten A, van Honk J, Kessels RP, Thijssen J. Effects of testosterone administration on selective aspects of object-location memory in healthy young women. Psychoneuroendocrinology 2000;25(6):563–575.
88. Shute VJ, Pellegrino JW, Hubert L, Reynolds RW. The relationship between androgen levels and human spatial abilities. Bull Psychonomic Soc 1983;21(6):465–468.
89. Hogervorst E. Serum levels of estradiol and testosterone and performance in different cognitive domains in healthy elderly men and women. Psychoneuroendocrinology 2004;29(3):404–421.
90. Thilers PP, Macdonald SWS, Herlitz A. The association between endogenous free testosterone and cognitive performance: a population-based study in 35 to 90 year-old men and women. Psychoneuroendocrinology 2006;31(5):565–576.
91. Schattmann L, Sherwin BB. Testosterone levels and cognitive functioning in women with polycystic ovary syndrome and in healthy young women. Hormones and Behavior 2007;51(5):587–596.
92. Abbasi F, Brown B, Lamendola C, McLaughlin T, Reaven G. Relationship between obesity, insulin resistance, and coronary heart risk. J Am Coll Cardiol 2002;40:937–943.
93. Schattmann L, Sherwin BB. Effects of the pharmacologic manipulation of testosterone on cognitive functioning in women with polycystic ovary syndrome: a randomized, placebo-controlled treatment study. Hormones and Behavior 2007;51(5):579–586.

94. Keettel WC, Bradbury JT, Stoddard FJ. Observations on the PCO syndrome. Am J Obstet Gynecol 1957;73:954–965.
95. Yen SS, Vela P, Rankin J. Inappropriate secretion of follicle stimulating hormone and luteinizing hormone in polycystic ovarian disease. J Clin Endocrinol Metab 1970;30:435–442.
96. Waldstreicher J, Santoro NF, Hall JE, Filicori M, Crowley WF. Hyperfunction of the hypothalamic pituitary axis in women with polycystic ovarian disease: indirect evidence for partial gonadotroph desensitization. J Clin Endocrinol Metab 1988;66:165–172.
97. Barnard L, Balen AH, Ferriday D, Tiplady B, Dye L. Cognitive functioning in polycystic ovary syndrome. Psychoneuroendocrinology 2007;32(8–10):906–914.
98. Potter GG, Steffens DC. Contribution of depression to cognitive impairment and dementia in older adults. Neurologist 2007;13(3):105–117.
99. Osei K. Insulin resistance and systemic hypertension. Am J Cardiol 1999;84(1A):33 J–36 J.
100. Cannon-Spoor HE, Levy JA, Zubenko GS, et al. Effects of previous major depressive illness on cognition in Alzheimer disease patients. Am J Geriatr Psychiatry 2005;13(4):312–318.
101. Alexopoulos GS, Meyers BS, Young RC, Mattis S, Kakuma T. The course of geriatric depression with "reversible dementia": a controlled study. Am J Psychiatry 1993;150(11):1693–1699.
102. Alexopoulos GS, Young RC, Meyers BS. Geriatric depression: age of onset and dementia. Biol Psychiatry 1993;34(3): 141–145.
103. Broe GA, Henderson AS, Creasey H, et al. A case-control study of Alzheimer's disease in Australia. Neurology 1990;40(11):1698–1707.
104. Buntinx F, Kester A, Bergers J, Knottnerus JA. Is depression in elderly people followed by dementia? A retrospective cohort study based in general practice. Age Ageing 1996;25(3):231–233.
105. Chen P, Ganguli M, Mulsant BH, DeKosky ST. The temporal relationship between depressive symptoms and dementia: a community-based prospective study. Arch Gen Psychiatry 1999;56(3):261–266.
106. Devanand DP, Sano M, Tang MX, et al. Depressed mood and the incidence of Alzheimer's disease in the elderly living in the community. Arch Gen Psychiatry 1996;53(2):175–182.
107. Geerlings MI, Schoevers RA, Beekman AT, et al. Depression and risk of cognitive decline and Alzheimer's disease. Results of two prospective community-based studies in The Netherlands. Br J Psychiatry 2000;176:568–575.
108. Reding M, Haycox J, Blass J. Depression in patients referred to a dementia clinic. A three-year prospective study. Arch Neurol 1985;42(9):894–896.
109. Ownby RL, Crocco E, Acevedo A, John V, Loewenstein D. Depression and risk for Alzheimer disease: systematic review, meta-analysis, and metaregression analysis. Arch Gen Psychiatry 2006;63(5):530–538.
110. Austin MP, Mitchell P, Goodwin GM. Cognitive deficits in depression: possible implications for functional neuropathology. Br J Psychiatry 2001;178:200–206.
111. Green RC, Cupples LA, Kurz A, et al. Depression as a risk factor for Alzheimer disease: the MIRAGE study. Arch Neurol 2003;60(5):753–759.
112. Kessing LV, Andersen PK. Does the risk of developing dementia increase with the number of episodes in patients with depressive disorder and in patients with bipolar disorder? J Neurol Neurosurg Psychiatry 2004;75(12):1662–1666.
113. Kessing LV, Nilsson FM, Siersma V, Andersen PK. Increased risk of developing diabetes in depressive and bipolar disorders? J Psychiatr Res 2004;38(4):395–402.
114. Palsson S, Aevarsson O, Skoog I. Depression, cerebral atrophy, cognitive performance and incidence of dementia. Population study of 85-year-olds. Br J Psychiatry 1999;174:249–253.
115. Arvanitakis Z, Wilson RS, Bienias JL, Evans DA, Bennett DA. Diabetes mellitus and risk of Alzheimer disease and decline in cognitive function. Arch Neurol 2004;61(5):661–666.
116. Kalmijn S, Feskens EJ, Launer LJ, Stijnen T, Kromhout D. Glucose intolerance, hyperinsulinaemia and cognitive function in a general population of elderly men. Diabetologia 1995;38(9):1096–1102.
117. Kilander L, Nyman H, Boberg M, Hansson L, Lithell H. Hypertension is related to cognitive impairment: a 20-year follow-up of 999 men. Hypertension 1998;31(3):780–786.
118. Kuusisto J, Koivisto K, Mykkanen L, et al. Essential hypertension and cognitive function. The role of hyperinsulinemia. Hypertension 1993;22(5):771–779.
119. Leibson CL, O'Brien PC, Atkinson E, Palumbo PJ, Melton LJ. Relative contributions of incidence and survival to increasing prevalence of adult-onset diabetes mellitus: a population-based study. Am J Epidemiol 1997;146(1):12–22.
120. Ott A, Stolk R, van Harskamp F, Pols HA, Hofman A, Breteler MM. Diabetes mellitus and the risk of dementia: the Rotterdam Study. Neurology 1999;53(9):1937–1942.
121. Peila R, Rodriguez BL, Launer LJ. Type 2 diabetes, APOE gene, and the risk for dementia and related pathologies: the Honolulu-Asia aging study. Diabetes 2002;51(4):1256–1262.
122. Stolk RP, Breteler MM, Ott A, et al. Insulin and cognitive function in an elderly population. The Rotterdam study. Diabetes Care 1997;20(5):792–795.
123. Vanhanen M, Koivisto K, Kuusisto J, et al. Cognitive function in an elderly population with persistent impaired glucose tolerance. Diabetes Care 1998;21(3):398–402.
124. Beeri MS, Silverman JM, Davis KL, et al. Type 2 diabetes is negatively associated with Alzheimer's disease neuropathology. J Gerontol A Biol Sci Med Sci 2005;60(4):471–475.

125. Steen E, Terry BM, Rivera EJ, et al. Impaired insulin and insulin-like growth factor expression and signaling mechanisms in Alzheimer's disease – is this type 3 diabetes? J Alzheimers Dis 2005;7(1):63–80.
126. Kuusisto J, Koivisto K, Mykkanen L, et al. Association between features of the insulin resistance syndrome and Alzheimer's disease independently of apolipoprotein E4 phenotype: cross sectional population based study. BMJ 1997;315(7115): 1045–1049.
127. Luchsinger JA, Tang M-X, Shea S, Mayeux R. Hyperinsulinemia and risk of Alzheimer disease. Neurology 2004;63(7): 1187–1192.
128. Gustafson D, Rothenberg E, Blennow K, Steen B, Skoog I. An 18-year follow-up of overweight and risk of Alzheimer disease. Arch Intern Med 2003;163(13):1524–1528.
129. Curb JD, Rodriguez BL, Abbott RD, et al. Longitudinal association of vascular and Alzheimer's dementias, diabetes, and glucose tolerance. Neurology 1999;52(5):971–975.
130. Kalmijn S, Foley D, White L, et al. Metabolic cardiovascular syndrome and risk of dementia in Japanese-American elderly men: the Honolulu-Asia aging study. Arterioscler Thromb Vasc Biol 2000;20(10):2255–2260.
131. McLaughlin T, Allison G, Abbasi F, Lamendola C, Reaven G. Prevalence of insulin resistance and associated cardiovascular disease risk factors among normal weight, overweight, and obese individuals. Metabolism 2004;53(4):495–499.
132. Petersen KF, Dufour S, Savage DB, et al. Inaugural Article: The role of skeletal muscle insulin resistance in the pathogenesis of the metabolic syndrome. Proc Natl Acad Sci 2007;104(31):12587–12594.

Chapter 15
Psychological Issues and Their Treatment

Melissa J. Himelein and Samuel S. Thatcher

Most physicians recognize that common features of PCOS, from menstrual irregularities and infertility to hirsutism and obesity, can be highly distressing. However, relatively few researchers have systematically studied the psychological consequences of PCOS: Of nearly 2900 PubMed citations on PCOS appearing since 2000, only about 2% focused on mental health issues. In this chapter, we aim to heighten awareness of the disruptive impact of PCOS on adjustment and to suggest treatment approaches that incorporate the psychological domain.

15.1 Psychological Consequences

15.1.1 Depression

Recent research on depression among women with PCOS leaves little doubt that women with PCOS are at significant risk not only of depressive symptoms, based on their elevated scores on standardized measures of depression[1–5], but also of depressive disorders [6–7], as defined by the guidelines of the Diagnostic and Statistical Manual IV [DSM-IV] [8]. Women with PCOS are over three times as likely to experience depression than women without PCOS: Hollinrake et al. found that 35% of women with PCOS met criteria for depressive disorders, versus 11% of controls [6]. A follow-up investigation revealed that most women diagnosed with depression at the outset of the study received treatment and were no longer depressed 2 years later (75%). Although an encouraging success rate, a number of new cases of depression were identified at follow-up [conversion rate = 19%], indicating that the presence of PCOS both substantially and persistently elevates the risk of clinical depression.

What aspects of PCOS are most associated with depression? Obesity has been linked to depression in women overall [9], and among women with PCOS, obesity is frequent [10]. It is also an area of considerable concern for women with PCOS. Weight difficulties have consistently been shown to be the symptom dimension of PCOS most strongly associated with reduced quality of life [5,11–13]. As might be expected, therefore, higher body mass among PCOS patients has been associated with greater depressive symptomatology [4]. Examined somewhat differently, depressed women with PCOS have also been found to have significantly greater body mass than nondepressed women with PCOS [6]. However, obesity alone does not account for greater depression among women with PCOS. Among comparison group studies of PCOS, the difference in depression levels among women with and without PCOS was reduced, though not eliminated, when body mass group differences were controlled [1,3].

Efforts to identify other features of PCOS that might contribute to depressive symptoms have been largely unsuccessful. Androgen levels have not been found to be related to depression [4,6], and although hirsutism is clearly very upsetting to women [14], among women with PCOS it appears more linked with anxiety than depression [14,15]. Infertility, a frequent consequence of PCOS, has also failed to account for depression [3,6].

M.J. Himelein (✉)
Professor of Psychology, University of North Carolina at Asheville, Licensed Psychologist, Center for Applied Reproductive Science, Johnson City, TN, & Asheville, NC, USA
e-mail: himelein@unca.edu

N.R. Farid, E. Diamanti-Kandarakis (eds.), *Diagnosis and Management of Polycystic Ovary Syndrome*,
DOI 10.1007/978-0-387-09718-3_15,

Only insulin resistance, associated with depressive symptoms or depression in two studies [4,6], may prove to be influential. However, because insulin resistance is also associated with obesity, the independent influence of insulin resistance on depression is not yet clear.

15.1.2 Body Dissatisfaction and Eating Disorders

In developing an instrument to assess quality of life among PCOS patients, researchers interviewed 100 women with PCOS about aspects of the syndrome they considered most problematic. Perhaps not surprisingly, all of the ten characteristics viewed by women as having the greatest impact were related to appearance, e.g., "difficulties staying at a weight you would like or "growth of visible hair on face [16]. Even when the effect of weight on body image is removed from consideration, women with PCOS are more dissatisfied with their bodies than comparison samples of women without PCOS [2,3,15].

Perhaps because body dissatisfaction is so prevalent among women overall that it can be considered normative [17], mental health professionals have been slow to recognize its pernicious impact. In fact, poor body image has numerous unhappy psychological consequences. In adolescent females, body dissatisfaction and depression are not merely correlated; longitudinal research has established that poor body image is significantly, causally predictive of later depression [18–19]. It is possible that body dissatisfaction also mediates, at least in part, the relationship between PCOS and depression [3]. In women overall, poor body image is also associated with low self-esteem, anxiety, and lowered satisfaction with sexual functioning [20–22].

An especially devastating consequence of body dissatisfaction is the potential onset of an eating disorder. Poor body image is not only the most consistent predictor of eating pathology in longitudinal studies; it is also thought by many scholars to be the *core* feature of eating disorders [17]. Women with PCOS have been found to have higher rates of both bulimia [23] and binge eating disorder [7]. Interestingly, successful treatment of bulimia has been shown to be followed by normalization of previously polycystic ovaries [24].

Body dissatisfaction may also help explain the relationship between PCOS and eating disorders. Women who gain weight as a consequence of PCOS might become progressively more concerned about their appearance. In the effort to reduce body weight, they may resort to increasingly pathological dieting behaviors, for example, severe caloric restriction, laxative use, or bingeing and purging – all precursors for an eating disorder. Physiological mechanisms, such as the reduced secretion of a satiety peptide, may also play a role in the onset of eating pathology [25]. However, because the causal direction of the relationship between PCOS and eating disorders is not yet established, it should be noted that bulimia or binge eating disorder could underlie polycystic ovaries, rather than the reverse [24].

15.1.3 Other Mental Health Correlates

Although depression, body dissatisfaction, and pathological eating are the mental health problems most strongly and consistently associated with PCOS, women with PCOS are also vulnerable to other emotional difficulties. Approximately 15% of women with PCOS scored in the "marked psychological distress range of a standardized psychiatric screening tool, with multiple areas of psychopathology affected [26]. Greater body mass was a significant contributor to the likelihood of psychological symptoms.

Quality of life is clearly compromised in women with PCOS [1,26–28]. In comparison with patients with other medical problems such as asthma or diabetes, psychological symptoms are more pronounced among women with PCOS [28], and obesity does not appear to account for this greater impact [27]. As noted previously, anxiety, like depression, has been reported to be more prevalent among women with PCOS [1,14,15]. However, increased anxiety may be the consequence of negative affect overall rather than a unique problem area [2].

PCOS also appears to negatively affect women s sexual functioning. Compared with normative data or comparison group women, women with PCOS report diminished sexual satisfaction [1,27,29]. Specifically, women with PCOS have been found to view themselves as less sexually attractive, as well as to perceive their partners as less sexually attracted to them [1]. Obesity and hirsutism may feed these negative perceptions [27], suggesting that appearance-related aspects of PCOS suppress sexual self-confidence, and in turn, overall sexual satisfaction [1].

15.2 Treating Psychological Aspects of PCOS

Because women with PCOS are at significant risk of mental health problems, treatment of PCOS must encompass psychological, as well as physical, concerns. Predicting which PCOS patients might be prone to greater psychological consequences is a nearly impossible task, as specific physical symptoms of PCOS are not strongly correlated with either the type or the severity of distress experienced by patients [27]. Consequently, physicians must attempt to assess and oversee the treatment of psychological symptoms in *all* PCOS patients.

15.2.1 Screening for Psychological Symptoms

At a minimum, women with PCOS should be evaluated for the presence of the most frequently occurring psychological symptoms, i.e., depression, body dissatisfaction, and pathological eating. Screening instruments could be combined into a single questionnaire, to be completed in the waiting room by all patients diagnosed with PCOS. Measures can be scored by office staff, and treating professionals could then use the findings to introduce discussion of specific symptoms or disorders of concern.

To assess depression, the nine-item Patient Health Questionnaire-9 [PHQ-9] is a recommended tool that specifically measures the DSM-IV diagnostic criteria for depressive disorders. Though brief, the PHQ-9 has sound psychometric properties, and it has also been found to be sensitive to change [30], essential if patients progress over time is to be tracked. The PHQ-9 is especially suited for screening in populations of patients presumed at particular risk of depression [31], as is the case with PCOS.

Body dissatisfaction is most commonly operationalized as global unhappiness with one s physical appearance, which can be measured via the seven-item Appearance Evaluation subscale of the well-validated Body-Self Relations Questionnaire [32]. Because body dissatisfaction in adolescent females is so strongly linked to later depression and eating disorders, body image assessment is imperative in this age group. A simple interview question such as "Are you happy with the way you look? can suffice. Currently, just over half of female adolescents report discussing feelings about their bodies with their primary care or pediatric physicians [33], though it is likely that most would be interested in doing so.

Undetected eating abnormalities among women with PCOS are likely to further jeopardize physical health. Again, screening in adolescent girls is especially important, a practice that national guidelines suggest should occur annually [33]. Moreover, prompt identification of eating pathology is critical to treatment success. If early signs go unnoticed, full-blown eating disorders are much more likely to result, which, over time, become more severe and resistant to treatment [34]. To screen for pathological eating patterns as well as eating disorders, Morgan and colleagues developed the 5-item SCOFF questionnaire, a measure with proven validity and reliability [34–36]. Direct questioning from clinicians may be a necessary additional step, as women who engage in abnormal eating behaviors are unlikely to divulge this information to a physician unless directly asked [34].

15.2.2 Management of Depression

Providing primary care clinicians with feedback about the results of their patients depression screening substantially increases the identification of depression. Although such feedback also lowers the risk of persistent depression, the benefit is not as large as might be assumed [37]. Optimal care requires treatment and monitoring of depressive symptoms as well as ongoing follow-up, strategies that may call for system-level changes in clinic policies. In primary care, a promising strategy is the use of in-house mental health-care coordinators, who oversee care plans and provide updates to treating physicians [38].

Health-care providers who do not wish to manage the treatment of depression themselves should arrange for ready referral to mental health specialists, ideally well-coordinated arrangements that allow for periodic feedback. Even providers who are comfortable initiating antidepressant therapy should consider whether concurrent psychological support may also be necessary. Not only is a combination of psychotherapy and pharmacotherapy more effective in treating depression than medication alone [39], but given the range of emotional difficulties that may affect women with PCOS, talking therapy can provide an opportunity for women to address multiple issues.

In any case, treatment of depression is critical not only in alleviating depressive symptoms but also in improving the management of certain physical aspects of PCOS. For example, relief of depression may result in improvements in weight and insulin resistance, and in greater motivation to comply with treatment regimens [40].

15.2.3 Management of Body Dissatisfaction and Eating Disorders

Because poor body image is associated with many emotional consequences of PCOS, clinicians should address identified body dissatisfaction concerns with patients. Even in the absence of weight loss, successful treatment of severe body dissatisfaction is possible [17], indicating that referral to a mental health specialist could be helpful.

In addition, appearance-related symptoms of PCOS must be viewed as a serious matter, as more than "cosmetic annoyances. Their relief should be considered an important goal of overall PCOS management and can pay off in lessened psychological distress. Treatment of hirsutism, for example, a significant contributor to poor body image [15], can result in increased overall psychological well-being. Laser therapy to reduce unwanted hair has been demonstrated to lower depression and anxiety levels in women with PCOS [41]. Likewise, acne can elicit strongly negative emotional states. Such reactions have been shown to subside when skin appearance is improved through medical intervention [42]. A variety of effective treatments for both hirsutism and acne are currently available, including oral contraceptives, antiandrogens, and topical medications [43]. Clinicians should familiarize themselves with the most up-to-date treatment options in the effort to alleviate this source of emotional distress.

If screening for pathological eating behaviors suggests the presence of an eating disorder, a patient should be referred for full evaluation with a qualified mental health professional. Effective management of eating disorders requires multidisciplinary teamwork, including, at a minimum, treatment by a counselor, nutritionist, and psychiatrist [44].

15.2.4 Lifestyle Modification

Because obesity is so common among women with PCOS, treating clinicians must be familiar with evidence-based strategies for weight management. The National Institutes of Health advocates a lifestyle modification approach, viewing obesity as a chronic disease requiring ongoing alterations in diet and exercise; behavior change therapies are recommended to assist patients in making these changes [45]. Given the success of lifestyle modification trials in reducing diabetes and the metabolic syndrome in at-risk populations, this approach would seem ideal for women with PCOS. Initial studies support its effectiveness not only in terms of physical benefits (e.g., weight decreases, pregnancy and ovulation rate increases) but also in terms of psychological improvements [46]. In addition to diet and exercise adjustments, PCOS-specific recommendations include reducing psychosocial stressors or improving coping abilities, eliminating smoking, and moderating alcohol and caffeine consumption. Group programs, which can provide the camaraderie and support necessary to effect difficult changes, are especially encouraged [46,47].

Of course, most clinicians do not have ready access to established lifestyle modification programs, particularly not programs targeting women with PCOS. Without such resources available, it must be emphasized that most diet programs result in only short-term weight reduction. Maintenance of weight loss past 1 year continues to be an elusive goal [48,49]. The authors of a recent comprehensive review of long-term diet studies, which followed individuals on calorie-restrictive diets from 2 to 5 years, concluded, "The benefits of dieting are simply too small and the potential harms of dieting are too large for it to be recommended as a safe and effective treatment for obesity [49, p. 230]. Consequently, although achieving a healthy weight is clearly desirable for optimal physical and psychological well-being, vague admonitions to lose weight may be counterproductive. Because women with PCOS may be prone to unhealthy eating behaviors, unsupervised dieting could even exacerbate harmful binge-purge tendencies [24].

Nonetheless, the hazards of obesity are clear, and medical encouragement to lose weight is strongly associated with patients initiating attempts to do so [50]. How can health professionals most responsibly navigate this challenging issue? One strategy may be to emphasize exercise – rather than dietary restriction – in advising patients. Exercise is viewed by some researchers as the most important component of lifestyle modification programs [46] and may well emerge as the most critical variable overall in the treatment of obesity [49].

Exercise has extensive health benefits beyond weight stabilization, a point that should be stressed when recommending it to patients. In fact, trying exercise to weight reduction may ultimately discourage exercise if weight loss is slow. Likewise, the quantity and intensity of activity required for weight control – up to 60 minutes per day of moderate-intensity exercise [51] – may be off-putting to some women.

Exercise should, however, be encouraged as a means of improving overall health, psychological as well as physical. In general populations, the effects of exercise on mental health include improved mood, decreased symptoms of depression and anxiety, increased quality of life and psychological well-being, and enhanced self-image [52]. The mental health consequences of PCOS suggest that exercise is likely to be an especially important remedy in this group. Moreover, body dissatisfaction, widespread among women with PCOS, is positively affected by participation in exercise. Exercise intervention studies demonstrate that the body satisfaction levels of exercisers increase as a result of physical activity, and exercisers emerge significantly more body-satisfied than control group participants [53]. Both aerobic exercise and weight training participation are linked to improvements in body image. Regardless of the type of activity, exercise must be moderate or strenuous in intensity for improvements in body image to be achieved [53].

Although more research on the efficacy of physicians advice to exercise is needed [54], available evidence suggests that prescribing exercise can successfully motivate activity in previously sedentary individuals. For example, a prescription for walking at either hard intensity or high frequency was shown to produce significant, long-term gains in cardiorespiratory fitness, maintained over 24 months [55]. Recommended strategies for improving maintenance of exercise include [a] referring patients to specific community exercise programs or opportunities; [b] encouraging patients to set concrete, realistic goals, anticipating barriers to success; and [c] following up to ensure compliance and to assist in problem solving [54]. Because research indicates that patients are likely to engage in significantly less amounts of exercise than are advised, suggestions about intensity and frequency should not be presented at a minimal level [55]. However, previously inactive overweight or obese women should be advised to initiate exercise at a low duration, building up over time [51]. Finally, self-monitoring, an important tool of behavior therapy, can be facilitated through use of a pedometer. Increasingly affordable, large clinical practices might consider purchasing pedometers wholesale and handing them out to patients along with daily steps goals.

15.3 Conclusions

The clinical spectrum of PCOS may be viewed as including not only its physiological hallmarks but also risk of a wide range of mental health difficulties. While depression, body dissatisfaction, and pathological eating behaviors are not psychological symptoms unique to PCOS, it is important that clinicians be aware of their prevalence among this patient group. Screening for and managing such concerns must be construed as essential to holistic PCOS treatment. Such attention is likely to be highly appreciated and valued by patients, who frequently rate the quality of information about PCOS that they receive as less than optimal – and not surprisingly, poorer quality of information receipt is associated with lower quality of life [56]. Although medical treatment of PCOS may relieve some emotional as well as physiological symptoms [57], most often patients psychological difficulties will require psychological treatments.

References

1. Elsenbruch S, Hahn S, Kowalsky D, et al. Quality of life, psychosocial well-being, and sexual satisfaction in women with polycystic ovary syndrome. J Clin Endocrinol Metab 2003;88:5801–5807.
2. Weiner CL, Primeau M, Ehrmann DA. Androgens and mood dysfunction in women: comparison of women with polycystic ovarian syndrome to healthy controls. Psychosom Med 2004;66:356–362.
3. Himelein MJ, Thatcher SS. Depression and body image among women with polycystic ovary syndrome. J Health Psychol 2006;11:613–625.
4. Rasgon NL, Rao RC, Hwang S, et al. Depression in women with polycystic ovary syndrome: clinical and biochemical correlates. J Affect Disord 2003;74:299–304.
5. Barnard L, Ferriday D, Guenther N, et al. Quality of life and psychological well being in polycystic ovary syndrome. Hum Reprod 2007;22:2279–2286.
6. Hollinrake E, Abreu A, Maifeld M, et al. Increased risk of depressive disorders in women with polycystic ovary syndrome. Fertil Steril 2007;87:1369–1376.
7. Kerchner A, Lester W, Stuart SP, et al. Risk of depression and other mental health disorders in women with polycystic ovary syndrome: a longitudinal study. Fertil Steril 2008 Feb 2;[Epub ahead of print].
8. American Psychiatric Association. Diagnostic and Statistical Manual of Mental Disorders, fourth edition-text revision (DSM-IV-TR). Washington, DC: American Psychiatric Association, 2000.
9. Stunkard AJ, Faith MS, Allison KC. Depression and obesity. Biol Psychiatry 2003; 54: 330–337.
10. Martínez-Bermejo E, Luque-Ramírez M, Escobar-Morreale HF. Obesity and the polycystic ovary syndrome. Minerva Endocrinol. 2007 Sep;32(3):129–140.
11. Guyatt G, Weaver B, Cronin L, et al. Health-related quality of life in women with polycystic ovary syndrome, a self-administered questionnaire, was validated. J Clin Epidemiol 2004;57:1279–1287.
12. Jones GL, Benes K, Clark TL, et al. The Polycystic Ovary Syndrome Health-Related Quality of Life Questionnaire (PCOSQ): a validation. Hum Reprod 2004;19:371–377.
13. McCook JG, Reame NE, Thatcher SS. Health-related quality of life issues in women with polycystic ovary syndrome. J Obstet Gynecol Neonatal Nurs 2005;34:12–20.
14. Lipton MG, Sherr L, Elford J, et al. Women living with facial hair: the psychological and behavioral burden. J Psychosom Res 2006;61:161–168.
15. Keegan A, Liao LM, Boyle M. Hirsutism : a psychological analysis. J Health Psychol 2003;8:327–345.
16. Cronin L, Guyatt G, Griffith L, et al. Development of a health-related quality-of-life questionnaire (PCOSQ) for women with polycystic ovary syndrome (PCOS). J Clin Endocrinol Metab 1998;83:1976–1987.
17. Thompson JK, Heinberg LJ, Altabe M, et al. Exacting Beauty: Theory, Assessment, and Treatment of body image disturbance. Washington, DC: American Psychological Association, 1999.
18. Stice E, Hayward C, Cameron RP, et al. Body-image and eating disturbances predict onset of depression among female adolescents: a longitudinal study. J Abnorm Psychol 2000; 109: 438–444.
19. Seiffge-Krenke I, Stemmler M. Factors contributing to gender differences in depressive symptoms: a test of three developmental models. J Youth Adolescence 2002;31:405–417.
20. Cash TF. Women s body images. In: Wingood GM, editor. Handbook of women s sexual and reproductive health. New York: Kluwer Academic/Plenum Publishers, 2002:175–194.
21. Davison TE, McCabe M. Adolescent body image and psychosocial functioning. J Soc Psychol 2006; 146:15–30.
22. Weaver AD, Byers ES. The relationships among body image, body mass index, exercise, and sexual functioning in heterosexual women. Psychol Women Q 2006; 30:333–339.
23. McCluskey S, Evans C, Lacey JH, et al. Polycystic ovaries and bulimia. Fertil Steril 1991;55:287–291.
24. Morgan JF, McCluskey SE, Brunton JN, et al. Polycystic ovarian morphology and bulimia nervosa: a 9-year follow-up study. Fertil Steril 2002;77:928–931.
25. Hirschberg AL, Naessen S, Stridsberg M, et al. Impaired cholecystokinin secretion and disturbed appetite regulation in women with polycystic ovary syndrome. Gynecol Endocrinol 2004;19:79–87.
26. Elsenbruch S, Benson S, Hahn S, et al. Determinants of emotional distress in women with polycystic ovary syndrome. Hum Reprod 2006;21:1092–1099.
27. Hahn S, Janssen OE, Tan S, et al. Clinical and psychological correlates of quality-of-life in polycystic ovary syndrome. Eur J Endocrinol 2005;153:853–860.

28. Coffey S, Bano G, Mason HD. Health-related quality of life in women with polycystic ovary syndrome: a comparison with the general population using the Polycystic Ovary Syndrome Questionnaire (PCOSQ) and the Short Form-36 (SF-36). Gynecol Endocrinol 2006;22:80–86.
29. Conaglen HM, Conaglen JV. Sexual desire in women presenting for antiandrogen therapy. J Sex Marital Ther 2003;29: 255–267.
30. Lowe B, Kroenke K, Herzog W, et al. Measuring depression outcome with a brief self-report instrument: sensitivity to change of the Patient Health Questionnaire (PHQ-9). J Affect Disord 2004;81:61–66.
31. Wittkampf KA, Naeije L, Schene AH, et al. Diagnostic accuracy of the mood module of the Patient Health Questionnaire: a systematic review. Gen Hosp Psychiatry 2007;29:388–395.
32. Cash TF. The Multidimensional Body-Self Relations Questionnaire Users Manual, third edition. Norfolk, VA: Old Dominion University, 2000.
33. Klein JD, Postle CK, Kreipe RE. Do physicians discuss needed diet and nutrition health topics with adolescents? J Adolesc Health 2006;38:608.e1–e6.
34. Parker SC, Lyons J, Bonner J. Eating disorders in graduate students: Exploring the SCOFF questionnaire as a simple screening tool. J Am Coll Health 2005;54:103–107.
35. Morgan JF, Reid F, Lacey JH. The SCOFF questionnaire: assessment of a new screening tool for eating disorders. BMJ 1999;319:1467–1468.
36. Luck AJ, Morgan JF, Reid F, et al. The SCOFF questionnaire and clinical interview for eating disorders in general practice: comparative study. BMJ 2002;325:755–756.
37. Pignone MP, Gaynes BN, Rushton JL, et al. Screening for depression in adults: a summary of the evidence for the U.S. Preventive Services Task Force. Ann Intern Med 2002;136:765–776.
38. Kates N, Mach M. Chronic disease management for depression in primary care: a summary of the current literature and implications for practice. Can J Psychiatry 2007;52:77–85.
39. Pampallona S, Bollini P, Tibaldi G, et al. Combined pharmacotherapy and psychological treatment for depression: a systematic review. Arch Gen Psychiatry 2004;61:714–719.
40. Barnard L, Ferriday D, Guenther N. Quality of life and psychological well being in polycystic ovary syndrome. Hum Reprod 2007;22:2279–2286.
41. Clayton WJ, Lipton M, Elford J, et al. A randomized controlled trial of laser treatment among hirsute women with polycystic ovary syndrome. Br J Dermatol 2005;152:986–992.
42. Fried RG, Wechsler A. Psychological problems in the acne patient. Dermatol Ther 2006;19:237–240.
43. Archer JS, Chang RJ. Hirsutism and acne in polycystic ovary syndrome. Best Pract Res Clin Obstet Gynaecol 2004;18: 737–754.
44. Zerbe KJ. Eating disorders in the 21st century: identification, management, and prevention in obstetrics and gynecology. Best Pract Res Clin Obstet Gynaecol 2007;21:331–343.
45. National Institutes of Health. The Practical Guide: Identification, Evaluation, and Treatment of Overweight and Obesity in Adults. Bethesda, MD: North American Association for the Study of Obesity, National Heart, Lung, and Blood Institute; 2000. NIH publication 00-4084. Available at http://www.nhlbi.nih.gov/guidelines/obesity/practgde.htm
46. Moran LJ, Brinkworth G, Noakes M, et al. Effects of lifestyle modification in polycystic ovarian syndrome. Reprod Biomed Online 2006;12:569–578.
47. Norman RJ, Davies MJ, Lord J, et al. The role of lifestyle modification in polycystic ovary syndrome. Trends Endocrinol Metab 2002;13:251–257.
48. Curioni CC, Lourenco PM. Long-term weight loss after diet and exercise: a systematic review. Int J Obes (Lond) 2005;29:1168–1174.
49. Mann T, Tomiyama AJ, Westling E, et al. Medicare s search for effective obesity treatments: diets are not the answer. Am Psychol 2007;62:220–233.
50. Bish CL, Blanck HM, Serdula MK, et al. Diet and physical activity behaviors among Americans trying to lose weight: 2000 Behavioral Risk Factor Surveillance System. Obes Res 2005;13:596–607.
51. Warburton DE, Nicol CW, Bredin SS. Prescribing exercise as preventive therapy. CMAJ 2006;174:961–974.
52. Penedo FJ, Dahn JR. Exercise and well-being: a review of mental and physical health benefits associated with physical activity. Curr Opin Psychiatry 2005;18:189–193.
53. Hausenblas HA, Fallon EA. Exercise and body image: a meta-analysis. Psychol Health 2006;21:33–47.
54. Estabrooks PA, Glasgow RE, Dzewaltowski DA. Physical activity promotion through primary care. JAMA 2003;289: 2913–2916.
55. Duncan GE, Anton SD, Sydeman SJ, et al. Prescribing exercise at varied levels of intensity and frequency: a randomized trial. Arch Intern Med 2005;165:2362–2369.
56. Ching HL, Burke V, Stuckey BGA. Quality of life and psychological morbidity in women with polycystic ovary syndrome: body mass index, age and the provision of patient information are significant modifiers. Clin Endocrinol 2007;66:373–379.
57. Hahn S, Benson S, Elsenbruch S, et al. Metformin treatment of polycystic ovary syndrome improves health-related quality-of-life, emotional distress and sexuality. Hum Reprod 2006;21:1925–1934.

Part IV
Management

Chapter 16
Dietary Management of PCOS

Kate Marsh

16.1 Introduction

The majority of women with PCOS, regardless of weight, have a form of insulin resistance that is intrinsic to the syndrome. For this reason, lifestyle changes that improve insulin sensitivity should be the first line of treatment for women with PCOS, particularly for those who are overweight. Lifestyle interventions should also accompany pharmacological treatment [1, 2].

Beyond this general consensus, there is much confusion about the most appropriate dietary advice for women with PCOS and no specific dietary recommendations have been published. In fact, although many studies have shown the benefits of weight loss for these women, few have explored different types of diet in the management of PCOS. There is, however, a significant amount of nutrition research in the areas of weight management and chronic disease prevention, which provides an evidence base for the development of nutrition recommendations for this condition.

16.2 Obesity and Weight Loss in PCOS

Approximately 50% of women with PCOS are obese and have an added burden of obesity-related insulin resistance, with a greater degree of insulin resistance, hyperinsulinaemia, lipid abnormalities, hyperandrogenism, hirsutism and menstrual irregularities [3–9]. There is also a higher prevalence of abdominal body fat distribution in women with PCOS, even in those with a normal body weight. This increase in visceral fat has been shown to be associated with glucose intolerance, dyslipidaemia and a greater degree of insulin resistance and hyperinsulinaemia [9–14].

Women with PCOS often report difficulties losing weight, although some studies have not shown this to be the case [15, 16]. However, a study comparing dietary intake and physical activity levels in women with PCOS and age-matched controls found no overall differences between the groups despite women with PCOS having a higher BMI, suggesting that dietary intake and physical activity alone are not sufficient to explain the differences in weight between women with and without PCOS [17]. The normal weight PCOS women in this study reported significantly lower energy intakes than normal weight women without PCOS, suggesting that women with PCOS may need to restrict energy intake significantly in order to maintain a normal weight. A recent study found that women with PCOS, with or without insulin resistance, had a significantly lower basal metabolic rate (BMR) compared with non-PCOS women [18].

Impairments in appetite regulation have also been demonstrated in women with PCOS which may contribute to difficulties controlling weight. Levels of ghrelin and cholecystokinin (CCK), hormones which play an impor-

K. Marsh (✉)
Advanced Accredited Practising Dietitian (AdvAPD) and Credentialled Diabetes Educator (CDE), The PCOS Health & Nutrition Centre, Sydney, Australia,
e-mail: kate@nnd.com.au

N.R. Farid, E. Diamanti-Kandarakis (eds.), *Diagnosis and Management of Polycystic Ovary Syndrome*,
DOI 10.1007/978-0-387-09718-3_16, © Springer Science+Business Media, LLC 2009

tant role in appetite regulation, have been found to be impaired in women with PCOS [19–21]. In one of these studies, overweight women with PCOS experienced more hunger and were less satiated following a test meal than non-PCOS women, both before and after weight loss [20].

16.3 Lifestyle Changes Effective in Women with PCOS

Lifestyle modifications including diet, exercise and weight loss are effective in women with PCOS, with a reduction in weight of as little as 5% of total body weight having been shown to reduce insulin levels, improve menstrual function, reduce testosterone levels, improve symptoms of hirsutism and acne and increase ovulation and fertility [3, 6, 15, 16, 22–39].

Furthermore, research suggests that diet and lifestyle changes may be more effective in women with PCOS than the insulin-lowering medication metformin, which is now commonly prescribed. One study found that while the addition of metformin to a hypocaloric diet improved menstrual function, there was no improvement in insulin sensitivity and hyperinsulinaemia [29]. Similarly, no benefits on insulin sensitivity or glucose metabolism were found with the addition of metformin to lifestyle changes, although the combination did result in a greater weight loss and reduction in androgen levels compared to lifestyle changes or metformin alone [40]. Tang et al., on the other hand, found that metformin did not improve weight loss, menstrual frequency, insulin sensitivity or lipid profiles when added to a hypocaloric diet [34]. A recent study comparing a hypocaloric diet with metformin treatment found similar improvements in weight loss, menstrual cyclicity and reproductive outcomes in both groups [32]. Finally, a meta-analysis of the effects of metformin use in PCOS found that while metformin does improve ovulation rate, both alone and in combination with clomiphene, equal or better ovulation rates have been achieved using lifestyle modification [41].

These findings are consistent with those of the Diabetes Prevention Program (DPP), which found that lifestyle modification (diet and exercise) in people with impaired glucose tolerance (IGT) produced a greater reduction in risk of developing type 2 diabetes than metformin [42].

16.4 Dietary Management of PCOS – More Than Just Weight Loss

Most of the studies of dietary intervention in women with PCOS have focused on energy restriction rather than dietary composition per se, yet the weight loss seen in most of these studies has been small in comparison to the outcomes achieved. And while the incidence of insulin resistance is higher in women with PCOS who are obese, and weight loss clearly improves outcomes for these women, not all women with PCOS who have insulin resistance are overweight or obese. Studies have demonstrated a higher than normal incidence of insulin resistance, IGT and type 2 diabetes in women with PCOS of normal weight [43–45], suggesting that dietary management of this condition must go beyond weight loss.

Two studies investigating the effects of a reduced carbohydrate diet in women with PCOS (40% vs. 55% CHO) have failed to show any significant benefits on weight loss, endocrine or metabolic characteristics [33, 37]. A short-term study comparing a reduced carbohydrate (43% energy) and a monounsaturated fatty acid (MUFA)-rich diet (17% energy) with a standard low-fat, high-carbohydrate diet found lower fasting insulin levels following the reduced carbohydrate diet compared to a standard diet but no significant changes in fasting glucose, insulin sensitivity or reproductive hormones [46]. A polyunsaturated fatty acid (PUFA)-rich diet was found to significantly increase urinary pregnanediol 3-glucuronide in women with PCOS, although only 2 of the 17 subjects showed signs of ovulation [47]. LH, FSH, SHBG, DHEAS and testosterone levels did not change. Energy restriction alone, independent of weight loss, has also been shown to improve reproductive parameters [37].

In most of the dietary studies in women with PCOS, improvements in metabolic and reproductive outcomes have been closely related to improvements in insulin sensitivity, suggesting that dietary modification designed to improve insulin resistance may produce benefits greater than those achieved by energy restriction alone.

16.5 What Should You Recommend to Your Patients with PCOS?

While further research looking specifically at the dietary management of PCOS is needed, there is now a significant amount of research looking at the role of diet in reducing diabetes, cardiovascular disease and cancer risk, all of which are relevant to women with PCOS. Based on these findings, the following recommendations can be made.

16.5.1 Encourage the Use of Low GI, Wholegrain Breads and Cereals Over High GI, Processed Grain Products

There is now a significant body of evidence demonstrating the benefits of low GI diets. While many of the features of insulin resistance, including postprandial glycaemia and insulinaemia, hypertriglyceridaemia, low HDL levels and fibrinolysis may be worsened by a high-carbohydrate diet, there is increasing evidence that the type of carbohydrate in the diet is important. In particular, many studies show that low and high glycemic index (GI) foods have significantly different effects on metabolism [48]. Low GI diets can improve insulin resistance and many of its metabolic consequences [49–58] while a high GI diet has been shown to worsen postprandial insulin resistance [55, 59, 60].

Epidemiological studies have associated a low GI diet with reduced risk of cardiovascular disease, type 2 diabetes, insulin resistance and the metabolic syndrome [61–67]. Low GI diets have also been associated with a reduced risk of endometrial cancer [68], breast cancer [69], colon cancer [70, 71] and ovarian cancer [72], all of which may be linked with high insulin levels.

There is now convincing evidence that low GI diets may assist in weight management via effects on appetite and fuel partitioning. In a review of 16 studies, Ludwig found that low GI foods increased satiety, delayed return of hunger or reduced ad libitum food intake in all but one [73]. Two studies have found that low GI or low GL weight loss diets result in a smaller decrease in energy expenditure when compared to higher GI diets, despite similar weight loss [74, 75]. A low GI meal prior to exercise has been found to increase the rate of fat oxidation and lower oxidation of carbohydrate compared with a higher GI meal [76–79]. Finally, a number of clinical studies have found greater loss of body fat with a lower GI diet [80–83].

This research is also supported by the findings of a number of observational studies showing a relationship between dietary GI and body weight, waist circumference, body fat levels and weight gain [84–86]. And a recent meta-analysis published in the *Cochrane Database of Systematic Reviews* supports the use of a low GI diet in weight management, with the combined results of six randomized controlled studies showing significantly greater reductions in body mass, fat mass, body mass index, total cholesterol and LDL cholesterol with a low GI diet [87]. Even when ad libitum low GI diets were compared to conventional low-fat energy-restricted diets, the low GI dieters achieved the same or better results.

Surprisingly, there are no published studies of low GI diets in women with PCOS. We are nearing completion of a clinical trial of two higher carbohydrate diets (low GI and conventional low fat high fibre) in the management of PCOS. To date, 96 overweight women with PCOS have been recruited and followed until they lose 7% of their starting body weight, which has taken up to 12 months in some cases. They are assessed for changes in body fat, glucose and insulin levels during an OGTT, cardiovascular risk factors, reproductive hormone levels and self-reported menstrual cyclicity. Preliminary analyses show that women who consumed the low GI diet had greater improvements in 2 hour post-load insulin levels, inflammatory markers, and menstrual cyclicity.

Higher intakes of fibre, cereal fibre and wholegrains have been associated with a reduced risk of type 2 diabetes in a number of studies [61, 63, 64, 88–92]. In support of this finding, Pereira et al. demonstrated improved insulin sensitivity in overweight subjects, independent of body weight, when refined grains were replaced with wholegrains over a 6 week period [93], and Liese et al. found a higher intake of wholegrains to be associated with increased insulin sensitivity in a study of 978 subjects with normal or impaired glucose tolerance [94]. Intake of high-fibre, wholegrain foods has also been shown to be inversely associated with weight gain in middle-aged women [95].

While some advocate the use of low-carbohydrate diets in women with PCOS, there is little evidence to support such a recommendation. As discussed earlier, only two studies have assessed the effects of a reduced carbohydrate diet in women with PCOS (40% vs. 55% CHO) and both failed to show any significant benefits on weight loss, endocrine or metabolic characteristics [33, 37]. Furthermore, several studies have found no association between total carbohydrate intake and risk of diabetes, insulin resistance or prevalence of the metabolic syndrome [63, 64, 66, 91, 96, 97], while others have found that a lower fat, higher carbohydrate diet can reduce the progression to diabetes in those with IGT [98, 99] and reduce the development of glucose intolerance in pregnancy [100].

The DASH study (Dietary Approaches to Stop Hypertension) [101] showed a significant improvement in blood lipids and blood pressure with a relatively high (57%) carbohydrate diet based on a high intake of fruit, vegetables, wholegrains and low-fat dairy products. The effects of this dietary pattern on insulin sensitivity was subsequently tested in the PREMIER Interventions on Insulin Sensitivity study, finding that the DASH diet resulted in great improvements in insulin sensitivity than a comprehensive behavioural intervention alone (incorporating weight loss, reduced sodium intake, increased physical activity and moderate alcohol intake) [102].

Finally, the third National Health and Nutrition Examination Survey (NHANES III) found that carbohydrate intakes were not associated with HbA1c, plasma glucose or serum insulin concentrations but were inversely associated with the risk of elevated serum C-peptide [103] while the Strong Heart Study demonstrated that a higher intake of total fat, saturated fat and protein and a lower intake of carbohydrate and dietary fibre was associated with poorer blood glucose control in adults with diabetes [104].

The type of carbohydrate in the diet, not the total intake, it appears, is what is most important for metabolic health.

16.5.2 Advise Limiting Intake of Saturated and Trans Fats and Favouring Monounsaturated and Omega-3 Fats

Diets high in fat, particularly saturated fat, are associated with reduced insulin sensitivity [90, 105–109] and an increased risk of developing type 2 diabetes [96, 97, 110, 111]. Furthermore, subjects with insulin resistance and type 2 diabetes have been found to have changes in the fatty acid pattern in serum cholesterol esters (a marker of dietary fat intake) with a higher proportion of saturated fatty acids and lower proportions of linoleic acid [112–116].

Research has also linked a higher intake of trans fats with an increased risk of diabetes, obesity and metabolic syndrome [117, 118]. The consumption of trans fats has been found to worsen blood lipid profiles (increase total and LDL cholesterol and reduce HDL cholesterol), increase inflammatory markers and negatively impact endothelial function [119–121]. A recent study particularly relevant to women with PCOS found that consumption of trans fats is associated with a significantly increased risk of ovulatory infertility [122].

Diets high in unsaturated fats, on the other hand, are associated with a reduced risk of cardiovascular disease and type 2 diabetes [118]. In particular, diets higher in monounsaturated and omega-3 fatty acids may improve many of the metabolic risk factors seen in women with PCOS (including blood lipids, insulin sensitivity and endothelial function) and are associated with a reduced risk of cardiovascular disease and diabetes [123].

16.5.3 Caution Against High-Protein Diets and Favour Plant Protein Over Animal Protein

Recent times have seen a renewed interest in high-protein diets for weight loss, diabetes management and for women with PCOS. To date, however, there is little evidence to suggest benefits of high-protein diets on insulin resistance and some evidence that this type of diet may worsen insulin resistance and impair glucose metabolism [124–128].

A number of studies in women with PCOS, overweight and obese subjects as well as those with hyperinsulinaemia and type 2 diabetes have failed to show significant long-term benefits of a high-protein diet on weight loss or insulin sensitivity [33, 37, 129–133].

Two studies in women with PCOS have shown that while a hypocaloric diet results in significant weight loss and consequent improvement in metabolic and reproductive abnormalities, a high-protein (HP) diet is no more effective that a high-carbohydrate (HC) diet [20, 33, 37].

While not increasing blood glucose levels to the same extent as carbohydrate foods, protein foods do elicit an insulin response and the impact of this in those with insulin resistance is not clear. There are also concerns about the safety of high-protein, low-carbohydrate diets including the effects on kidney function, bone mineral density and the reduction in intake of protective foods such as fruits, vegetables and wholegrains. Several studies have now shown a positive association between dietary haem iron intake and haem iron intake from red meat and the risk of type 2 diabetes [134–137]. A positive association between intake of red meat, processed meats and animal protein and incidence of type 2 diabetes in women has also been demonstrated [137, 138]. In addition, there is evidence to suggest an association between iron stores and type 2 diabetes risk [136, 139]. Finally, the ATTICA study found that red meat consumption was positively associated with hyperglycaemia, hyperinsulinaemia and HOMA levels after adjusting for BMI and various other potential confounders [140]. While the findings of these studies need to be confirmed, they provide further evidence that diets high in animal protein may be detrimental to those with insulin resistance.

It is also important to consider that a high intake of fruits, vegetables and wholegrains have been shown to protect against cardiovascular disease, diabetes and cancer, while some studies showing a high intake of animal protein may increase cancer risk [141]. Risk of endometrial cancer, in particular, has been shown to be inversely associated with a higher intake of plant foods, wholegrains and soy products and positively associated with a higher intake of energy, fat and animal foods [142–146].

16.5.4 Promote Low Energy Density

Diets with a low energy density are associated with a reduced energy intake and have been shown to be effective for weight loss [147–152]. One study of almost 100 obese women followed over 12 months found that reducing energy density by combining an increase in fruit and vegetable intake with a reduced fat intake was more effective for weight loss than a reduced fat diet alone, and resulted in less hunger [153], while another study found that energy density influenced energy intake in both lean and obese women across a range of fat intakes [150].

Considering the findings of research showing that women with PCOS may have impaired appetite regulation [19, 20] and may require less energy to maintain a normal weight [17] consuming a diet with a low energy density may be particularly important for these women.

Furthermore, diets rich in foods with a low energy density such as fruit and vegetables are generally associated with a lower risk of metabolic syndrome [154], type 2 diabetes [155], CVD [156] and cancer.

Table 16.1 provides practical guidelines to assist women with PCOS to encompass these dietary changes. However, referral to a dietitian with experience in the dietary management of PCOS is recommended, as research has shown that only intensive dietary and lifestyle intervention is effective for providing significant health benefits [157].

16.6 Evidence in Support of These Recommendations

These recommendations are supported by the findings of three studies, which while not specifically conducted in women with PCOS, are of particular relevance to this group.

The first study, in postmenopausal women with high testosterone levels, found that a comprehensive dietary change designed to reduce insulin resistance resulted in a significant increase in sex hormone-binding globulin (SHBG) and a significant decrease in testosterone, body weight, waist to hip ratio (WHR), total cholesterol (TC),

Table 16.1 Practical dietary advice for women with PCOS

- Choose oat-based cereals such as porridge or natural muesli
- Choose wholegrain breads (with intact grains) in place of white or brown varieties
- Aim to fill half of your plate at lunch and dinner with a variety of vegetables or salad vegetables
- Include low GI grains in your meals including barley, cracked wheat (bulgur), quinoa and buckwheat
- Choose lean cuts of meat and alternate red meat with lean poultry, fish, seafood, tofu and legumes
- Avoid processed foods high in fat and added sugar, particularly those made with hydrogenated vegetable oils
- Snack on fresh fruit, raw nuts, yoghurt or wholegrain crackers
- Replace butter on bread with avocado, tahini or pure nut spreads
- Use olive or canola oil in cooking and olive oil or flaxseed oil in salad dressings
- Replace salt in cooking with fresh or dried herbs and spices

fasting blood glucose (FBG) and insulin [158]. The diet focused on lowering intake of animal fats and increasing intake of fibre, low GI carbohydrates (with total CHO intake approximately 51% of energy), monounsaturated and omega-3 polyunsaturated fats and phytoestrogens.

The second study found that a diet designed to evoke a low insulin response (with a focus on low GI carbohydrates) reduced insulin concentrations and weight in obese hyperinsulinaemic females significantly more than a conventional diet with the same energy and macronutrient content [60]. Carbohydrate intake in this study was 50% of energy.

Finally, recent findings from the Nurses Health Study II (investigating more than 17,500 women without a history of infertility) found that over an 8 year period, the risk of ovulatory infertility was significantly less in women who ate less trans fat and sugar, more low GI carbohydrates and more protein from vegetable sources rather than from animals [159].

Numerous studies have also found an association between dietary patterns rich in fruit, vegetables, grains, legumes, fish, nuts and olive oil and low in red meat and processed grains for reducing the risk of chronic disease including obesity, diabetes, cardiovascular disease and the metabolic syndrome [155, 156, 159–162].

16.7 Conclusion

The recognition of the link between PCOS and IR offers an excellent opportunity for the early intervention to prevent or delay the onset of type 2 diabetes and cardiovascular disease in these women. While the dietary management of PCOS should focus on weight reduction for those who are overweight, consideration also needs to be given to the role of varying dietary composition in increasing insulin sensitivity. The optimal diet for women with PCOS is one which is low in saturated fat with moderate amounts of monounsaturated and omega-3 fats, high in fibre from wholegrains, legumes and vegetables and which contains predominantly low GI carbohydrate foods. Such a diet may help short term in improving the symptoms of this condition, as well as long term, in reducing the risk of diseases linked with insulin resistance.

16.8 Practice Points

- Lifestyle changes including diet and exercise should be the first line of treatment of women with PCOS and should accompany pharmacologic or surgical treatments.
- Weight loss of as little as 5% of body weight can improve symptoms of PCOS.
- This degree of weight loss, accompanied by lifestyle changes, has also been shown to reduce diabetes risk.
- The dietary management of PCOS should focus on reducing saturated and trans fats, choosing low GI carbohydrate foods, basing meals around vegetables, legumes and wholegrains, eating more plant protein rather than animal protein and avoiding processed carbohydrate foods and concentrated sugars.
- Dietary changes should be accompanied by other lifestyle changes including regular physical activity, managing stress and obtaining adequate sleep.

References

1. Norman, R.J., et al., The role of lifestyle modification in polycystic ovary syndrome. *Trends Endocrinol Metab*, 2002;. 13(6): 251–7.
2. Norman, R.J., et al., Lifestyle choices, diet, and insulin sensitizers in polycystic ovary syndrome. *Endocrine*, 2006;. 30(1): 35–43.
3. Andersen, P., et al., Increased insulin sensitivity and fibrinolytic capacity after dietary intervention in obese women with polycystic ovary syndrome. *Metabolism*, 1995;. 44(5): 611–6.
4. Ciaraldi, T.P., et al., Cellular insulin resistance in adipocytes from obese polycystic ovary syndrome subjects involves adenosine modulation of insulin sensitivity. *J Clin Endocrinol Metab*, 1997;. 82(5): 1421–5.
5. Gambineri, A., et al., Obesity and the polycystic ovary syndrome. *Int J Obes Relat Metab Disord*, 2002;. 26(7): 883–96.
6. Kiddy, D.S., et al., Improvement in endocrine and ovarian function during dietary treatment of obese women with polycystic ovary syndrome. *Clin Endocrinol (Oxf)*, 1992;. 36(1): 105–11.
7. Pasquali, R. and F. Casimirri, The impact of obesity on hyperandrogenism and polycystic ovary syndrome in premenopausal women. *Clin Endocrinol (Oxf)*, 1993;. 39(1): 1–16.
8. Pasquali, R., et al., Insulin and androgen relationships with abdominal body fat distribution in women with and without hyperandrogenism. *Horm Res*, 1993. 39(5–6): 179–87.
9. Pasquali, R., et al., Body fat distribution has weight-independent effects on clinical, hormonal, and metabolic features of women with polycystic ovary syndrome. *Metabolism*, 1994;. 43(6): 706–13.
10. Yildirim, B., N. Sabir, and B. Kaleli, Relation of intra-abdominal fat distribution to metabolic disorders in nonobese patients with polycystic ovary syndrome. *Fertil Steril*, 2003;. 79(6): 1358–64.
11. Douchi, T., et al., Body fat distribution in women with polycystic ovary syndrome. *Obstet Gynecol*, 1995. 86(4 Pt 1): 516–9.
12. Kirchengast, S. and J. Huber, Body composition characteristics and body fat distribution in lean women with polycystic ovary syndrome. *Hum Reprod*, 2001;. 16(6): 1255–60.
13. Carmina, E., et al., Abdominal fat quantity and distribution in women with polycystic ovary syndrome and extent of its relation to insulin resistance. *J Clin Endocrinol Metab*, 2007;. 92(7): 2500–5.
14. Cascella, T., et al., Visceral fat is associated with cardiovascular risk in women with polycystic ovary syndrome. *Hum Reprod*, 2007.
15. Jakubowicz, D.J. and J.E. Nestler, 17 alpha-Hydroxyprogesterone responses to leuprolide and serum androgens in obese women with and without polycystic ovary syndrome offer dietary weight loss. *J Clin Endocrinol Metab*, 1997;. 82(2): 556–60.
16. Pasquali, R., et al., Effect of long-term treatment with metformin added to hypocaloric diet on body composition, fat distribution, and androgen and insulin levels in abdominally obese women with and without the polycystic ovary syndrome. *J Clin Endocrinol Metab*, 2000;. 85(8): 2767–74.
17. Wright, C.E., et al., Dietary intake, physical activity, and obesity in women with polycystic ovary syndrome. *Int J Obes Relat Metab Disord*, 2004;. 28(8): 1026–32.
18. Georgopoulos, N.A., et al., Basal metabolic rate is decreased in women with polycystic ovary syndrome and biochemical hyperandrogenemia and is associated with insulin resistance. *Fertil Steril*, 2008.
19. Hirschberg, A.L., et al., Impaired cholecystokinin secretion and disturbed appetite regulation in women with polycystic ovary syndrome. *Gynecol Endocrinol*, 2004;. 19(2): 79–87.
20. Moran, L.J., et al., Ghrelin and measures of satiety are altered in polycystic ovary syndrome but not differentially affected by diet composition. *J Clin Endocrinol Metab*, 2004;. 89(7): 3337–44.
21. Pagotto, U., et al., Plasma ghrelin, obesity, and the polycystic ovary syndrome: correlation with insulin resistance and androgen levels. *J Clin Endocrinol Metab*, 2002;. 87(12): 5625–9.
22. Pasquali, R., et al., Clinical and hormonal characteristics of obese amenorrheic hyperandrogenic women before and after weight loss. *J Clin Endocrinol Metab*, 1989;. 68(1): 173–9.
23. Kiddy, D.S., et al., Diet-induced changes in sex hormone binding globulin and free testosterone in women with normal or polycystic ovaries: correlation with serum insulin and insulin-like growth factor-I. *Clin Endocrinol (Oxf)*, 1989;. 31(6): 757–63.
24. Guzick, D.S., et al., Endocrine consequences of weight loss in obese, hyperandrogenic, anovulatory women. *Fertil Steril*, 1994;. 61(4): 598–604.
25. Clark, A.M., et al., Weight loss results in significant improvement in pregnancy and ovulation rates in anovulatory obese women. *Hum Reprod*, 1995;. 10(10): 2705–12.
26. Clark, A.M., et al., Weight loss in obese infertile women results in improvement in reproductive outcome for all forms of fertility treatment. *Hum Reprod*, 1998;. 13(6): 1502–5.
27. Crave, J.C., et al., Effects of diet and metformin administration on sex hormone-binding globulin, androgens, and insulin in hirsute and obese women. *J Clin Endocrinol Metab*, 1995;. 80(7): 2057–62.
28. Crosignani, P.G., et al., Overweight and obese anovulatory patients with polycystic ovaries: parallel improvements in anthropometric indices, ovarian physiology and fertility rate induced by diet. *Hum Reprod*, 2003;. 18(9): 1928–32.
29. Gambineri, A., et al., Effect of flutamide and metformin administered alone or in combination in dieting obese women with polycystic ovary syndrome. *Clin Endocrinol (Oxf)*, 2004;. 60(2): 241–9.

30. Holte, J., et al., Restored insulin sensitivity but persistently increased early insulin secretion after weight loss in obese women with polycystic ovary syndrome. *J Clin Endocrinol Metab*, 1995;. 80(9): 2586–93.
31. Huber-Buchholz, M.M., D.G. Carey, and R.J. Norman, Restoration of reproductive potential by lifestyle modification in obese polycystic ovary syndrome: role of insulin sensitivity and luteinizing hormone. *J Clin Endocrinol Metab*, 1999;. 84(4): 1470–4.
32. Qublan, H.S., et al., Dietary intervention versus metformin to improve the reproductive outcome in women with polycystic ovary syndrome. A prospective comparative study. *Saudi Med J*, 2007;. 28(11): 1694–9.
33. Stamets, K., et al., A randomized trial of the effects of two types of short-term hypocaloric diets on weight loss in women with polycystic ovary syndrome. *Fertil Steril*, 2004;. 81(3): 630–7.
34. Tang, T., et al., Combined lifestyle modification and metformin in obese patients with polycystic ovary syndrome. A randomized, placebo-controlled, double-blind multicentre study. *Hum Reprod*, 2006;. 21(1): 80–9.
35. Van Dam, E.W., et al., Increase in daily LH secretion in response to short-term calorie restriction in obese women with PCOS. *Am J Physiol Endocrinol Metab*, 2002. 282(4): E865–72.
36. Wahrenberg, H., et al., Divergent effects of weight reduction and oral anticonception treatment on adrenergic lipolysis regulation in obese women with the polycystic ovary syndrome. *J Clin Endocrinol Metab*, 1999;. 84(6): 2182–7.
37. Moran, L.J., et al., Dietary composition in restoring reproductive and metabolic physiology in overweight women with polycystic ovary syndrome. *J Clin Endocrinol Metab*, 2003;. 88(2): 812–9.
38. Moran, L.J., et al., C-reactive protein before and after weight loss in overweight women with and without polycystic ovary syndrome. *J Clin Endocrinol Metab*, 2007;. 92(8): 2944–51.
39. Moran, L.J., et al., Short-term meal replacements followed by dietary macronutrient restriction enhance weight loss in polycystic ovary syndrome. *Am J Clin Nutr*, 2006;. 84(1): 77–87.
40. Hoeger, K.M., et al., A randomized, 48-week, placebo-controlled trial of intensive lifestyle modification and/or metformin therapy in overweight women with polycystic ovary syndrome: a pilot study. *Fertil Steril*, 2004;. 82(2): 421–9.
41. Lord, J.M., I.H. Flight, and R.J. Norman, Metformin in polycystic ovary syndrome: systematic review and meta-analysis. *BMJ*, 2003;. 327(7421): 951–3.
42. Diabetes Prevention Program Research Group, Reduction in the incidence of type 2 diabetes with lifestyle intervention or metformin. *N Engl J Med*, 2002. 346: 393–403.
43. Chang, R.J., et al., Insulin resistance in nonobese patients with polycystic ovarian disease. *J Clin Endocrinol Metab*, 1983;. 57(2): 356–9.
44. Dunaif, A., et al., Profound peripheral insulin resistance, independent of obesity, in polycystic ovary syndrome. *Diabetes*, 1989;. 38(9): 1165–74.
45. Jialal, I., et al., Evidence for insulin resistance in nonobese patients with polycystic ovarian disease. *J Clin Endocrinol Metab*, 1987;. 64(5): 1066–9.
46. Douglas, C.C., et al., Role of diet in the treatment of polycystic ovary syndrome. *Fertil Steril*, 2006;. 85(3): 679–88.
47. Kasim-Karakas, S.E., et al., Metabolic and endocrine effects of a polyunsaturated fatty acid-rich diet in polycystic ovary syndrome. *J Clin Endocrinol Metab*, 2004;. 89(2): 615–20.
48. Jenkins, D.J., et al., Glycemic index: overview of implications in health and disease. *Am J Clin Nutr*, 2002;. 76(1): 266S–73S.
49. Luscombe, N., M. Noakes, and P. Clifton, Diets high and low in glycemic index versus high monounsaturated fat diets: effects on glucose and lipid metabolism in NIDDM. *Eur J Clin Nutr*, 1999;. 53(6): 473–8.
50. Rizkalla, S.W., et al., Improved plasma glucose control, whole-body glucose utilization, and lipid profile on a low-glycemic index diet in type 2 diabetic men: a randomized controlled trial. *Diabetes Care*, 2004;. 27(8): 1866–72.
51. Frost, G., et al., Glycaemic index as a determinant of serum HDL-cholesterol concentration. *Lancet*, 1999;. 353(9158): 1045–8.
52. Jenkins, D., et al., Low glycemic index carbohydrate foods in the management of hyperlipidemia. *Am J Clin Nutr*, 1985;. 42(4): 604–17.
53. Jenkins, D.J., et al., Low-glycemic index diet in hyperlipidemia: use of traditional starchy foods. *American Journal of Clinical Nutrition*, 1987;. 46(1): 66–71.
54. Jrvi, A.E., et al., Improved glycemic control and lipid profile and normalized fibrinolytic activity on a low-glycemic index diet in type 2 diabetic patients. *Diabetes Care*, 1999;. 22(1): 10–8.
55. Wolever, T., et al., Beneficial effect of a low glycaemic index diet in type 2 diabetes. *Diabet Med*, 1992. 9: 451–8.
56. Wolever, T., et al., Beneficial effect of low-glycemic index diet in overweight NIDDM subjects. *Diabetes Care*, 1992;. 15(4): 562–4.
57. Ebbeling, C.B., et al., Effects of an ad libitum low-glycemic load diet on cardiovascular disease risk factors in obese young adults. *Am J Clin Nutr*, 2005;. 81(5): 976–82.
58. Fontvieille, A., et al., The use of low glycaemic index foods improves metabolic control of diabetic patients over five weeks. *Diabet Med*, 1992;. 9(5): 444–50.
59. Brynes, A., et al., A randomised four-intervention crossover study investigating the effect of carbohydrates on daytime profiles of insulin, glucose, non-esterified fatty acids and triacylglycerols in middle-aged men. *Br J Nutr*, 2003. 89: 207–18.

60. Slabber, M., et al., Effects of a low-insulin-response, energy-restricted diet on weight loss and plasma insulin concentrations in hyperinsulinemic obese females. *Am J Clin Nutr*, 1994;. 60(1): 48–53.
61. Krishnan, S., et al., Glycemic index, glycemic load, and cereal fiber intake and risk of type 2 diabetes in US black women. *Arch Intern Med*, 2007;. 167(21): 2304–9.
62. Liu, S., et al., A prospective study of dietary glycemic load, carbohydrate intake, and risk of coronary heart disease in US women. *Am J Clin Nutr*, 2000;. 71(6): 1455–61.
63. Salmeron, J., et al., Dietary fiber, glycemic load, and risk of NIDDM in men. *Diabetes Care*, 1997;. 20(4): 545–50.
64. Salmeron, J., et al., Dietary fiber, glycemic load, and risk of non-insulin-dependent diabetes mellitus in women. *JAMA*, 1997;. 277(6): 472–7.
65. Villegas, R., et al., Prospective study of dietary carbohydrates, glycemic index, glycemic load, and incidence of type 2 diabetes mellitus in middle-aged Chinese women. *Arch Intern Med*, 2007;. 167(21): 2310–6.
66. McKeown, N., et al., Carbohydrate nutrition, insulin resistance, and the prevalence of the metabolic syndrome in the Framingham offspring cohort. *Diabetes Care*, 2004. 27: 538–46.
67. Murakami, K., et al., Dietary glycemic index and load in relation to metabolic risk factors in Japanese female farmers with traditional dietary habits. *Am J Clin Nutr*, 2006;. 83(5): 1161–9.
68. Augustin, L.S., et al., Glycemic index and glycemic load in endometrial cancer. *Int J Cancer*, 2003;. 105(3): 404–7.
69. Augustin, L.S., et al., Dietary glycemic index and glycemic load, and breast cancer risk: a case-control study. *Ann Oncol*, 2001;. 12(11): 1533–8.
70. Franceschi, S., et al., Dietary glycemic load and colorectal cancer risk. *Ann Oncol*, 2001;. 12(2): 173–8.
71. Slattery, M., et al., Dietary sugar and colon cancer. *Cancer Epidemiol Biomarkers Prev*, 1997;. 6(9): 677–85.
72. Augustin, L.S., et al., Dietary glycemic index, glycemic load and ovarian cancer risk: a case-control study in Italy. *Ann Oncol*, 2003;. 14(1): 78–84.
73. Ludwig, D., Dietary glycemic index and obesity. *J Nutr*, 2000. 130(2S Suppl): 280S–283S.
74. Agus, M., et al., Dietary composition and physiologic adaptations to energy restriction. *Am J Clin Nutr*, 2000;. 71(4): 901–7.
75. Pereira, M., et al., Effects of a low – glycemic load diet on resting energy expenditure and heart disease risk factors during weight loss. *JAMA*, 2004. 292: 2482–2490.
76. Febbraio, M., et al., Preexercise carbohydrate ingestion, glucose kinetics, and muscle glycogen use: effect of the glycemic index. *J Appl Physiol*, 2000;. 89(5): 1845–51.
77. Stevenson, E., C. Williams, and M. Nute, The influence of the glycaemic index of breakfast and lunch on substrate utilisation during the postprandial periods and subsequent exercise. *Br J Nutr*, 2005. 93: 885–893.
78. Wee, S.L., et al., Ingestion of a high-glycemic index meal increases muscle glycogen storage at rest but augments its utilization during subsequent exercise. *J Appl Physiol*, 2005;. 99(2): 707–14.
79. Wu, C.L., et al., The influence of high-carbohydrate meals with different glycaemic indices on substrate utilisation during subsequent exercise. *Br J Nutr*, 2003;. 90(6): 1049–56.
80. Bahadori, B., et al., Low-fat, high-carbohydrate (low-glycaemic index) diet induces weight loss and preserves lean body mass in obese healthy subjects: results of a 24-week study. *Diabetes, Obesity and Metabolism*, 2005. 7: 290–293.
81. Bouché, C., et al., Five-week, low–glycemic index diet decreases total fat mass and improves plasma lipid profile in moderately overweight nondiabetic men. *Diab Care*, 2003. 2: 822–28.
82. McMillan-Price, J., et al., Comparison of 4 diets of varying glycemic load on weight loss and cardiovascular risk reduction in overweight and obese young adults: a randomised controlled trial. *Archives Internal Medicine*, 2006. 166: 1466–75.
83. Dumesnil, J.G., et al., Effect of a low-glycaemic index–low-fat–high protein diet on the atherogenic metabolic risk profile of abdominally obese men. *Br J Nutr*, 2001. 86(5): p. 557–68.
84. Hare-Bruun, H., A. Flint, and B.L. Heitmann, Glycemic index and glycemic load in relation to changes in body weight, body fat distribution, and body composition in adult Danes. *Am J Clin Nutr*, 2006;. 84(4): 871–9; quiz 952–3.
85. Ma, Y., et al., Association between dietary carbohydrates and body weight. *Am J Epidemiol*, 2005. 161: 359–367.
86. Buyken, A., et al., Glycemic index in the diet of European outpatients with type 1 diabetes: relations to glycated hemoglobin and serum lipids. *Am J Clin Nutr*, 2001;. 73(3): 574–81.
87. Thomas, D.E., E.J. Elliott, and L. Baur, Low glycaemic index or low glycaemic load diets for overweight and obesity. *Cochrane Database Syst Rev*, 2007(3): CD005105.
88. Boeing, H., et al., Association between glycated hemoglobin and diet and other lifestyle factors in a nondiabetic population: cross-sectional evaluation of data from the Potsdam cohort of the European Prospective Investigation into Cancer and Nutrition Study. *Am J Clin Nutr*, 2000;. 71(5): 1115–22.
89. Liu, S., et al., A prospective study of whole-grain intake and risk of type 2 diabetes mellitus in US women. *Am J Public Health*, 2000;. 90(9): 1409–15.
90. Marshall, J.A., D.H. Bessesen, and R.F. Hamman, High saturated fat and low starch and fibre are associated with hyperinsulinaemia in a non-diabetic population: the San Luis Valley Diabetes Study. *Diabetologia*, 1997;. 40(4): 430–8.
91. Meyer, K., et al., Carbohydrates, dietary fiber, and incident type 2 diabetes in older women. *Am J Clin Nutr*, 2000. 71: 921–930.
92. Montonen, J., et al., Whole-grain and fiber intake and the incidence of type 2 diabetes. *Am J Clin Nutr*, 2003;. 77(3): 622–9.
93. Pereira, M., et al., Effect of whole grains on insulin sensitivity in overweight hyperinsulinemic adults. *Am J Clin Nutr*, 2002. 75: 848–855.

94. Liese, A.D., et al., Whole-grain intake and insulin sensitivity: the Insulin Resistance Atherosclerosis Study. *Am J Clin Nutr*, 2003;. 78(5): 965–71.
95. Liu, S., et al., Relation between changes in intakes of dietary fiber and grain products and changes in weight and development of obesity among middle-aged women. *Am J Clin Nutr*, 2003. 78: 920–927.
96. Marshall, J.A., R.F. Hamman, and J. Baxter, High-fat, low-carbohydrate diet and the etiology of non-insulin-dependent diabetes mellitus: the San Luis Valley Diabetes Study. *Am J Epidemiol*, 1991;. 134(6): 590–603.
97. Marshall, J.A., et al., Dietary fat predicts conversion from impaired glucose tolerance to NIDDM. The San Luis Valley Diabetes Study. *Diabetes Care*, 1994;. 17(1): 50–6.
98. Schulze, M.B., et al., Carbohydrate intake and incidence of type 2 diabetes in the European Prospective Investigation into Cancer and Nutrition (EPIC)-Potsdam Study. *Br J Nutr*, 2007: 1–10.
99. Swinburn, B.A., P.A. Metcalf, and S.J. Ley, Long-term (5-year) effects of a reduced-fat diet intervention in individuals with glucose intolerance. *Diabetes Care*, 2001;. 24(4): 619–24.
100. Saldana, T.M., A.M. Siega-Riz, and L.S. Adair, Effect of macronutrient intake on the development of glucose intolerance during pregnancy. *Am J Clin Nutr*, 2004;. 79(3): 479–86.
101. Appel, L.J., et al., A clinical trial of the effects of dietary patterns on blood pressure. DASH Collaborative Research Group. *N Engl J Med*, 1997;. 336(16): 1117–24.
102. Ard, J.D., et al., The effect of the PREMIER interventions on insulin sensitivity. *Diabetes Care*, 2004;. 27(2): 340–7.
103. Yang, E.J., et al., Carbohydrate intake and biomarkers of glycemic control among US adults: the third National Health and Nutrition Examination Survey (NHANES III). *Am J Clin Nutr*, 2003;. 77(6): 1426–33.
104. Xu, J., et al., Macronutrient intake and glycemic control in a population-based sample of American Indians with diabetes: the Strong Heart Study. *Am J Clin Nutr*, 2007;. 86(2): 480–7.
105. Feskens, E.J. and D. Kromhout, Habitual dietary intake and glucose tolerance in euglycaemic men: the Zutphen Study. *Int J Epidemiol*, 1990;. 19(4): 953–9.
106. Lovejoy, J. and M. DiGirolamo, Habitual dietary intake and insulin sensitivity in lean and obese adults. *Am J Clin Nutr*, 1992;. 55(6): 1174–9.
107. Mayer, E.J., et al., Usual dietary fat intake and insulin concentrations in healthy women twins. *Diabetes Care*, 1993;. 16(11): 1459–69.
108. Mayer-Davis, E.J., et al., Dietary fat and insulin sensitivity in a triethnic population: the role of obesity. The Insulin Resistance Atherosclerosis Study (IRAS). *Am J Clin Nutr*, 1997;. 65(1): 79–87.
109. Parker, D.R., et al., Relationship of dietary saturated fatty acids and body habitus to serum insulin concentrations: the Normative Aging Study. *Am J Clin Nutr*, 1993;. 58(2): 129–36.
110. Colditz, G., et al., Diet and risk of clinical diabetes in women. *Am J Clin Nutr*, 1992. 55: 1018–1023.
111. Tsunehara, C.H., D.L. Leonetti, and W.Y. Fujimoto, Diet of second-generation Japanese-American men with and without non-insulin-dependent diabetes. *Am J Clin Nutr*, 1990;. 52(4): 731–8.
112. Ohrvall, M., et al., The serum cholesterol ester fatty acid composition but not the serum concentration of alpha tocopherol predicts the development of myocardial infarction in 50-year-old men: 19 years follow-up. *Atherosclerosis*, 1996;. 127(1): 65–71.
113. Salomaa, V., et al., Fatty acid composition of serum cholesterol esters in different degrees of glucose intolerance: a population-based study. *Metabolism*, 1990;. 39(12): 1285–91.
114. Vessby, B., et al., The risk to develop NIDDM is related to the fatty acid composition of the serum cholesterol esters. *Diabetes*, 1994;. 43(11): 1353–7.
115. Vessby, B., S. Tengblad, and H. Lithell, Insulin sensitivity is related to the fatty acid composition of serum lipids and skeletal muscle phospholipids in 70-year-old men. *Diabetologia*, 1994;. 37(10): 1044–50.
116. Wang, L., et al., Plasma fatty acid composition and incidence of diabetes in middle-aged adults: the Atherosclerosis Risk in Communities (ARIC) Study. *Am J Clin Nutr*, 2003;. 78(1): 91–8.
117. Stender, S. and J. Dyerberg, Influence of trans fatty acids on health. *Ann Nutr Metab*, 2004;. 48(2): 61–6.
118. Grundy, S.M., N. Abate, and M. Chandalia, Diet composition and the metabolic syndrome: what is the optimal fat intake? *Am J Med*, 2002. 113(Suppl 9B): 25S–29S.
119. Tricon, S., et al., Opposing effects of cis-9,trans-11 and trans-10,cis-12 conjugated linoleic acid on blood lipids in healthy humans. *Am J Clin Nutr*, 2004;. 80(3): 614–20.
120. Mozaffarian, D., Trans fatty acids – effects on systemic inflammation and endothelial function. *Atheroscler Suppl*, 2006;. 7(2): 29–32.
121. Lopez-Garcia, E., et al., Consumption of trans fatty acids is related to plasma biomarkers of inflammation and endothelial dysfunction. *J Nutr*, 2005;. 135(3): 562–6.
122. Chavarro, J.E., et al., Dietary fatty acid intakes and the risk of ovulatory infertility. *Am J Clin Nutr*, 2007;. 85(1): 231–7.
123. Zivkovic, A.M., J.B. German, and A.J. Sanyal, Comparative review of diets for the metabolic syndrome: implications for nonalcoholic fatty liver disease. *Am J Clin Nutr*, 2007;. 86(2): 285–300.
124. Krebs, M., et al., Mechanism of amino acid-induced skeletal muscle insulin resistance in humans. *Diabetes*, 2002;. 51(3): 599–605.
125. Larivire, F., et al., Effects of dietary protein restriction on glucose and insulin metabolism in normal and diabetic humans. *Metabolism*, 1994;. 43(4): 462–7.

126. Linn, T., et al., Effect of dietary protein intake on insulin secretion and glucose metabolism in insulin-dependent diabetes mellitus. *J Clin Endocrinol Metab*, 1996;. 81(11): 3938–43.
127. Linn, T., et al., Effect of long-term dietary protein intake on glucose metabolism in humans. *Diabetologia*, 2000;. 43(10): 1257–65.
128. Rossetti, L., et al., Effect of dietary protein on in vivo insulin action and liver glycogen repletion. *Am J Physiol*, 1989. 257(2 Pt 1): E212–9.
129. Farnsworth, E., et al., Effect of a high-protein, energy-restricted diet on body composition, glycemic control, and lipid concentrations in overweight and obese hyperinsulinemic men and women. *Am J Clin Nutr*, 2003;. 78(1): 31–9.
130. Foster, G.D., et al., A randomized trial of a low-carbohydrate diet for obesity. *N Engl J Med*, 2003;. 348(21): 2082–90.
131. Parker, B., et al., Effect of a high-protein, high-monounsaturated fat weight loss diet on glycemic control and lipid levels in type 2 diabetes. *Diabetes Care*, 2002;. 25(3): 425–30.
132. Stern, L., et al., The effects of low-carbohydrate versus conventional weight loss diets in severely obese adults: one-year follow-up of a randomised trial. *Ann Intern Med*, 2004. 140: 778–785.
133. Tay, J., et al., Metabolic effects of weight loss on a very-low-carbohydrate diet compared with an isocaloric high-carbohydrate diet in abdominally obese subjects. *J Am Coll Cardiol*, 2008;. 51(1): 59–67.
134. Jiang, R., et al., Dietary iron intake and blood donations in relation to risk of type 2 diabetes in men: a prospective cohort study. *Am J Clin Nutr*, 2004;. 79(1): 70–5.
135. Lee, D.H., A.R. Folsom, and D.R. Jacobs, Dietary iron intake and Type 2 diabetes incidence in postmenopausal women: the Iowa Women s Health Study. *Diabetologia*, 2004;. 47(2): 185–94.
136. Luan, D.C., et al., Body Iron Stores and Dietary Iron Intake in Relation to Diabetes in Adults in North China. *Diabetes Care*, 2007; 31(2): 285–6.
137. Song, Y., et al., A prospective study of red meat consumption and type 2 diabetes in middle-aged and elderly women: the women s health study. *Diabetes Care*, 2004;. 27(9): 2108–15.
138. Schulze, M.B., et al., Processed meat intake and incidence of Type 2 diabetes in younger and middle-aged women. *Diabetologia*, 2003;. 46(11): 1465–73.
139. Jiang, R., et al., Body iron stores in relation to risk of type 2 diabetes in apparently healthy women. *JAMA*, 2004;. 291(6): 711–7.
140. Panagiotakos, D.B., et al., The relationship between dietary habits, blood glucose and insulin levels among people without cardiovascular disease and type 2 diabetes; the ATTICA study. *Rev Diabet Stud*, 2005;. 2(4): 208–15.
141. WCRF/AICR, *Food, Nutrition, Physical Activity and the Prevention of Cancer: a Global Perspective.* 2007, World Cancer Research Fund and American Institute for Cancer Research Washington DC, USA.
142. Goodman, M.T., et al., Association of soy and fiber consumption with the risk of endometrial cancer. *Am J Epidemiol*, 1997;. 146(4): 294–306.
143. Littman, A.J., S.A. Beresford, and E. White, The association of dietary fat and plant foods with endometrial cancer (United States). *Cancer Causes Control*, 2001;. 12(8): 691–702.
144. McCann, S.E., et al., Diet in the epidemiology of endometrial cancer in western New York (United States). *Cancer Causes Control*, 2000;. 11(10): 965–74.
145. Petridou, E., et al., Diet in relation to endometrial cancer risk: a case-control study in Greece. *Nutr Cancer*, 2002;. 44(1): 16–22.
146. Zheng, W., et al., Dietary intake of energy and animal foods and endometrial cancer incidence. The Iowa women s health study. *Am J Epidemiol*, 1995;. 142(4): 388–94.
147. Ledikwe, J.H., et al., Reductions in dietary energy density are associated with weight loss in overweight and obese participants in the PREMIER trial. *Am J Clin Nutr*, 2007;. 85(5): 1212–21.
148. Ledikwe, J.H., et al., Dietary energy density is associated with energy intake and weight status in US adults. *Am J Clin Nutr*, 2006;. 83(6): 1362–68.
149. Rolls, B.J., L.S. Roe, and J.S. Meengs, Reductions in portion size and energy density of foods are additive and lead to sustained decreases in energy intake. *Am J Clin Nutr*, 2006;. 83(1): 11–17.
150. Bell, E.A. and B.J. Rolls, Energy density of foods affects energy intake across multiple levels of fat content in lean and obese women. *Am J Clin Nutr*, 2001;. 73(6): 1010–1018.
151. Ello-Martin, J.A., J.H. Ledikwe, and B.J. Rolls, The influence of food portion size and energy density on energy intake: implications for weight management. *Am J Clin Nutr*, 2005;. 82(1): 236S–41S.
152. Kral, T.V.E., L.S. Roe, and B.J. Rolls, Combined effects of energy density and portion size on energy intake in women. *Am J Clin Nutr*, 2004;. 79(6): 962–968.
153. Ello-Martin, J.A., et al., Dietary energy density in the treatment of obesity: a year-long trial comparing 2 weight-loss diets. *Am J Clin Nutr*, 2007;. 85(6): 1465–1477.
154. Baxter, A.J., T. Coyne, and C. McClintock, Dietary patterns and metabolic syndrome–a review of epidemiologic evidence. *Asia Pac J Clin Nutr*, 2006;. 15(2): 134–42.
155. Hodge, A.M., et al., Dietary patterns and diabetes incidence in the Melbourne Collaborative Cohort Study. *Am J Epidemiol*, 2007;. 165(6): 603–10.
156. Harriss, L.R., et al., Dietary patterns and cardiovascular mortality in the Melbourne Collaborative Cohort Study. *Am J Clin Nutr*, 2007;. 86(1): 221–9.

157. Norris, S.L., et al., Long-term non-pharmacological weight loss interventions for adults with prediabetes. *Cochrane Database Syst Rev*, 2005(2): CD005270.
158. Berrino, F., et al., Reducing bioavailable sex hormones through a comprehensive change in diet: the diet and androgens (DIANA) randomized trial. *Cancer Epidemiol Biomarkers Prev*, 2001;. 10(1): 25–33.
159. Chavarro, J.E., et al., Diet and lifestyle in the prevention of ovulatory disorder infertility. *Obstet Gynecol*, 2007;. 110(5): 1050–8.
160. Giugliano, D. and K. Esposito, Mediterranean diet and metabolic diseases. *Curr Opin Lipidol*, 2008;. 19(1): 63–8.
161. Bull, M., et al., Inflammation, obesity and comorbidities: the role of diet. *Public Health Nutr*, 2007. 10(10A): 1164–72.
162. Esmaillzadeh, A., et al., Dietary patterns, insulin resistance, and prevalence of the metabolic syndrome in women. *Am J Clin Nutr*, 2007;. 85(3): 910–8.

Chapter 17
Exercise in the Treatment of PCOS

Emma Stevenson

17.1 Introduction

The prevalence of insulin resistance, overweight and obesity are increasing at alarming rates world wide but are problems which are extremely prevalent in women with PCOS. A decline in energy expenditure through reduced daily activity and physical exercise (accompanied by an increase in energy intake) is a major contributor to increases in obesity and insulin resistance. Lifestyle interventions that alter energy balance are therefore essential in the treatment and prevention of these epidemics. The combination of exercise, diet and other lifestyle interventions should be promoted however, this chapter aims to highlight the important role that exercise can play in the prevention and treatment of PCOS not only through the management of body weight but also through its effects on the metabolic and hormonal environment associated with PCOS.

17.2 Exercise and Weight Loss

It has already been well documented in this book that a large proportion of women who suffer from PCOS are overweight or obese and that weight loss significantly improves the symptoms associated with the syndrome. The role of exercise in the management of body weight is an important one but there are still few large-scale randomised controlled trials assessing the effects of exercise alone on weight loss. There is also little data for the quantification of exercise and its relationship to obesity in PCOS and as a result there are limited studies exploring exercise as a treatment option for women with PCOS [1].

The studies that have been carried out investigating the effects of exercise programmes alone on weight loss have shown only modest changes as the energy deficit produced by exercise alone is very small compared to the deficit that can result from changes in both physical activity patterns and dietary intake.

The majority of studies that have shown a reduction in weight following an exercise programme compared with a control group have not focussed on weight loss as their primary outcome and the type and duration of exercise has varied significantly between studies [2–5]. Although most of these studies have shown that exercise alone can result in weight reduction, the changes are usually small ($\sim$3 kg).

A study carried out by Ross and colleagues [6] in Canada investigated the effect of equivalent diet- or exercise-induced weight loss and exercise without weight loss on subcutaneous fat, visceral fat and insulin sensitivity in obese women. The study reported that caloric deficit, whether achieved by exercise or diet, resulted in similar weight loss. The results therefore suggest that weight loss can be achieved without changes to dietary intake however, adherence to the exercise programme was poor in this study questioning the relevance of the results to long-term interventions.

E. Stevenson (✉)
School of Psychology and Sports Sciences, Northumbria University, Newcastle Upon Tyne, NE1 8ST, UK
e-mail: e.stevenson@unn.ac.uk

N.R. Farid, E. Diamanti-Kandarakis (eds.), *Diagnosis and Management of Polycystic Ovary Syndrome*,
DOI 10.1007/978-0-387-09718-3_17,

More data is available on the use of exercise to maintain weight loss following a successful weight reduction programme and it appears that the amount of exercise undertaken in the weight maintenance phase correlates well with the amount of weight regained over time [7, 8]. However, the type and duration of exercise programmes varies greatly in research studies and there is still a large amount of research to be carried out in this area to be able to provide accurate practical recommendations. The challenge, of course, is improving adherence to exercise programmes to ensure maintenance of weight loss is achieved.

Relatively few studies have looked at the effects of chronic training programmes on weight loss in the PCOS population. Of those which have, exercise training has been shown to be beneficial in the treatment of PCOS and its symptoms. One large-scale study reported that a 3-month training programme (bicycle training, three times per week for 30 min) resulted in 4.5% reduction in body weight in 45 women with PCOS compared with healthy controls [9]. Improvements in waist-to-hip ratios have been reported following a 6-month training programme in overweight or obese women (BMI: 35.49 ± 7.57 kg/m^2) with PCOS [10].

Although the metabolic benefits of weight loss are clear, there is still little information regarding the effects of weight loss through exercise in women with PCOS. Further research is required to examine both the negative and the positive effects of exercise in reproductive improvements in PCOS and also further information on the amount and duration of exercise required to have an effect on different aspects of the syndrome [11].

17.3 Exercise and Insulin Resistance

Insulin resistance and compensatory hyperinsulinaemia appear to be one of key features in the majority of cases of PCOS [12]. Insulin sensitivity is enhanced by physical activity, and low levels of physical activity are related to most of the abnormalities associated with insulin resistance. Several epidemiological studies have tested the hypothesis that insulin resistance is more prevalent in those who are unfit or do not partake in any physical activity [13–15].

Intervention studies have also shown improvements in insulin resistance following an exercise programme. In the study described in the previous section by Ross and colleagues [6], improvements in insulin sensitivity were only observed in the exercise weight-loss group and not in any of the groups that did not include an exercise intervention.

How much exercise needs to be done to see an improvement in insulin sensitivity? The results of studies show conflicting results and therefore intensity and duration of exercise required is still unclear. In a study from Otago University in New Zealand [16], normoglycemic, insulin resistant men and women were randomised to a control group or ‘modest’ or ‘intense’ exercise and dietary intervention group. The ‘modest’ group were provided with a diet commonly recommended by health authorities and were required to exercise for 30 min five times a week. The ‘intense’ group had stricter dietary recommendations and were asked to exercise for at least 20 min five times a week at 80–90% HRmax. Only the ‘intensive’ group showed a significant improvement in their insulin sensitivity and this was associated with a significant improvement in aerobic fitness. Although diet composition may have played a role in determining insulin sensitivity, the results from this study would suggest that current exercise recommendations may not be sufficient to have a significant impact on insulin sensitivity. A study by Houmard and colleagues [17] reported that an exercise prescription that incorporated approximately 170 min of exercise/wk improved insulin sensitivity more substantially than a program utilising approximately 115 min of exercise/wk, regardless of exercise intensity and volume. The authors concluded that total exercise duration is therefore more important when designing training programmes to improve insulin action.

Studies on the impact of exercise on insulin sensitivity in women with PCOS are very limited. In a randomised controlled trial investigating the effect of a 3-month exercise programme in young women with PCOS [9], a significant improvement in insulin sensitivity was observed in those who undertook three 30 min exercise sessions a week compared to sedentary controls. The authors concluded that exercise programmes represent a simple, therapeutic option that can be safely and routinely performed to reduce cardiovascular risk profiles in young women with PCOS. Further research is however required in older populations that may find exercise more challenging.

17.4 Exercise, Diet and PCOS

Although it is clear that exercise can have a beneficial effect on insulin sensitivity and obviously plays an important role in weight loss, the combination of exercise and a healthy diet has additive benefits and the two should be promoted as effective lifestyle changes. Although studies in PCOS patients are limited, studies have investigated the effects of exercise programmes versus dietary intervention and also the combination of exercise and diet in the treatment of PCOS.

An early study investigating the effects of the combination of exercise and diet reported a 6-month exercise and diet programme resulted in improved reproductive function as well as a 71% improvement in insulin sensitivity, 33% fall in fasting insulin levels and 11% reduction in central fat in young obese PCOS sufferers [18]. It is interesting to note that these changes were observed despite minimal weight loss in the patients (~ 2%) suggesting that changes in insulin sensitivity may be the metabolic mediator for the changes.

Bruner and colleagues carried our study to investigate the effect of a programme of resistance and endurance exercise plus nutritional counselling versus nutritional counselling only for 12 wk on hormonal, menstrual and reproductive function in women with PCOS [19]. Following the 12 wk intervention, greater reductions in sum of two skinfolds were seen in the exercise group however, significant decreases in waist girth and insulin concentrations were seen in both groups. The results of this study were therefore unable to claim that one treatment was superior to the other however suggest that exercise may provide an additional benefit than nutritional changes alone.

Recently, a study carried out in Italy compared the efficacy on reproductive functions of a 24-wk-structured exercise programme with a hypocaloric, hyperproteic diet programme in obese PCOS patients [20]. Although both the exercise and the diet programmes improved menstrual cyclicity and fertility in overweight PCOS patients, greater improvements in body weight, BMI, waist circumference and insulin resistance indexes were seen in the exercising group. Although the results of this study indicate that exercise can have additional benefits compared to dietary intervention alone, it does not tell us the additive benefits of exercise when combined with energy restriction.

A group of researchers from the Commonwealth Scientific and Industrial Research Organisation in Australia have recently addressed this question and investigated the additional benefits of exercise training when combined with a moderate hypocaloric weight-loss diet on body composition, cardiometabolic and hormonal profiles on overweight and obese women with PCOS [21]. Subjects in the study consumed an energy restricted, high-protein diet (5000–6000 kJ/d) for 20 weeks and took part in no exercise, aerobic or aerobic-resistance training. Weight loss via energy restriction resulted in improved reproductive function, cardiometabolic abnormalities and hormonal parameters in overweight and obese women with PCOS. However, the addition of exercise provided no additional improvement in these parameters. The additional exercise did result in more favourable changes in body composition.

It would therefore appear that the combination of exercise and diet is more favourable in the treatment of PCOS but further research is required in this area in lean individuals with PCOS and also to investigate the effects of different modes and duration of exercise on different parameters of the syndrome.

17.5 Other Potential Benefits of Exercise in PCOS Patients

As well as obesity and insulin resistance, women with PCOS may have other cardiovascular risk factors such as lipid abnormalities, hypertension and high homocysteine concentrations. It is clear that the major impact of exercise in the treatment of PCOS is through effects on insulin sensitivity and weight loss however, exercise can have many other potential benefits which can help in the treatment of the disease.

Regular exercise has been shown to significantly lower plasma homocysteine concentrations in young overweight or obese women with PCOS [10]. Subjects in the study were instructed to complete three walks per week of 20–60 min duration for 6 months. Volume of walking was prescribed by means of fortnightly targets, which increased from 120 min in the first fortnight to 420 min in fortnight 6 and thereafter. A significant decrease in plasma total homocysteine concentrations, waist-to-hip ratio and a significant increase in maximal oxygen consumption were recorded in the exercise group with no changes in any of the variables observed in the no exercise group.

Abnormal post-exercise heart rate recovery (HRR) have been reported in women with PCOS and abnormal HRR has also been significantly correlated to markers of insulin sensitivity and BMI [22], suggesting a close relationship between autonomic function and glucose metabolism in patients with PCOS [22]. In a recent study, Giallauria and colleagues [23] investigated the effect of exercise training on autonomic function and inflammatory markers. Young women with PCOS undertook either a 3-month exercise programme or no exercise. As well as reducing BMI and improving insulin sensitivity, exercise resulted in significant improvements in autonomic function (as expressed by HRR) and inflammatory patterns (C-reactive protein levels [CRP] and white blood cell count [WBC]) compared to the no exercise group. Cross-sectional studies have linked HRR and WBC's to the metabolic syndrome and many of its components [24] and inflammatory markers such as WBC and CRP are strong predictors of cardiovascular events [25]. It is therefore evident that exercise can play an important role in improving cardiovascular risk profile in women with PCOS [23].

17.6 Practical Recommendations

Although convincing evidence exists for the benefits of physical activity and/or exercise training for treatment of PCOS, dose–response relationships remain tentative. This is partly attributable to discrepancies over the optimal and minimum volume for treatment of this condition, in particular, the effects of intensity (moderate versus vigorous) on health status. The general consensus at the moment appears that chronic exercise training lasting 3–6 months is beneficial for PCOS patients to manage weight loss. Both aerobic exercise and resistance training seem to be equally effective in reducing central adiposity, which is the most common fat distribution in PCOS.

There are currently no specific physical activity guidelines that focus specifically on PCOS but given the associations between PCOS, insulin resistance and cardiovascular risk factors and the evidence reported in this chapter, the following recommendations based on the American Diabetes Association (ADA) [26] exercise recommendations should be followed for exercise prescription:

- At least 150 min per week of moderate to high-intensity exercise.
- Distribute exercise over 3 days with no more than two consecutive days without activity.
- Reduce sedentary activities (watching television and playing computer games) as much as possible.

17.7 Conclusions

Although there appears to be a lack of data relating to the effects of exercise specifically on PCOS, there is evidence that exercise has benefits on many of the metabolic disturbances related to the syndrome. Regular exercise is an important part of a healthy lifestyle, and in combination with a healthy diet, can significantly improve insulin sensitivity, aid weight loss and weight maintenance and significantly improve cardiovascular risk factors. Further research is required to specifically investigate the effect of exercise on the prevention and treatment of PCOS with specific attention on the intensity and duration of exercise required so that practical recommendations can be provided.

References

1. Clark, A.M., et al., *Weight loss in obese infertile women results in improvement in reproductive outcome for all forms of fertility treatment.* Hum Reprod, 1998. **13**(6): 1502–5.
2. Irwin, M.L., et al., *Effect of exercise on total and intra-abdominal body fat in postmenopausal women: a randomized controlled trial.* Jama, 2003. **289**(3): 323–30.

3. Ready, A.E., et al., *Walking program reduces elevated cholesterol in women postmenopause.* Can J Cardiol, 1995. **11**(10): 905–12.
4. Wood, P.D., et al., *Changes in plasma lipids and lipoproteins in overweight men during weight loss through dieting as compared with exercise.* N Engl J Med, 1988. **319**(18): 1173–9.
5. Stewart, K.J., et al., *Exercise and risk factors associated with metabolic syndrome in older adults.* Am J Prev Med, 2005. **28**(1): 9–18.
6. Ross, R., et al., *Exercise-induced reduction in obesity and insulin resistance in women: a randomized controlled trial.* Obes Res, 2004. **12**(5): 789–98.
7. Wadden, T.A., et al., *Exercise and the maintenance of weight loss: 1-year follow-up of a controlled clinical trial.* J Consult Clin Psychol, 1998. **66**(2): 429–33.
8. Wing, R.R., et al., *Exercise in a behavioural weight control programme for obese patients with Type 2 (non-insulin-dependent) diabetes.* Diabetologia, 1988. **31**(12): 902–9.
9. Vigorito, C., et al., *Beneficial effects of a three-month structured exercise training program on cardiopulmonary functional capacity in young women with polycystic ovary syndrome.* J Clin Endocrinol Metab, 2007. **92**(4): 1379–84.
10. Randeva, H.S., et al., *Exercise decreases plasma total homocysteine in overweight young women with polycystic ovary syndrome.* J Clin Endocrinol Metab, 2002. **87**(10): 4496–501.
11. Hoeger, K.M., *Exercise therapy in polycystic ovary syndrome.* Semin Reprod Med, 2008. **26**(1): 93–100.
12. Dunaif, A., *Insulin resistance and the polycystic ovary syndrome: mechanism and implications for pathogenesis.* Endocr Rev, 1997. **18**(6): 774–800.
13. Brunner, E.J., et al., *Social inequality in coronary risk: central obesity and the metabolic syndrome. Evidence from the Whitehall II study.* Diabetologia, 1997. **40**(11): 1341–9.
14. Whaley, M.H., et al., *Physical fitness and clustering of risk factors associated with the metabolic syndrome.* Med Sci Sports Exerc, 1999. **31**(2): 287–93.
15. Thune, I., et al., *Physical activity improves the metabolic risk profiles in men and women: the Tromso Study.* Arch Intern Med, 1998. **158**(15): 1633–40.
16. McAuley, K.A., et al., *Intensive lifestyle changes are necessary to improve insulin sensitivity: a randomized controlled trial.* Diabetes Care, 2002. **25**(3): 445–52.
17. Houmard, J.A., et al., *Effect of the volume and intensity of exercise training on insulin sensitivity.* J Appl Physiol, 2004. **96**(1): 101–6.
18. Huber-Buchholz, M.M., D.G. Carey, and R.J. Norman, *Restoration of reproductive potential by lifestyle modification in obese polycystic ovary syndrome: role of insulin sensitivity and luteinizing hormone.* J Clin Endocrinol Metab, 1999. **84**(4): 1470–4.
19. Bruner, B., K. Chad, and D. Chizen, *Effects of exercise and nutritional counseling in women with polycystic ovary syndrome.* Appl Physiol Nutr Metab, 2006. **31**(4): 384–91.
20. Palomba, S., et al., *Structured exercise training programme versus hypocaloric hyperproteic diet in obese polycystic ovary syndrome patients with anovulatory infertility: a 24-week pilot study.* Hum Reprod, 2008. **23**(3): 642–50.
21. Thomson, R.L., et al., *The effect of a hypocaloric diet with and without exercise training on body composition, cardiometabolic risk profile, and reproductive function in overweight and obese women with polycystic ovary syndrome.* J Clin Endocrinol Metab, 2008.
22. Giallauria, F., et al., *Abnormal heart rate recovery after maximal cardiopulmonary exercise stress testing in young overweight women with polycystic ovary syndrome.* Clin Endocrinol (Oxf), 2008. **68**(1): 88–93.
23. Giallauria, F., et al., *Exercise training improves autonomic function and inflammatory pattern in women with polycystic ovary syndrome.* Clin Endocrinol (Oxf), 2008.
24. Lind, L. and B. Andren, *Heart rate recovery after exercise is related to the insulin resistance syndrome and heart rate variability in elderly men.* Am Heart J, 2002. **144**(4): 666–72.
25. Brown, D.W., W.H. Giles, and J.B. Croft, *White blood cell count: an independent predictor of coronary heart disease mortality among a national cohort.* J Clin Epidemiol, 2001. **54**(3): 316–22.
26. Sigal, R.J., et al., *Physical activity/exercise and type 2 diabetes: a consensus statement from the American Diabetes Association.* Diabetes Care, 2006. **29**(6): 1433–8.

Chapter 18
Medical Treatment

Jean-Patrice Baillargeon and Nadir R. Farid

18.1 Introduction

The polycystic ovary syndrome (PCOS) is a very common disorder, affecting 6–10% of women of reproductive age [1–5], that significantly reduces the quality of life of affected women [6–11] and greatly increases the risk for the metabolic syndrome [12–14], type 2 diabetes [15–23] and probably cardiovascular diseases [14,24–31]. It is therefore not only an infertility or cosmetic issue but also a disabling condition with serious long-term consequences. In order to provide the best quality of care, physicians should consider both immediate and long-term issues when managing women with PCOS.

18.2 Role of Insulin Resistance and Insulin Action in Polycystic Ovary Syndrome

18.2.1 PCOS Insulin Resistance

PCOS is associated with the long-term consequences of insulin resistance syndrome. It has been recognized for 20 years that most women with PCOS are indeed insulin resistant. Insulin resistance is classically defined as the reduced ability of insulin to stimulate glucose disappearance in peripheral tissues [32], mainly skeletal muscles. According to this definition, Dunaif et al. [33,34] were among the first to found that both obese and lean women with PCOS were both more insulin resistant than body mass index (BMI)-matched normal controls. This pioneering study was subsequently confirmed by many others (see Chapter by E. Diamanti-Kandarakis). Moreover, both female [35–38] and male [35,37–39] siblings of women with PCOS are affected by higher degree of insulin resistance and parameters of the metabolic syndrome than were controls of similar ages and BMIs. Numerous studies have showed that treatments improving insulin resistance in lean and obese women with PCOS reduce androgen levels, improve ovulatory function and decrease the exaggerated androgenic response to LH [40–45] and ACTH [46–51], supporting a key role of insulin resistance or insulin action in the pathophysiology of PCOS.

Hyperandrogenemia is also improved in hyperinsulinemic PCOS women after interventions that only decrease insulin levels. Testosterone decreased significantly in obese PCOS women after 10 days of treatment with diazoxide, which directly suppresses insulin secretion [52]. A randomized-controlled trial (RCT) found that reduction of serum insulin for 6 months with acarbose reduced testosterone levels in obese PCOS women [53], confirming a previous uncontrolled 3-month study [54]. Thus, these studies suggest that insulin directly modulates androgen production in vivo.

J.-P. Baillargeon (✉)
Associate Professor, Departments of Medicine and Physiology/Biophysics, Director, Program of Endocrinology and Metabolism, University of Sherbrooke, Sherbrooke, QC J1H 5N4, Canada
e-mail: Jean-Patrice.Baillargeon@USherbrooke.ca

N.R. Farid, E. Diamanti-Kandarakis (eds.), *Diagnosis and Management of Polycystic Ovary Syndrome*,
DOI 10.1007/978-0-387-09718-3_18,

18.2.2 Role of Insulin Action in PCOS Hyperandrogenemia

However, only a minority of women with insulin resistance, such as most of those who are obese, develop PCOS. Furthermore, Morin-Papunen et al. [55] and Vrbikova et al. [56] confirmed the presence of metabolic insulin resistance in obese PCOS women, but not in lean PCOS women as compared to BMI-matched controls. Ciampelli et al. [57] also found that lean PCOS women with normal insulin levels have perfectly normal insulin sensitivity, in contrast with lean PCOS women with hyperinsulinemia. Thus, although insulin action seems to play an important role in PCOS pathogenesis, metabolic insulin resistance and compensatory hyperinsulinemia are not necessary to develop PCOS. Does that mean that the etiology of PCOS differs between insulin-sensitive and insulin-resistant PCOS women? We have tried to answer this question by performing two clinical studies in normo-insulinemic PCOS women.

We first conducted a randomized-controlled trial using two insulin-sensitizing drugs (metformin and rosiglitazone, a PPARγ agonist) in 100 non-obese women with PCOS and normal insulin levels [58]. Despite normal baseline insulin, insulin sensitization significantly decreased testosterone levels and improved ovulation frequencies in these women compared to placebo. Metformin reduced insulin, but not rosiglitazone. Thus, metformin might have improved hyperandrogenemia in part by decreasing insulin levels, which suggests that hyperandrogenemia was indeed related to enhanced insulin action even in these normo-insulinemic women. PPARγ agonists increase metabolic insulin actions in adipose, muscle and hepatic tissues, but insulin sensitivity and levels remain unchanged in subjects with normal insulin sensitivity [59,60]. Since rosiglitazone improved hyperandrogenemia without decreasing insulin in our lean PCOS women, PPARγ agonists may directly restore normal androgen production in these women.

Second, we assessed directly the effect of insulin on androgen levels in PCOS women with normal insulin levels and sensitivity (measured with insulin–glucose clamps) [61]. Diazoxide-induced lowering of insulin secretion in these women was associated with a significant decrease in free testosterone and androstenedione levels; whereas it did not alter testosterone levels in healthy, non-obese women [62]. Thus insulin contributes to hyperandrogenemia even in PCOS women with normal insulin sensitivity, probably due to enhanced androgenic insulin action.

18.2.3 PCOS: A Syndrome of Androgenic Insulin Hypersensitivity?

Insulin's actions are mediated via two major pathways: the phosphatidyl-inositol 3-kinase (PI-3 K)/Akt pathway implicated in the metabolic effects of insulin, like cellular glucose transport, glycogen synthesis, etc., and the MEK/ERK pathway, responsible for the proliferative effects of insulin [63]. However, these insulin-signaling pathways may express *divergent* activity. Indeed, Wu et al. [64] found a decrease in glucose metabolism associated with an *increase* in proliferative activity in ovarian luteinizing granulosa cells from PCOS women. The same group also found in cultured porcine theca cells that dexamethasone induces resistance to insulin-mediated glucose transport concomitant with increased testosterone production and P450c17 expression [65]. These observations support the possibility that altered insulin action may be a causal factor in PCOS, with increased activity for androgen production concomitant with normal or reduced metabolic activity. Moreover, the same studies found that troglitazone, another PPARγ agonist, corrects these increased proliferative and androgenic activities, along with improvement of glucose metabolism. Apparently, PPARγ agonists may directly improve the hypothesized androgenic insulin hypersensitivity.

In summary, the foregoing studies suggest that women develop PCOS in part because of a selective androgenic insulin *hyper*sensitivity [66] (see Fig. 18.1). In some women, this defect may be sufficiently severe to cause typical PCOS in the absence of insulin resistance and hyperinsulinemia. These women's PCOS consequences will improve after interventions reducing insulin levels (acarbose, diazoxide and metformin) or improving specifically androgenic insulin hypersensitivity (PPARγ-agonists?). However, in most women with PCOS, development of compensatory hyperinsulinemia is probably necessary for expression of the syndrome. In these women, interventions that improve insulin resistance and compensatory hyperinsulinemia (weight loss, insulin-sensitizing drugs), decrease directly insulin levels (acarbose, diazoxide) or improve specifically androgenic insulin hypersensitivity (PPARγ-agonists?) would improve their PCOS manifestations.

18.3 Insulin Sensitization Through Weight Loss and Exercise

18.3.1 Obesity and PCOS

Based on a recent study from the United States [67], the proportion of obesity among women with PCOS, defined as a BMI of 30 kg/m^2 or greater, increased from 51% in 1987–1990 to 74% in 2000–2002. These proportions are higher in PCOS as compared to non-PCOS women from the same population (10–14% obesity rate in 1987–1990 and 25% in 2000–2002), but the progression of obesity in PCOS women over time likely reflects weight increase in the background population. Interestingly, this study found that obesity did not increase the risk of developing PCOS: the prevalence of PCOS was 9.8% in normal, 9.9% of overweight and 9.0% of obese women. These results support the hypothesis that a predisposition to PCOS is necessary in order to develop the syndrome, regardless of obesity (Fig. 18.1). However, clinical manifestations and endocrine features of the syndrome are greatly worsen in obese compared to lean women with PCOS, which is probably due to the superimposed insulin resistance and compensatory hyperinsulinemia induced by excess body weight (Fig. 18.1). Although most studies only assessed BMI, it is important to underscore that the obesity associated with PCOS is characterized by a central distribution, as reported in most [68,69] but not all studies [70]. This explains why some non-obese women with PCOS (as defined by the BMI) display insulin resistance and hyperinsulinemia. Indeed, when matched for BMI, these women still have a higher percentage of body fat and a larger waist-to-hip ratio (WHR) [69,71].

18.3.2 Benefits of Weight Loss and Exercise in Women with PCOS

This essential aspect of the management of women with PCOS is discussed in detailed in Kate Marsh's Chapter, but a summary of studies assessing the benefits of lifestyle intervention specifically in women with PCOS is presented in Table 18.1. Most were short term (=24 weeks) or included a relatively small number of PCOS women (6–90), and few were randomized to standard lifestyle intervention alone (4 out of 23). However, they almost all found that weight loss or exercise training in obese or overweight women with PCOS was associated

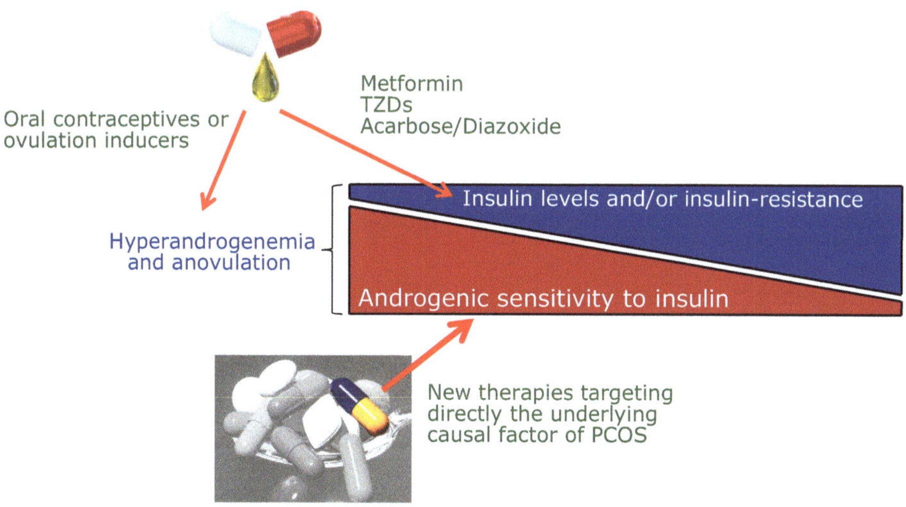

Fig. 18.1 An unifying metabolic hypothesis of polycystic ovary syndrome's pathogenesis. Both increased insulin action on androgen biosynthesis and hyperinsulinemia, which is secondary to insulin resistance, are required at different degree for the development of polycystic ovary syndrome (PCOS). This hypothesis explains why some PCOS are not insulin resistant and, conversely, why most insulin-resistant women do not develop PCOS. Drugs are available to control pituitary–ovarian function and insulin resistance, but the discovery of specific drugs targeting the hypothesized androgenic hypersensitivity to insulin may prove useful in the medical management of PCOS

Table 18. 1 Results of lifestyle intervention studies specifically performed in women with PCOS

Author	Year	Number of subjects	Intervention	Duration	Results
Harlass et al. [193]	1984	6	500 kcal/d diet	16–24 weeks	↓Total testosterone, ↑SHBG, ↓LH
Pasquali et al. [194]	1989	20	1000–1500 kcal/d diet	6–12 months	↓Insulin, ↓total testosterone, ↓hirsutism; Ovulation: 70%, pregnancies: 20%
Kiddy et al. [195]	1992	24 (19 anovulatory)	350 kcal/d diet × 4 weeks, then 1000 kcal/d	28 weeks	↓Insulin, ↓free testosterone; regular cycles: 50%, pregnancies: 32% (6/19)
Hamilton-Fairley et al. [196]	1993	6	350 kcal/d diet	4 weeks	↓Insulin, ↑SHBG
Guzick et al. [197]	1994	6 treated vs. 6 untreated	400 kcal/d diet (randomized)	12 weeks	↓Insulin, ↓non SHBG-bound testosterone, ↑SHBG (treated vs. untreated); ovulation: 67% (of treated)
Holte et al. [198]	1995	13 treated, 23 untreated, 21 non-PCOS controls	1200 kcal/d diet	14.9 months	↓Insulin, ↓total testosterone, ↑SHBG (treated vs. untreated); ovulation: 54% (of treated)
Andersen et al. [199]	1995	9	400 kcal/d diet × 4 weeks, then 1000-1500 kcal/d	24 weeks	No change in total testosterone and SHBG
Jackubowicz and Nestler [42]	1997	12 obese PCOS + 11 obese controls	1000–1200 kcal/d diet	8 weeks	↓Insulin, ↓total and free testosterone, ↑SHBG (PCOS)
Huber-Buchholz et al. [72]	1999	18	Lifestyle modifications	24 weeks	↓Insulin, ↓free androgen index; ovulation: 50%
Wahrenberg et al. [200]	1999	20 diet vs. OCPs	Very-low calorie diet vs. OCPs	12 weeks	↓Insulin and ↓free testosterone only in diet group
Pasquali et al. [201]	2000	20 obese PCOS + 20 obese controls	1200–1400 kcal/d diet + metformin or placebo	24 weeks	↓Insulin (both interventions), ↓total testosterone (metformin only)
Randeva et al. [202]	2002	12 exercisers vs. 9 nonexercisers	20–60-min walks, 3 times/week	24 weeks	↓WHR, ↓homocystein (exercisers only); no change in weight, insulin and testosterone
Moran et al. [203]	2003	28	High protein vs. low protein diet (randomized): ≈1430 kcal/d	12 weeks	↓Insulin, ↑insulin sensitivity index, ↓total testosterone, ↓free androgen index (no difference between diets); improvement of menstrual cycles: 44% (11/25)
Hoeger et al. [204]	2004	38	Metformin (1.5 g/d), lifestyle modification + metformin, lifestyle modification + placebo or placebo alone (randomized)	48 weeks	↓Weight (all except placebo), ↓total testosterone, ↓free androgen index (only in lifestyle + metformin group)
Jayagopal et al. [205]	2005	21	Diet advices × 8 weeks, then orlistat (360 mg/d) vs. metformin (1.5 g/d) (randomized)	20 weeks	↓Weight (orlistat>metformin), ↓total testosterone (both interventions)

Table 18. 1 (continued)

Author	Year	Number of subjects	Intervention	Duration	Results
Eid et al. [206]	2005	24	Laparoscopic gastric bypass surgery	27.5 months	↓BMI (from 50 to 30 kg/m^2), resolution of type 2 diabetes: 100% (11/11) and dyslipidemia: 92% (11/12); regular cycles: 100%, pregnancies: 21% (without treatment)
Moran et al. [207]	2006	23 completers (on 43)	Low-carbohydrate vs. low-fat diet (randomized): 1170 kcal/d diet (mean) × 8 weeks, then maintenance	8 months	↓Weight, ↓total and free testosterone, ↓insulin, ↑insulin sensitivity index (no difference between diets); improvement of menstrual cycles: 57% (16/28)
Diamanti-Kandarakis et al. [75]	2007	29 PCOS + 18 controls	Orlistat + hypocaloric diet	24 weeks	↓Total testosterone (PCOS), ↓weight, ↓WHR, ↓Insulin, ↑Insulin sensitivity indexes (both groups)
Vigorito et al. [208]	2007	45 treated vs. 45 untreated	30-min exercise training, 3 times/week (randomized)	12 weeks	↓weight, ↓WHR, ↓insulin, ↑insulin sensitivity indexes (treated vs. untreated); no change in total testosterone and SHBG; regular cycles: 60% (of treated)
Palomba et al. [209]	2008	20 exercise vs. 20 diet	Exercise training vs. hypocaloric hyperproteic diet (randomized)	24 weeks	↓Total testosterone, ↓insulin, ↑insulin sensitivity indexes (both groups); ovulation: 100% (both interventions), ↑ovulation frequency (exercise vs. diet), pregnancies: 35% (exercise) vs. 10% (diet) (P=0.06)
Panidis et al. [76]	2008	18 PCOS + 14 controls	Orlistat + hypocaloric diet	24 weeks	↓Total testosterone (PCOS), ↓insulin, ↑insulin sensitivity indexes (both groups)
Lindholm et al. [77]	2008	21 treated vs. 20 placebo	Sibutramine 15 mg daily or placebo (randomized)	24 weeks	↑Weight loss (treated vs. placebo), ↓free androgen index, ↓triglycerides (treated only); ↑menstrual periods (treated vs. placebo)
Sathyapalan et al. [78]	2008	10 (rimonabant) vs. 10 (metformin)	Rimonabant (20 mg/d) vs. metformin (1.5 g/d) (randomized, open labelled)	12 weeks	↓weight, ↓WHR, ↓total testosterone, ↓free androgen index, ↑insulin sensitivity index (rimonabant only)

with improvement in ovulation rates and menstrual cycles, as well as decrease in testosterone levels (mainly free testosterone). These benefits are probably due to the reduction of insulin resistance and insulin levels in these PCOS women, as observed in many studies where such parameters were measured (Table 18.1). Increased pregnancy rates were also achieved with weight loss in many studies, but this parameter is difficult to estimate because studies were not all performed in women seeking fertility. Importantly, in many studies a loss of only 5–10% of initial body weight was enough to achieve reported benefits, including the restoration of fertility [72]. Indeed, this weight loss objective, which is realistic for most PCOS women, is associated with significant decrease in visceral adipose tissues (≈30% loss) and important benefits on insulin resistance [73,74].

Table 18.1 also reports the results of two uncontrolled prospective studies with orlistat [75,76] and one randomized-controlled study with sibutramine [77]. These two drugs are approved in many countries for promoting weight loss in obese individuals, in combination with a lifestyle intervention. There is essentially no risk with the use of orlistat, but this drug reduce fat absorption (by 30%) and is thus associated with oily stools, urgent bowel movements, diarrhea, abdominal pain or discomfort and incontinence. These side effects are reduced or alleviated by reducing fat consumption below 60 g per day. By inhibiting the reuptake of noradrenaline and serotonin in the central nervous system, sibutramine enhances satiety signals and potentiates energy expenditure by stimulating thermogenesis. Sibutramine is generally well tolerated, with most common side effects being constipation, inability to sleep, headache and dry mouth, but should not be used in women with uncontrolled hypertension or tachycardia. Rimonabant is another weight-loss drug that is approved in some European countries, but not in North America. A small randomized-controlled trial has compared the effects of this weight-loss drug to metformin in PCOS women [78]. As shown in Table 18.1, these drugs induce enough weight loss to decrease testosterone levels, along with insulin levels and indices of insulin resistance, in women with PCOS as compared to baseline [75,76,78] or placebo [77]. However, none of these drugs is approved for use during pregnancy and therefore an effective contraceptive method should be recommended when these drugs are prescribed. If used to improve fertility, they should be stopped before conception is desired.

There are no long-term studies assessing the benefits of lifestyle intervention or weight-loss drugs on the chronic metabolic outcomes of PCOS, namely the development of type 2 diabetes mellitus (DM) and cardiovascular diseases. However, two large initial studies, the Diabetes Prevention Program (DPP) [79] and the Finnish Diabetes Prevention Study [80], assessed the effects of lifestyle modification on the development of type 2 DM in overweight individuals with impaired glucose tolerance (IGT). Both studies found a 58% reduction of the incidence of DM in the lifestyle intervention as compared to the control group, after a mean follow-up of 2.8 [79] and 3.2 years [80], respectively. These significant results were confirmed in two subsequent studies by Ramachandran et al. [81] and Pan et al. [82] that found 28.5% and 38% reductions in the relative risk of developing DM after 3 and 6 years of lifestyle intervention in 531 and 577 subjects with IGT, respectively. The smaller benefit in these last studies may be explained by the Asiatic origin of both populations and lower mean BMIs. Regarding anti-obesity drugs, the XENDOS randomized trial [83] reported significant relative risk reductions for developing DM of 37% in all obese subjects and 45% in obese subjects with IGT after 4-year intervention with lifestyle modifications plus orlistat, as compared to lifestyle changes plus placebo.

In summary, lifestyle modification is recommended as first-line therapy for all women with PCOS and excess body weight [84]. This is especially important for women seeking pregnancy because weight loss will not only improve their fertility but also reduce adverse pregnancy outcomes associated with obesity (as discussed above, see Chapter by Homburg). When lifestyle counselling is not effective, with poor reduction of weight or waist circumference, weight-loss drugs may be considered.

18.4 Insulin-Sensitizing Drugs

When lifestyle intervention fails to control PCOS symptoms or long-term cardiometabolic risk factors, or if symptoms require rapid intervention, pharmacologic treatment needs to be considered. For years, the only treatment of PCOS was oral contraceptives (OCPs), when fertility is not an issue. They remain the mainstay for the treatment of PCOS because they effectively regulate menstrual cycles, decrease the risk of endometrial cancer and improve acne and hirsutism, while assuring a reliable reversible contraceptive method. However, OCPs have well known increased risks of thrombo-embolism, hypertension and hypertriglyceridemia. Moreover, OCPs decrease insulin sensitivity and glucose tolerance in the short term [85] and may therefore increase the long-term risk of type DM [86,87]. Finally, OCs may potentially increase cardiovascular risks in these women [88–90]. Therefore, for women with PCOS, especially those who do not need contraception, OCPs may not be the optimal treatment since they are already at higher risks for DM and cardiovascular diseases than the general population and they will have to use OCPs for a longer period of time. Since insulin action plays a key role in the pathophysiology of PCOS, growing interest was given in the past 10 years to the use of insulin sensitizers as a metabolically suited alternative for PCOS management. We will thus review in this section the potential benefits of these drugs, although none of them have received approval for specific use in PCOS by governmental regulatory agencies.

18.4.1 Agents

18.4.1.1 Metformin

Metformin is a biguanide approved for diabetes control (since 1982 in United Kingdom), whose primary mechanism of action is the reduction of hepatic gluconeogenesis, via activation of the LKB1–AMPK pathway [91], along with other systemic insulin-sensitizing effects. Metformin is not a pure insulin sensitizer because it will reduce gluconeogenesis and insulin levels in all individuals, even those without insulin resistance and hyperinsulinemia. Importantly, metformin does not cause hypoglycemia. Regular formulation of metformin was beneficial at dosages between 1275 and 2550 mg per day in well-designed RCTs assessing ovulation in women with PCOS [92] and in prospective studies on hyperandrogenism (see Tables 18.3–18.4). Furthermore, it was shown recently that a higher dose of metformin (2.5 g/day) is more effective on waist circumference and weight loss than a lower dose (1.5 g/day) [93]. Therefore, since metformin tends to be more effective in non-obese as compared to obese women with PCOS [94,95], it is probably advisable to prescribe initially the highest dosage in obese patients (1000 mg twice daily) and use a lower dosage in non-obese ones (875 mg twice daily), in order to minimize side effects. Based on the dose–response curve of metformin described for HbA1c in type 2 diabetics [96], there is probably no benefit in increasing the dose above 2000 mg per day.

The most serious risk with the use of metformin is lactic acidosis, which has been reported rarely and almost exclusively in populations at high risk, such as individuals with renal insufficiency (creatinine clearance <30 mL/min), liver disease, or congestive heart failure (left ventricular ejection fraction <30%). The most common side effects are gastrointestinal disturbance. A meta-analysis of three studies found that the incidence of nausea and vomiting was 3.8-fold higher in women with PCOS who were taking 1500–1750 mg per day of metformin as compared to placebo [97]. But in most RCTs, although not all [98], metformin was not more often stopped because of side effects than placebo. Side effects are usually self-limited in time and related to the dose, mainly the amount of metformin that is taken at once. This is why slow release formulations of metformin are associated with significantly less gastrointestinal side effects [99]. The only large RCT reporting side effects of metformin used such extended-release formulation [100]. The number of dropouts because of side effects was comparable between metformin and clomiphene, but metformin was associated with significantly more abdominal discomfort (59 vs. 53%), diarrhea (65 vs. 23%), nausea (62 vs. 39%), vomiting (30 vs. 13%) and decreased appetite (13 vs. 8%). Decreased appetite is in fact a frequent symptom reported by patients, although not as a side effect, and is probably the main reason for the weight loss often observed with the use of metformin [101]. When prescribing the regular formulation of metformin, it is important to increase the dose progressively to minimize side effects, i.e. by starting at 250 mg twice daily and increasing the dose by 500 mg per day every 7 days, based on tolerance. Another way to reduce side effects is splitting the dose to three or four times a day.

Metformin is classified as a Category B drug in pregnancy, which means that no teratogenic effects have been demonstrated in animal models or reported in humans. It crosses the placenta and could act directly on the fetus. But metformin was administered in a growing number of women with PCOS, gestational diabetes (GDM) or type 2 diabetes mellitus during the first trimester, the third trimester or throughout pregnancy. No teratogenic effects or adverse fetal outcomes were reported [102–109], except for higher unadjusted rates of perinatal loss and preeclampsia observed in 50 women (type 2 DM or GDM) treated with metformin as compared to a much less obese group of 42 women treated with insulin in a retrospective study [110]. Recently, a large RCT compared the use of metformin to insulin in 751 women with GDM and found that metformin was not associated with increased perinatal complications [102].

18.4.1.2 Thiazolidinediones (TZDs)

Thiazolidinediones (TZDs) are a class of insulin-sensitizing drugs approved for treatment of type 2 DM. These agents enhance glucose uptake in adipose and muscle tissues and decrease hepatic glucose output. TZDs act by activating gamma peroxisome proliferator activator receptors (PPAR? receptors) and are true insulin sensitizers because insulin levels will be maintained stable in individuals with normal insulin sensitivity. Similarly, these drugs do not cause hypoglycemia. Two drugs of the TZDs family are available: rosiglitazone (approved in the United States since 1999) and pioglitazone (approved in the United States since 2001). Rosiglitazone is usually prescribed at dosages of 4 or 8 mg per day, given in one or two doses, and pioglitazone at dosages of 15, 30 or 45 mg once daily. Due to their mechanism of action, the TZDs' actions increase progressively with maximal effects peaking only after 6–8 weeks of treatment. Therefore, after the initial prescription or a dose modification, further adjustment of the dosage should await at least 2 months.

There is much less experience with these drugs in women with PCOS, as well as in type 2 DM, as compared to metformin. But side effects with the use of TZDs in women with PCOS are rarely reported in studies. In diabetics, the most common side-effects include edema [111], which is increased with the concurrent use of insulin or insulin secretagogues, and weight gain [112]. In the large ACCORD trial, these side effects were reported in 14% and 7% of diabetic subjects, respectively [113]. This trial also revealed that after a median of 4 years of treatment with rosiglitazone, the risk of bone fractures in diabetic women of 56 years of age in average was 9%, which was increased by 83% as compared to metformin and 168% compared to glyburide. Pioglitazone treatment was followed by decreased lumbar and hip BMD and decreased measures of bone turnover even in women with PCOS, a premenopausal study population relatively protected from bone mineral loss [114]. These findings would be of concern in young girls who are acquiring their peak bone mass. Weight gain, which is partly water and partly true increase in adipose tissues, may also be a concern for obese PCOS women.

TZDs are classified as Category C drugs in pregnancy because they have been shown to cause decreased fetal maturation in animal models. Therefore, these drugs should be used with an effective contraceptive method and should be avoided in women seeking fertility. Very few pregnancies with the use of TZDs for ovulation induction in women with PCOS have been reported in the literature, without evidence of increased risk [115–120].

18.4.2 Clinical Benefits in Women with PCOS

18.4.2.1 Improving Menstrual Cyclicality and Fertility

Metformin

There are multiple RCTs assessing the clinical benefits of metformin on ovulation and pregnancy rates in women with PCOS. Most, but not all of these RCTs have shown higher frequencies with metformin as compared to placebo, either alone or in combination with clomiphene citrate (CC), an ovulation inducer. Since there are some discrepancies among study results and many studies observed non-statistically significant benefits of metformin, meta-analyses of these RCTs have been performed [92,97,121] and are presented in Table 18.2. As shown, these meta-analyses concluded to a significant improvement of ovulation and pregnancy rates with the use of metformin alone or in combination with CC, as compared to placebo. Metformin alone increased ovulation rates from 24–32% to 46–47%, based on summary statistics of the first two meta-analyses [97,121]; and metformin combined with CC increased ovulation rates from 21–42% to 64–76%. Benefits are more important with the addition of metformin to CC in CC-resistant women with PCOS, both for ovulation induction and for achieving pregnancy.

Table 18.2 Use of Metformin for ovulation induction and fertility in women with polycystic ovarian syndrome (PCOS): comparison of the results of three meta-analyses of randomized-controlled trials

	Lord et al. (2003) [97] rates metformin vs. placebo OR (95% CI)	Kashyap et al. (2004) [121] rates metformin vs. placebo RR (95% CI)	Creanga et al. (2008) [92] rates metformin vs. placebo OR (95% CI)
Ovulation rate			
Metformin vs. placebo	46% vs. 24% (7 trials) 3.88 (2.25–6.69)	47% vs. 32% (5 trials) Infertile : 1.50 (1.13–1.99) 75% vs. 52% (2 trials) Non infertile : 1.45 (1.11–1.90)	N/A (9 trials) 2.94 (1.43–6.02)
Metformin + CC	76% vs. 42% (3 trials) 4.41 (2.37–8.22)	64% vs. 21% (4 trials) 3.04 (1.77–5.24)	N/A (6 trials) 4.39 (1.94–9.96)
Pregnancy rate			
Metformin vs. placebo*	N/A (5 trials) 2.76 (0.85–8.98)	3.6% vs. 3.2% (2 trials) 1.07 (0.20–5.74)	N/A (11 trials) 1.56 (0.74–3.33)
Metformin + CC vs. CC	N/A (3 trials) 4.40 (1.96–9.85)	39% vs. 11% (2 trials) 3.65 (1.11–11.99)	N/A (10 trials) 2.67 (1.45–4.94)

*Not significant.
RR = relative risk; OR odds ratio; CI = confidence interval; CC = clomiphene citrate; non-infertile = patients with PCOS who were not complaining of infertility.

However, an even more important question is which therapy between metformin or CC should be used first in infertile women with PCOS. To answer this question, a first RCT was performed in non-obese anovulatory women with PCOS, which found that ovulation rates were not different between the groups, whereas the pregnancy rate was significantly higher in the metformin group (15.1 vs. 7.2%) [122]. Interestingly, in this trial ovulation and pregnancy rates increased progressively with the use of metformin, but declined over time with CC, such that metformin significantly outweighed CC from the fifth cycle. However, CC was used at a fix dose of 150 mg daily instead of a progressive dose as usually performed in clinical settings. Thus, the same authors repeated their RCT with a progressive increase of CC from 50 to 150 mg daily [123]. In this second trial, they reported that metformin resulted in a higher cumulative pregnancy rates after 6 months than CC, but the difference (63 vs. 49%) did not reach statistical significance. They found again a progressive increase of pregnancy rates with metformin over time as opposed to a progressive decline with CC. Such discrepant benefits over time with these drugs have also been reported in a retrospective study [124].

Although in favour of metformin, these trials did not have the power to assess differences in the rates of living newborn between metformin and CC when used as first-line therapies. The recent Pregnancy in Polycystic Ovarian Syndrome (PPCOS) study [100] was a large American study designed to answer this crucial question. In this study, 626 infertile women with PCOS received CC plus placebo, extended-release metformin plus placebo or a combination of both for 6 months. The results suggested that the live birth rate achieved with CC was higher for women who received CC alone (22.5%) or in combination with metformin (26.8%) than for women who received metformin alone (7.2%). Although not statistically significant, life-birth rate was 4.3% higher with the combination as compared to CC alone, which may be of importance to avoid more costly and demanding treatments.

However, this was the first study in PCOS that used an extended-release formulation of metformin, which demonstrated none of the expected metabolic benefits of this insulin sensitizer. Indeed, it did not decrease plasmac insulin and proinsulin levels or the homeostasis model assessment of insulin resistance (HOMA-IR) as compared to baseline. Furthermore, reduction in BMI with this metformin formulation was statistically significant but minor (–0.6 kg/m^2). Since metformin is not a non-specific ovulation inducer, it will improve ovulation in PCOS women only after reducing insulin resistance and levels. Therefore, in the absence of the expected metabolic improvements with metformin, it is not a surprise that fertility parameters did not improve, i.e. that the cumulative rate of ovulation after 6 months in the metformin group was only 29%, as compared with 55% and 63% in the two studies from Palomba and colleagues [122,123], and 46–47% after 3–6 months in two meta-analyses [97,121]. In fact, the cumulative ovulation rate with metformin was in the range observed with placebo in these meta-analyses (24–32%). Thus, due to unexpected minimal metabolic and ovulatory effects of the formulation of metformin used in the PPCOS study, it should probably not be considered the definitive study for the choice of the best pharmacologic first-line therapy in PCOS anovulatory women. Discrepancies in study results may also be explained by diet or genetic differences among populations. Indeed, it has been shown that a polymorphism in LKB1 (or STK11) was associated with ovulatory response to metformin treatment in the PPCOS trial [125].

Furthermore, the use of metformin during pregnancy [122,126–129] has been shown to reduce first trimester pregnancy loss, which can be as high as 30–50% in women with PCOS [130,131]. Indeed, we have shown that serum glycodelin and IGFPB-1, two important proteins for embryo implantation, were reduced in PCOS women during the first trimester of pregnancy [132] and were corrected with metformin [133]. It is still unclear if metformin should be continued after pregnancy is confirmed to reduce early fetal loss. Although some RCTs found reduced rates even after early discontinuation of metformin [122,126–129], others did not [98,100,123]. Finally, metformin induces normal ovulation, such that the risk of multiple gestation is no more than the general population [134], as confirmed in the PPCOS trial [100].

Thiazolidinediones (TZDs)

Some studies assessed the benefits of TZDs on fertility, but most did not report on pregnancy rates because subjects were advised not to get pregnant. Azziz et al. [135] conducted the largest RCT assessing the effects of TZDs on ovulation and menstrual regularity, for which they used troglitazone that is no longer on the market due to cases of severe liver failure. Results from 410 women with PCOS showed that troglitazone improved significantly ovulatory rates after 44 weeks of treatment as compared to women receiving placebo (42% and 58% at low and high dosages, respectively, vs. 32%). Smaller randomized placebo-controlled trials using rosiglitazone found significant improvement of menstrual cycle regularity after 4 months [136] and ovulation frequencies after 6 months [58], even in non-obese women with PCOS and normal insulin levels [58]. A 3-month randomized placebo-controlled trial also found higher rates of regular ovulatory cycles with pioglitazone than with placebo [137].

Few small studies also looked at the effect of TZDs in infertile women with PCOS resistant to CC. Indeed, TZDs in combination to CC were shown to achieve cumulative ovulation rates of 77% [120] and 83% [138] after 2 and 5 months, respectively, with a pregnancy rate of 39% after 5 months [138]. RCTs found significant improvement of ovulation rates [139] and menstrual pattern [140] with the combination of rosiglitazone with CC as compared to CC alone after 3 months. Interestingly, Rouzi and Ardawi [141] found a significantly higher ovulation rate after 3 months of rosiglitazone plus CC as compared to metformin plus CC (64 vs. 36%), which suggests that rosiglitazone may be superior to metformin, at least in combination with CC.

In summary, TZDs appear effective drugs in order to restore normal menstrual cyclicality and ovulation in women with PCOS, to a similar degree to metformin or even more. They are therefore potential drugs for treating oligoamenorrhea, but should not be used when fertility is desired before well-designed large trials can conclude on their role in restoring fertility and, particularly, on their safety for the foetus.

18.4.2.2 Benefits on Clinical Hyperandrogenism

Hirsutism

Most of published RCTs using insulin sensitizers in women with PCOS found a significant reduction of androgen levels in both obese and lean individuals [85]. However, only few of them were designed or powered to assess specifically clinical hyperandrogenesim, namely hirsutism and acne. Table 18.3summarizes results of published studies that were found to report on the effect of metformin on hirsutism in at least 10 women with PCOS. A chapter of this book on the management of hirsutism in women with PCOS by Salvatore Benvenga also summarizes the use of insulin-sensitizing drugs. Of note, hirsutism was a primary outcome only in the randomized placebo-controlled trial from Kelly et al. [142] and the prospective metformin arm of study by Horborne et al. [143]. They both demonstrated significant improvement of Ferriman–Gallwey (FG) scores, self-assessments and hair velocity or diameter after metformin treatment as compared to placebo [142] or baseline

Table 18.3 Summary of the results of prospective studies assessing the effect of metformin therapy on hirsutism specifically in women with polycystic ovary syndrome (PCOS) (studies with at least 10 PCOS women)

Citation	N	Study population	Dose and follow up period	Effect on hirsutism	Comments
Randomized placebo-controlled trials					
Moghetti et al. 2000 [170]	23	Overweight and obese, Italy	1500 mg/day, 6 months	No change	Clinical scores
Kelly et al. 2002 [142]	10*	Obese, United Kingdom	1500 mg/day, 6 months	Decreased	Hair velocities, FG scores and self-assessment scores; cross-over design
Maciel et al. 2004 [94]	29	Obese and non-obese, Brazil	1500 mg/day, 6 months	No change	Clinical scores; analyses by weight sub-groups (6–8 subjects per groups)
Prospective uncontrolled studies or study arms of a RCT that did not use placebo					
Kolodziejczyk et al. 2000 [144]	35	Obese, Poland	1500 mg/day, 12 weeks	Decreased	Clinical scores
Ibáñez et al. 2001 [145]	35	Non-obese, Spain	1275 mg/day, 6 months	Decreased	FG scores
Loverro et al. 2002 [146]	37	Overweight and obese, Spain	1500 mg/day, 6 months	No change	FG scores
Çiçek et al. 2003 [151]	22	Obese and non-obese, Turkey	1700 mg/day, 6 months	Decreased	FG scores
Harborne et al. 2003 [143]	18	Obese, Scotland	1500 mg/day, 52 weeks	Decreased	FG scores, hair diameter and self-assessments
Kazerooni et al. 2003 [147]	35	Obese and non-obese, Iran	1500 mg/day, 8 weeks	Decreased	FG scores
Aruna et al. 2004 [148]	41	Obese and non-obese, India	1000 mg/day, 6 months	No change	Clinical scores
Kriplani et al. 2004 [149]	66	Obese and non-obese, India	1500 mg/day, 6 months	No change	FG scores
Ganie et al. 2004 [153]	35	Obese and non-obese, India	1000 mg/day, 6 months	Decreased	FG scores
Yilmaz et al. 2005 [154]	48	Non-obese, Turkey	1700 mg/day, 6 months	Decreased	FG scores
Ortega-González et al. 2005 [117]	18	Obese, Mexico	2550 mg/day, 6 months	Decreased	FG scores
Orio et al. 2005 [156]	18	Normal-weight, Italy	1700 mg/day, 6 months	No change	FG scores
Gambineri et al. 2006 [158]	20	Obese, Italy	1700 mg/day (plus a hypocaloric diet), 6 and 12 months	Decreased	FG scores
Meyer et al. 2007 [155]	20	Obese, Australia	2000 mg/day, 6 months	Decreased	FG scores
Marcondes et al. 2007 [150]	15	Normal-weight, Brazil	2550 mg/day, 4 months	No change	FG scores

FG: Ferriman-Gallwey. * Cross-over design.

[143]. Even if Kelly's trial included a small number of subjects, the power of the study was doubled by the cross-over design, i.e. all women took both metformin and placebo.

The two other randomized placebo-controlled trials listed in Table 18.3 did not find a significant benefit of metformin over placebo for clinical hirsutism, but these trials were not specifically designed to evaluate hirsutism and were not appropriately powered. Out of fifteen prospective uncontrolled studies with metformin [144–150] or trials with a metformin treatment arm (but not compared to placebo) [117,143–155], only five did not find a significant improvement of hirsutism after the use of metformin as compared to baseline (Table 18.3). Of note, these studies assessed PCOS women with less hyperandrogenism [146], with a normal weight [150,156], using a lower dose of metformin (1000 mg per day) [148] or treated for a shorter period [150].

Of interest, Harborne's study [143], for which hirsutism was a primary outcome of interest, was in fact a RCT comparing the effects of metformin and ethinyl estradiol plus ciproterone acetate (EE/CA) in 52 PCOS women. The authors found that both treatments had comparable benefits on hirsutism after 52 weeks, except for the hirsutism self-assessment score that was more improved after metformin. Two other RCTs compared metformin to EE/CA and assessed hirsutism, although it was not their primary outcome of interest. The first randomized 67 obese women with PCOS, lasted 6 months, and found significant and similar decreases in the FG scores in both groups [155]. The second study revealed that EE/CA was significantly better for improving the FG score in 17 non-obese PCOS women after 6-month treatment [157]. However, this later trial enrolled fewer women, which may have introduced random variability in results, and there was baseline imbalance in hirsutism scores between groups. Also, women had lower mean hirsutism scores at baseline and were less insulin resistant than in the first two trials.

Regarding the combination of metformin with an anti-androgen drug, Gambineri et al. [158] published a 12-month RCT that compared the effects of metformin, flutamide, the combination of both and placebo, in addition to a hypocaloric diet, in 77 women with PCOS. The combination was no more effective than flutamide to decrease hirsutism, but was superior to metformin and placebo. Menstrual pattern improved more in the combination group than after metformin alone, which was better than flutamide alone and placebo. In addition, the combination decreased LDL cholesterol levels and improved insulin sensitivity significantly more than either treatment alone. These results confirmed those of a previous smaller 9-month RCT, which was not placebo-controlled [159]. This trial also found that combined flutamide and metformin treatment in 31 young, non-obese women with hyperinsulinemic PCOS had additive benefits on ovulation frequencies, insulin sensitivity, hyperandrogenemia and dyslipidemia, but not for hirsutism.

Collectively, these clinical studies suggest that metformin is an effective treatment for hirsutism, comparable to fourth generation oral contraceptives after at least 6 months of use. Metformin could be considered as first-line therapy for mild-to-moderate hirsutism in some women. However, severe hirsutism needs to be treated with anti-androgen drugs, supplemented with an appropriate contraceptive method. But for women who do not require hormonal contraception, the combination of metformin with an anti-androgen may be considered, although such combination was not tested for severe hirsutism in PCOS women.

The largest long-term randomized placebo-controlled trial with a TZD used troglitazone and demonstrated a significant reduction in hirsutism at the end of the 44-week study, as assessed by the FG score [135]. Two smaller placebo-controlled trials did not find a significant improvement of hirsutism after only 3 and 4 months of treatment with rosiglitazone [136] and pioglitazone [137], respectively. However, five 6- to 12-month uncontrolled studies found significant improvements in FG scores [117,154,160–162], but this was not the case after 6 months in a another study [163]. Furthermore, a small RCT found that rosiglitazone was significantly better than metformin to decrease FG scores [154], which was not the case for pioglitazone in another RCT [117]. Altogether, these studies suggest that TZDs improve hirsutism, probably at least as much as metformin.

Acne

Acne is a clinical outcome that is rarely assessed in studies with insulin sensitizers, and no RCT comparing an insulin sensitizer to placebo has reported this outcome. Table 18.4 summarizes the results of four published studies that were found to have assessed the effect of metformin on acne in at least 10 women with PCOS.

Table 18.4 Summary of the results of prospective studies assessing the effect of metformin therapy on acne specifically in women with polycystic ovary syndrome (PCOS) (studies with at least 10 PCOS women; all uncontrolled prospective studies or study arms of a RCT that did not use placebo)

Citation	N	Study population	Dose and follow up period	Effect on acne	Comments
Harborne et al. 2003 [143]	18	Obese, Scotland	1500 mg/day, 52 weeks	Improved	Self-assessment scores
Kazerooni et al. 2003 [147]	35	Obese and non-obese, Iran	1500 mg/day, 8 weeks	Improved	Clinical scores
Aruna et al. 2004 [148]	41	Obese and non-obese, India	1000 mg/day, 6 months	Not improved	Clinical scores
Kriplani et al. 2004 [149]	66	Obese and non-obese, India	1500 mg/day, 6 months	Not improved	Clinical scores

Accordingly, two studies on four have shown significant benefit of metformin for the control of acne. The study by Aruna et al. [148] did not find a significant improvement on acne but used a very low dosage of metformin. Furthermore, a prospective study evaluating the benefits of 6-month treatment with pioglitazone in 18 obese women with PCOS has demonstrated a significant improvement in clinical assessment of acne [160]. The paucity of literature and the lack of direct comparison with oral contraceptives, for example, do not support the recommendation of using insulin sensitizers as first-line therapy solely for acne.

18.4.2.3 Management of Long-Term Risks of Type 2 Diabetes and Cardiovascular Diseases

Since the PCOS is associated with significant long-term risks of type 2 diabetes and probably CVDs, its chronic management should not impact negatively on these risks and ideally reduce them. As discussed previously, classical therapy with OCPs has no beneficial effect on type 2 DM and CV risks in PCOS women and may even worsen these risks based on studies in the general population. On the contrary, insulin-sensitizing agents have shown in women with PCOS to increase glucose tolerance [164,165]; to improve endothelial function [156,166,167] and markers of established atherosclerosis [156,168]; and to reduce cardiovascular risk factors such as serum triglycerides [145,146,169], HDL-cholesterol [145,146,148,170,171], blood pressure [58,143,169], and serum PAI-1 [45], hsCRP [162,172] and endothelin-1 [156,173] concentrations. The use of insulin sensitizers for the prevention of cardiovascular diseases is already discussed in the previous chapter by Sharma and Nestler, in this book. In summary, cardioprotective effects of insulin-sensitizing drugs in PCOS women and other populations have been variable from study to study, but certainly no aggravation of glucose tolerance or cardiovascular risk factors has been reported, which is not the case for OCPs. Thus, insulin-sensitizing drugs do not appear to be harmful from a diabetes and cardiovascular risk perspective, and may be beneficial.

18.4.3 Indications

For women with PCOS seeking fertility, the first-line agent for improving fertility should be chosen by the physician after considering the discussed available data and consulting the patient's will. The decision should put safety, healthy pregnancy and rapidity issues in perspective in order to make a choice. If achieving rapid pregnancy is required by the couple, because of age or longstanding infertility, CC should probably be preferred as first-line therapy, along with lifestyle modifications. CC could be used in combination with metformin in order to maximize fertility. However, when the couple is willing to wait, metformin should probably be the first treatment because it will favour the return of normal ovulations, which carry the same risk of multiple pregnancy as the general population, and may decrease the risk of early pregnancy loss. Even more importantly, metformin acts more slowly and tends to reduce appetite, which allow for lifestyle changes and weight loss prior to pregnancy. As mentioned earlier, better weight control during pregnancy is essential in order to prevent adverse maternal and offspring outcomes.

When contraception is desired, the benefits of OCPs probably outweigh any potential risks in most women with PCOS. However, if a PCOS woman has IGT or type 2 DM or develop a metabolic complication following the use of OCP, she should probably be recommended another contraceptive method and prescribed an insulin sensitizer. If the OCP cannot be stopped, an insulin sensitizer should be prescribed to use in combination with the OCP. Indeed, the beneficial effects of these agents seem complementary, with insulin sensitizers appearing to counteract the deleterious effects of OCPs [163,174,175]. The preferred insulin-sensitizing drug should be metformin because of the weight of evidences favoring this drug and because metformin is associated with a significant weight loss in most women while TZDs can cause weight gain.

When fertility is not an issue and oral contraception is not required, the first-line therapy can consist of either OCP use or an insulin sensitizer. Fortunately, insulin-sensitizing drugs are new therapies that can give relieve to those women for whom OCPs are contra-indicated or not tolerated. Otherwise, because of long-term metabolic risks, insulin sensitizers should probably be preferred in women with PCOS who (a) have excess body weight (BMI > 25 kg/m^2) or central adiposity (waist circumference $>$88 cm); (b) display the metabolic syndrome [12]; (c) have another clinical evidence of insulin resistance, such as acanthosis nigricans, high insulin levels (during fasting or an OGTT) or low SHBG; or (d) have genetic predisposition to type 2 DM or cardiovascular diseases, such as a positive first-degree family history of type 2 diabetes or early cardiovascular disease or a strong second-degree family history. Of note, insulin-sensitizing agents have been shown to improve hyperandrogenemia, anovulation and acne in all PCOS women, regardless of pre-treatment degree of obesity or insulin resistance [58,176–178]. Thus, both alternatives should be discussed with the patient in order to help her choose the best individualized therapy, even in non-obese women with PCOS.

18.4.4 Monitoring of Clinical Outcomes

Baseline assessment of metabolic parameters is important in order to decide on the best long-term therapy, as discussed previously, but also for assessing the benefits of treatment. Thus, all women should be screened with a complete lipid profile and an oral glucose tolerance test (OGTT) [179]. Importantly, we have shown that fasting glucose is not appropriate in order to screen for abnormal glucose tolerance in women with PCOS [180]. It is also important to screen for IGT or DM in women seeking fertility, because any degree of abnormal glucose tolerance before pregnancy would translate in gestational diabetes when pregnancy occurs and should be managed as such.

After initial management provided to the patient, it is essential to offer an appropriate follow-up in order to ensure adherence to lifestyle modifications and medications, to verify weight changes and to assess responses to therapy and side effects. Women treated with metformin alone for fertility should be followed-up every 3–6 months, depending on the desired rapidity of the intervention. In general, the addition of CC should be discussed after 6 months if the woman is not yet pregnant, because maximal effects of the drug per se is probably achieved at that time, although progressive weight loss would provide subsequent improvement of fertility with time.

In women with PCOS who do not require fertility and are treated with insulin sensitizers for the long term, follow-up should probably be recommended initially at least every 6 months. An initial telephone availability or 3-month visit is required to discuss the side effects. If metformin is not tolerated, a slow-release formulation or a TZD should be considered. Since metformin and TZDs have additive effects on insulin sensitivity and glucose control in type 2 diabetics, it could be envisaged to combine these medications if the syndrome's manifestations are not improved enough by metformin alone [181]. In addition, evolution of weight (and waist circumference in overweight women), blood pressure and lipids should be assessed at every visits. Therapy should aim for non-deterioration and ideally improvement of these parameters. Furthermore, it is recommended that patients with normal glucose tolerance should be rescreened with an OGTT at least once every 2 years, or more frequently if additional risk factors are identified [179].

As previously mentioned, weight loss and exercise are effective means for restoring normal ovulatory menstrual cycles and androgen levels. It is also the best method for diabetes prevention. With adequate follow-up it is possible to achieve clinically significant and sustainable weight loss in women with PCOS, particularly with the combination of metformin [182]. Therefore, insulin sensitizers could be stopped if clinical outcomes, androgen levels and metabolic parameters are well controlled and the woman lost at least 10% of her initial body weight. Such degree of weight loss is expected to be associated with a significant proportion of subjects displaying resolution of symptoms and metabolic anomalies. If the likeliness of stopping the drug if she loses such amount of weight is explained to the patient, this may increase her motivation to engage in lifestyle modifications and provide her with a clear and realistic objective.

18.5 Insulin Sensitization During Pregnancy

As mentioned in Homburg's chapter, women with PCOS are among the populations at increased risk for GDM, which is estimated to be increased by two-fold [183]. Thus, when a woman with PCOS gets pregnancy, she should be monitored for the development of gestational diabetes mellitus (GDM). Based on many guidelines, including those from the American Diabetes Association [184], women at increased risk should be screened as soon as possible during pregnancy and those not found to have GDM at the initial screening should be tested between 24 and 28 weeks of gestation. Screening could follow a one- or two-step approach, but it is probably advisable to perform directly a 100-g or 75-g OGTT in these high-risk women in order to save time and decrease the risk of lost to follow-up. A PCOS woman diagnosed with IGT or DM shortly prior to pregnancy, as we recommended in the previous section, should be considered as being affected by GDM and managed as such when pregnancy is confirmed. Conversely, those who tested normal to the pre-pregnancy OGTT do not need to be re-tested early during pregnancy. Thus, performing an OGTT before pregnancy, when women consult for infertility, for example, avoids carrying out an OGTT during the first trimester, when women are particularly sensitive to the side effects of ingesting a high-glucose solution.

Although metformin is not approved during pregnancy (category B), increasing evidences suggest that its use in pregnant women is safe [102–109] and a large RCT have shown that metformin is as effective as insulin therapy to treat GDM in the general population [102]. This trial also found a lower maternal weight gain with metformin therapy. In women with PCOS, studies have shown that metformin was not associated with adverse maternal or neonatal outcomes when used for ovulation induction and continued during the first trimester [185], or throughout pregnancy [106,186]. A cohort study by Glueck et al. [187] also suggested that the use of metformin throughout pregnancy may prevent the development of GDM in women with PCOS.

Collectively, these evidences suggest that it may be appropriate to treat PCOS women throughout pregnancy in order to prevent early pregnancy loss (EPL), as discussed earlier, and to prevent or treat GDM. However, while awaiting appropriately controlled large trials, this approach cannot be recommended at large but it is probably advisable to limit the use of metformin during pregnancy. Accordingly, our practice is to stop metformin as soon as the woman knows she is pregnant if she did not experience a previous EPL. Otherwise, she will be advised to continue the metformin throughout the first trimester, which is the period at higher miscarriage risk in women with PCOS. If the women develop GDM during the pregnancy with criteria of pharmacological therapy, metformin could be used or re-introduced, based on clinical judgment. Since insulin resistance can be very high during pregnancy, especially in obese women, metformin dosage should be increased progressively up to the maximal dose of 2 g per day, as tolerated.

Pre-pregnancy body weight is another very important risk factor of many adverse maternal and neonatal outcomes [188]. For example, a meta-analysis has shown that women who are overweight and obesity before getting pregnant increase their risks of both caesarian delivery [189] and stillbirth [190] by 50% and 100%, respectively, and their risk of GDM by 2- and 3.5-fold, respectively [191], as compared to normal weight women. A recent large database study also found that pre-pregnancy obesity increase the length of hospital stay for delivery and use of health-care services [192]. It is therefore very important to encourage weight loss before pregnancy in all women seeking fertility. Since lifestyle interventions take time, obese women should be encouraged to postpone fertility treatments for as long as acceptable for the couple. As mentioned, this delay is an opportunity to use metformin because it will progressively favor fertility and, more importantly, reduce appetite in many women and thus help them lose weight.

18.6 Take Home Messages

The polycystic ovary syndrome is a frequent and serious condition that should be managed globally for both its current clinical issues and long-term metabolic consequences. The initial approach should target complaints while minimizing, and ideally improving, metabolic risks.

Accordingly, all women with PCOS should be advised for regular physical activities and obese women should receive minimal counseling for caloric restriction. Weight reduction in obese women is essential before getting pregnant, in order to nurture a healthier pregnancy, as well as lifelong, to achieve the best impact on cardiometabolic risks.

Together with lifestyle changes, insulin-sensitizing drugs are useful for managing fertility, menstrual cyclicality and hyperandrogenism, as well as reducing the risk of diabetes and cardiovascular events.

Metformin is recommended in infertile PCOS women resistant to clomiphene citrate or willing to wait the time required for achieving some weight loss before getting pregnant.

Metformin, or TZDs if metformin is not tolerated, is recommended in women with PCOS who do not tolerate OCPs or display abnormal glucose tolerance. Furthermore, these insulin sensitizers should probably be preferred to OCPs, and used alone or in combination with an anti-androgen, in a PCOS woman with excess adiposity, metabolic syndrome, another clinical evidence of insulin resistance (acanthosis nigricans, low SHBG or hyperinsulinemia) or genetic predisposition to type 2 DM.

Finally, when initial management is prescribed, an appropriate follow-up should be performed to ensure adherence to lifestyle modification and drugs, to re-enforce the importance of weight loss and favor motivation and to adjust treatment based on side effects and clinical evolution.

References

1. Asuncion M, Calvo RM, San Millan JL, Sancho J, Avila S, Escobar-Morreale HF. A prospective study of the prevalence of the polycystic ovary syndrome in unselected Caucasian women from Spain. J Clin Endocrinol Metab 2000; 85(7):2434–2438.
2. Knochenhauer ES, Key TJ, Kahsar-Miller M, Waggoner W, Boots LR, Azziz R. Prevalence of the polycystic ovary syndrome in unselected black and white women of the southeastern United States: a prospective study. J Clin Endocrinol Metab 1998; 83(9):3078–3082.
3. Diamanti-Kandarakis E, Kouli CR, Bergiele AT, Filandra FA, Tsianateli TC, Spina GG et al. A survey of the polycystic ovary syndrome in the Greek island of Lesbos: hormonal and metabolic profile. J Clin Endocrinol Metab 1999; 84(11):4006–4011.
4. Michelmore KF, Balen AH, Dunger DB, Vessey MP. Polycystic ovaries and associated clinical and biochemical features in young women. Clin Endocrinol (Oxf) 1999; 51(6):779–786.
5. Azziz R, Woods KS, Reyna R, Key TJ, Knochenhauer ES, Yildiz BO. The Prevalence and Features of the Polycystic Ovary Syndrome in an Unselected Population. J Clin Endocrinol Metab 2004; 89(6):2745–2749.
6. Coffey S, Mason H. The effect of polycystic ovary syndrome on health-related quality of life. [Review] [72 refs]. Gynecol Endocrinol 2003; 17(5):379–386.
7. Elsenbruch S, Hahn S, Kowalsky D, Offner AH, Schedlowski M, Mann K et al. Quality of life, psychosocial well-being, and sexual satisfaction in women with polycystic ovary syndrome. J Clin Endocrinol Metab 2003; 88(12):5801–5807.
8. Hahn S, Janssen OE, Tan S, Pleger K, Mann K, Schedlowski M et al. Clinical and psychological correlates of quality-of-life in polycystic ovary syndrome. Eur J Endocrinol 2005; 153(6):853–860.
9. McCook JG, Reame NE, Thatcher SS. Health-related quality of life issues in women with polycystic ovary syndrome. J Obstet Gynecol Neonatal Nurs 2005; 34(1):12–20.
10. Trent ME, Rich M, Austin SB, Gordon CM. Fertility concerns and sexual behavior in adolescent girls with polycystic ovary syndrome: implications for quality of life. Journal of Pediatric & Adolescent Gynecology 2003; 16(1):33–37.
11. Trent ME, Rich M, Austin SB, Gordon CM. Quality of life in adolescent girls with polycystic ovary syndrome. Archives of Pediatrics & Adolescent Medicine 2002; 156(6):556–560.
12. Executive Summary of the Third Report of the National Cholesterol Education Program (NCEP) Expert Panel on Detection, Evaluation, and Treatment of High Blood Cholesterol in Adults (Adult Treatment Panel III). JAMA 2001; 285(19): 2486–2497.
13. Glueck CJ, Papanna R, Wang P, Goldenberg N, Sieve-Smith L. Incidence and treatment of metabolic syndrome in newly referred women with confirmed polycystic ovarian syndrome. Metabolism 2003; 52(7):908–915.
14. Vural B, Caliskan E, Turkoz E, Kilic T, Demirci A. Evaluation of metabolic syndrome frequency and premature carotid atherosclerosis in young women with polycystic ovary syndrome. Hum Reprod 2005; 20(9):2409–2413.

15. Gambineri A, Pelusi C, Manicardi E, Vicennati V, Cacciari M, Morselli-Labate AM et al. Glucose intolerance in a large cohort of mediterranean women with polycystic ovary syndrome: phenotype and associated factors. Diabetes 2004; 53(9): 2353–2358.
16. Weerakiet S, Srisombut C, Bunnag P, Sangtong S, Chuangsoongnoen N, Rojanasakul A. Prevalence of type 2 diabetes mellitus and impaired glucose tolerance in Asian women with polycystic ovary syndrome. Int J Gynaecol Obstet 2001; 75(2): 177–184.
17. Legro RS, Kunselman AR, Dodson WC, Dunaif A. Prevalence and predictors of risk for type 2 diabetes mellitus and impaired glucose tolerance in polycystic ovary syndrome: a prospective, controlled study in 254 affected women. J Clin Endocrinol Metab 1999; 84(1):165–169.
18. Ehrmann DA, Barnes RB, Rosenfield RL, Cavaghan MK, Imperial J. Prevalence of impaired glucose tolerance and diabetes in women with polycystic ovary syndrome. Diabetes Care 1999; 22(1):141–146.
19. Palmert MR, Gordon CM, Kartashov AI, Legro RS, Emans SJ, Dunaif A. Screening for abnormal glucose tolerance in adolescents with polycystic ovary syndrome. J Clin Endocrinol Metab 2002; 87(3):1017–1023.
20. Legro RS, Gnatuk CL, Kunselman AR, Dunaif A. Changes in glucose tolerance over time in women with polycystic ovary syndrome: A controlled study. J Clin Endocrinol Metab 2005; 90(6):3236–3242.
21. Solomon CG, Hu FB, Dunaif A, Rich-Edwards J, Willett WC, Hunter DJ et al. Long or highly irregular menstrual cycles as a marker for risk of type 2 diabetes mellitus. JAMA 2001; 286(19):2421–2426.
22. Peppard HR, Marfori J, Iuorno MJ, Nestler JE. Prevalence of polycystic ovary syndrome among premenopausal women with type 2 diabetes. Diabetes Care 2001; 24(6):1050–1052.
23. Conn JJ, Jacobs HS, Conway GS. The prevalence of polycystic ovaries in women with type 2 diabetes mellitus. Clin Endocrinol (Oxf) 2000; 52(1):81–86.
24. Lakhani K, Hardiman P, Seifalian AM. Intima-media thickness of elastic and muscular arteries of young women with polycystic ovaries. Atherosclerosis 2004; 175(2):353–359.
25. Talbott EO, Zborowski JV, Rager JR, Boudreaux MY, Edmundowicz DA, Guzick DS. Evidence for an association between metabolic cardiovascular syndrome and coronary and aortic calcification among women with polycystic ovary syndrome. J Clin Endocrinol Metab 2004; 89(11):5454–5461.
26. Talbott EO, Guzick DS, Sutton-Tyrrell K, McHugh-Pemu KP, Zborowski JV, Remsberg KE et al. Evidence for association between polycystic ovary syndrome and premature carotid atherosclerosis in middle-aged women. Arterioscler Thromb Vasc Biol 2000; 20(11):2414–2421.
27. Shroff R, Kerchner A, Maifeld M, Van Beek EJ, Jagasia D, Dokras A. Young obese women with polycystic ovary syndrome have evidence of early coronary atherosclerosis. J Clin Endocrinol Metab 2007; 92(12):4609–4614.
28. Cascella T, Palomba S, De S, I, Manguso F, Giallauria F, De Simone B et al. Visceral fat is associated with cardiovascular risk in women with polycystic ovary syndrome. Hum Reprod 2008; 23(1):153–159.
29. Orio F, Jr., Palomba S, Cascella T, De Simone B, Di Biase S, Russo T et al. Early impairment of endothelial structure and function in young normal-weight women with polycystic ovary syndrome. J Clin Endocrinol Metab 2004; 89(9): 4588–4593.
30. Cibula D, Cifkova R, Fanta M, Poledne R, Zivny J, Skibova J. Increased risk of non-insulin dependent diabetes mellitus, arterial hypertension and coronary artery disease in perimenopausal women with a history of the polycystic ovary syndrome. Hum Reprod 2000; 15(4):785–789.
31. Solomon CG, Hu FB, Dunaif A, Rich-Edwards JE, Stampfer MJ, Willett WC et al. Menstrual cycle irregularity and risk for future cardiovascular disease. J Clin Endocrinol Metab 2002; 87(5):2013–2017.
32. DeFronzo RA, Tobin JD, Andres R. Glucose clamp technique: a method for quantifying insulin secretion and resistance. Am J Physiol 1979; 237(3):E214–E223.
33. Dunaif A, Segal KR, Futterweit W, Dobrjansky A. Profound peripheral insulin resistance, independent of obesity, in polycystic ovary syndrome. Diabetes 1989; 38(9):1165–1174.
34. Dunaif A. Insulin action in the polycystic ovary syndrome. Endocrinology & Metabolism Clinics of North America 1999; 28(2):341–359.
35. Yilmaz M, Bukan N, Ersoy R, Karakoc A, Yetkin I, Ayvaz G et al. Glucose intolerance, insulin resistance and cardiovascular risk factors in first degree relatives of women with polycystic ovary syndrome. Hum Reprod 2005; 20(9):2414–2420.
36. Legro RS, Bentley-Lewis R, Driscoll D, Wang SC, Dunaif A. Insulin resistance in the sisters of women with polycystic ovary syndrome: association with hyperandrogenemia rather than menstrual irregularity. J Clin Endocrinol Metab 2002; 87(5):2128–2133.
37. Yildiz BO, Yarali H, Oguz H, Bayraktar M. Glucose intolerance, insulin resistance, and hyperandrogenemia in first degree relatives of women with polycystic ovary syndrome. J Clin Endocrinol Metab 2003; 88(5):2031–2036.
38. Norman RJ, Masters S, Hague W. Hyperinsulinemia is common in family members of women with polycystic ovary syndrome. Fertil Steril 1996; 66(6):942–947.
39. Baillargeon JP, Carpentier AC. Brothers of women with polycystic ovary syndrome are characterised by impaired glucose tolerance, reduced insulin sensitivity and related metabolic defects. Diabetologia 2007; 50(12):2424–2432.
40. Koivunen RM, Morin-Papunen LC, Ruokonen A, Tapanainen JS, Martikainen HK. Ovarian steroidogenic response to human chorionic gonadotrophin in obese women with polycystic ovary syndrome: effect of metformin. Hum Reprod 2001; 16(12):2546–2551.

41. la Marca A, Egbe TO, Morgante G, Paglia T, Cianci A, De Leo V et al. Metformin treatment reduces ovarian cytochrome P-450c17alpha response to human chorionic gonadotrophin in women with insulin resistance-related polycystic ovary syndrome. Hum Reprod 2000; 15(1):21–23.
42. Jakubowicz DJ, Nestler JE. 17 alpha-Hydroxyprogesterone responses to leuprolide and serum androgens in obese women with and without polycystic ovary syndrome offer dietary weight loss. J Clin Endocrinol Metab 1997; 82(2):556–560.
43. Nestler JE, Jakubowicz DJ. Lean women with polycystic ovary syndrome respond to insulin reduction with decreases in ovarian P450c17 alpha activity and serum androgens. J Clin Endocrinol Metab 1997; 82(12):4075–4079.
44. Nestler JE, Jakubowicz DJ. Decreases in ovarian cytochrome P450c17 alpha activity and serum free testosterone after reduction of insulin secretion in polycystic ovary syndrome. N Engl J Med 1996; 335(9):617–623.
45. Ehrmann DA, Schneider DJ, Sobel BE, Cavaghan MK, Imperial J, Rosenfield RL et al. Troglitazone improves defects in insulin action, insulin secretion, ovarian steroidogenesis, and fibrinolysis in women with polycystic ovary syndrome. J Clin Endocrinol Metab 1997; 82(7):2108–2116.
46. Arslanian SA, Lewy V, Danadian K, Saad R. Metformin therapy in obese adolescents with polycystic ovary syndrome and impaired glucose tolerance: amelioration of exaggerated adrenal response to adrenocorticotropin with reduction of insulinemia/insulin resistance. J Clin Endocrinol Metab 2002; 87(4):1555–1559.
47. Vrbikova J, Hill M, Starka L, Cibula D, Bendlova B, Vondra K et al. The effects of long-term metformin treatment on adrenal and ovarian steroidogenesis in women with polycystic ovary syndrome. Eur J Endocrinol 2001; 144(6):619–628.
48. la Marca A, Morgante G, Paglia T, Ciotta L, Cianci A, De Leo V. Effects of metformin on adrenal steroidogenesis in women with polycystic ovary syndrome. [erratum appears in Fertil Steril 2000 Apr;73(4):874]. Fertil Steril 1999; 72(6): 985–989.
49. Romualdi D, Giuliani M, Draisci G, Costantini B, Cristello F, Lanzone A et al. Pioglitazone reduces the adrenal androgen response to corticotropin-releasing factor without changes in ACTH release in hyperinsulinemic women with polycystic ovary syndrome. Fertil Steril 2007; 88(1):131–138.
50. Guido M, Romualdi D, Suriano R, Giuliani M, Costantini B, Apa R et al. Effect of pioglitazone treatment on the adrenal androgen response to corticotrophin in obese patients with polycystic ovary syndrome. Hum Reprod 2004; 19(3):534–539.
51. Azziz R, Ehrmann DA, Legro RS, Fereshetian AG, O'Keefe M, Ghazzi MN. Troglitazone decreases adrenal androgen levels in women with polycystic ovary syndrome. Fertil Steril 2003; 79(4):932–937.
52. Nestler JE, Barlascini CO, Matt DW, Steingold KA, Plymate SR, Clore JN et al. Suppression of serum insulin by diazoxide reduces serum testosterone levels in obese women with polycystic ovary syndrome. J Clin Endocrinol Metab 1989; 68(6):1027–1032.
53. Penna IA, Canella PR, Reis RM, Silva de Sa MF, Ferriani RA. Acarbose in obese patients with polycystic ovarian syndrome: a double-blind, randomized, placebo-controlled study. Hum Reprod 2005; 20(9):2396–2401.
54. Ciotta L, Calogero AE, Farina M, De Leo V, la Marca A, Cianci A. Clinical, endocrine and metabolic effects of acarbose, an alpha-glucosidase inhibitor, in PCOS patients with increased insulin response and normal glucose tolerance. Hum Reprod 2001; 16(10):2066–2072.
55. Morin-Papunen LC, Vauhkonen I, Koivunen RM, Ruokonen A, Tapanainen JS. Insulin sensitivity, insulin secretion, and metabolic and hormonal parameters in healthy women and women with polycystic ovarian syndrome. Hum Reprod 2000; 15(6):1266–1274.
56. VrbIkova J, Cibula D, Dvorakova K, Stanicka S, Sindelka G, Hill M et al. Insulin Sensitivity in Women with Polycystic Ovary Syndrome. J Clin Endocrinol Metab 2004; 89(6):2942–2945.
57. Ciampelli M, Fulghesu AM, Cucinelli F, Pavone V, Caruso A, Mancuso S et al. Heterogeneity in beta cell activity, hepatic insulin clearance and peripheral insulin sensitivity in women with polycystic ovary syndrome. Hum Reprod 1997; 12(9):1897–1901.
58. Baillargeon JP, Jakubowicz DJ, Iuorno MJ, Jakubowicz S, Nestler JE. Effects of metformin and rosiglitazone, alone and in combination, in lean women with polycystic ovary syndrome and normal indices of insulin sensitivity. Fertil Steril 2004; 82(4):893–902.
59. Frias JP, Yu JG, Kruszynska YT, Olefsky JM. Metabolic effects of troglitazone therapy in type 2 diabetic, obese, and lean normal subjects. Diabetes Care 2000; 23(1):64–69.
60. Kruszynska YT, Yu JG, Olefsky JM, Sobel BE. Effects of troglitazone on blood concentrations of plasminogen activator inhibitor 1 in patients with type 2 diabetes and in lean and obese normal subjects. Diabetes 2000; 49(4):633–639.
61. Baillargeon JP, Carpentier A. Role of insulin in the hyperandrogenemia of lean women with polycystic ovary syndrome and normal insulin sensitivity. Fertil Steril 2007; 88(4):886–893.
62. Nestler JE, Singh R, Matt DW, Clore JN, Blackard WG. Suppression of serum insulin level by diazoxide does not alter serum testosterone or sex hormone-binding globulin levels in healthy, nonobese women. Am J Obstet Gynecol 1990; 163 (4 Pt 1):1243–1246.
63. Saltiel AR, Kahn CR. Insulin signalling and the regulation of glucose and lipid metabolism. Nature 2001; 414(6865): 799–806.
64. Wu XK, Zhou SY, Liu JX, Pollanen P, Sallinen K, Makinen M et al. Selective ovary resistance to insulin signaling in women with polycystic ovary syndrome. Fertil Steril 2003; 80(4):954–965.
65. Qu J, Wang Y, Wu X, Gao L, Hou L, Erkkola R. Insulin resistance directly contributes to androgenic potential within ovarian thecal cells. Fertil Steril 2008 Jul 29. [Epub ahead of print]; doi:10.1016/j.fertnstert.2008.02.167.

66. Baillargeon JP, Nestler JE. Polycystic ovary syndrome: A syndrome of ovarian hypersensitivity to insulin? J Clin Endocrinol Metab 2006; 91(1):22–24.
67. Yildiz BO, Knochenhauer ES, Azziz R. Impact of obesity on the risk for polycystic ovary syndrome. J Clin Endocrinol Metab 2008; 93(1):162–168.
68. Rebuffe-Scrive M, Cullberg G, Lundberg PA, Lindstedt G, Bjorntorp P. Anthropometric variables and metabolism in polycystic ovarian disease. Horm Metab Res 1989; 21(7):391–397.
69. Yildirim B, Sabir N, Kaleli B. Relation of intra-abdominal fat distribution to metabolic disorders in nonobese patients with polycystic ovary syndrome. Fertil Steril 2003; 79(6):1358–1364.
70. Barber TM, Golding SJ, Alvey C, Wass JA, Karpe F, Franks S et al. Global adiposity rather than abnormal regional fat distribution characterizes women with polycystic ovary syndrome. J Clin Endocrinol Metab 2008; 93(3):999–1004.
71. Michelmore K, Ong K, Mason S, Bennett S, Perry L, Vessey M et al. Clinical features in women with polycystic ovaries: relationships to insulin sensitivity, insulin gene VNTR and birth weight. Clin Endocrinol (Oxf) 2001; 55(4):439–446.
72. Huber-Buchholz MM, Carey DGP, Norman RJ. Restoration of Reproductive potential by lifestyle modification in obese polycystic ovary syndrome: Role of insulin sensitivity and luteinizing hormone. J Clin Endocrinol Metab 1999; 84(4): 1470–1474.
73. Hoeger KM. Role of lifestyle modification in the management of polycystic ovary syndrome. Best Pract Res Clin Endocrinol Metab 2006; 20(2):293–310.
74. Despres JP, Lemieux I, Prud'homme D. Treatment of obesity: Need to focus on high risk abdominally obese patients. BMJ 2001; 322(7288):716–720.
75. Diamanti-Kandarakis E, Katsikis I, Piperi C, Alexandraki K, Panidis D. Effect of long-term orlistat treatment on serum levels of advanced glycation end-products in women with polycystic ovary syndrome. Clin Endocrinol (Oxf) 2007; 66(1):103–109.
76. Panidis D, Farmakiotis D, Rousso D, Kourtis A, Katsikis I, Krassas G. Obesity, weight loss, and the polycystic ovary syndrome: effect of treatment with diet and orlistat for 24 weeks on insulin resistance and androgen levels. Fertil Steril 2008; 89(4):899–906.
77. Lindholm A, Bixo M, Bjorn I, Wolner-Hanssen P, Eliasson M, Larsson A et al. Effect of sibutramine on weight reduction in women with polycystic ovary syndrome: a randomized, double-blind, placebo-controlled trial. Fertil Steril 2008; 89(5): 1221–1228.
78. Sathyapalan T, Cho L, Kilpatrick ES, Coady AM, Atkin SL. A comparison between rimonabant and metformin in reducing biochemical hyperandrogenaemia and insulin resistance in patients with polycystic ovary syndrome: a randomised open labelled parallel study. Clin Endocrinol (Oxf) 2008; [Epub ahead of print].
79. Knowler WC, Barrett-Connor E, Fowler SE, Hamman RF, Lachin JM, Walker EA et al. Reduction in the incidence of type 2 diabetes with lifestyle intervention or metformin. N Engl J Med 2002; 346(6):393–403.
80. Tuomilehto J, Lindstrom J, Eriksson JG, Valle TT, Hamalainen H, Ilanne-Parikka P et al. Prevention of type 2 diabetes mellitus by changes in lifestyle among subjects with impaired glucose tolerance. N Engl J Med 2001; 344(18):1343–1350.
81. Ramachandran A, Snehalatha C, Mary S, Mukesh B, Bhaskar AD, Vijay V. The Indian Diabetes Prevention Programme shows that lifestyle modification and metformin prevent type 2 diabetes in Asian Indian subjects with impaired glucose tolerance (IDPP-1). Diabetologia 2006; 49(2):289–297.
82. Pan XR, Li GW, Hu YH, Wang JX, Yang WY, An ZX et al. Effects of diet and exercise in preventing NIDDM in people with impaired glucose tolerance. The Da Qing IGT and Diabetes Study. Diabetes Care 1997; 20(4):537–544.
83. Torgerson JS, Hauptman J, Boldrin MN, Sjostrom L. XENical in the prevention of diabetes in obese subjects (XENDOS) study: a randomized study of orlistat as an adjunct to lifestyle changes for the prevention of type 2 diabetes in obese patients. Diabetes Care 2004; 27(1):155–161.
84. Revised 2003 consensus on diagnostic criteria and long-term health risks related to polycystic ovary syndrome. Fertil Steril 2004; 81(1):19–25.
85. Baillargeon JP, Iuorno MJ, Nestler JE. Insulin sensitizers for polycystic ovary syndrome. Clin Obstet Gynecol 2003; 46(2):325–340.
86. Rimm EB, Manson JE, Stampfer MJ, Colditz GA, Willett WC, Rosner B et al. Oral contraceptive use and the risk of type 2 (non-insulin-dependent) diabetes mellitus in a large prospective study of women. Diabetologia 1992; 35(10):967–972.
87. Chasan-Taber L, Willett WC, Stampfer MJ, Hunter DJ, Colditz GA, Spiegelman D et al. A prospective study of oral contraceptives and NIDDM among U.S. women. Diabetes Care 1997; 20(3):330–335.
88. Baillargeon JP, McClish DK, Essah PA, Nestler JE. Association between the current use of low-dose oral contraceptives and cardiovascular arterial disease: A meta-analysis. J Clin Endocrinol Metab 2005; 90(7):3863–3870.
89. Beral V, Hermon C, Kay C, Hannaford P, Darby S, Reeves G. Mortality associated with oral contraceptive use: 25 year follow up of cohort of 46 000 women from Royal College of General Practitioners' oral contraception study. BMJ 1999; 318(7176):96–100.
90. Stampfer MJ, Willett WC, Colditz GA, Speizer FE, Hennekens CH. A prospective study of past use of oral contraceptive agents and risk of cardiovascular diseases. N Engl J Med 1988; 319(20):1313–1317.
91. Shaw RJ, Lamia KA, Vasquez D, Koo SH, Bardeesy N, Depinho RA et al. The kinase LKB1 mediates glucose homeostasis in liver and therapeutic effects of metformin. Science 2005; 310(5754):1642–1646.
92. Creanga AA, Bradley HM, McCormick C, Witkop CT. Use of metformin in polycystic ovary syndrome: a meta-analysis. Obstet Gynecol 2008; 111(4):959–968.

93. Bruno RV, de Avila MA, Neves FB, Nardi AE, Crespo CM, Sobrinho AT. Comparison of two doses of metformin (2.5 and 1.5 g/day) for the treatment of polycystic ovary syndrome and their effect on body mass index and waist circumference. Fertil Steril 2007; 88(2):510–512.
94. Maciel GA, Soares Junior JM, Alves da Motta EL, Abi HM, de Lima GR, Baracat EC. Nonobese women with polycystic ovary syndrome respond better than obese women to treatment with metformin. Fertil Steril 2004; 81(2):355–360.
95. Palomba S, Falbo A, Orio F, Jr., Tolino A, Zullo F. Efficacy predictors for metformin and clomiphene citrate treatment in anovulatory infertile patients with polycystic ovary syndrome. Fertil Steril 2008; [Epub ahead of print].
96. Garber AJ, Duncan TG, Goodman AM, Mills DJ, Rohlf JL. Efficacy of metformin in type II diabetes: results of a double-blind, placebo-controlled, dose-response trial. Am J Med 1997; 103(6):491–497.
97. Lord JM, Flight IH, Norman RJ. Metformin in polycystic ovary syndrome: systematic review and meta-analysis. BMJ 2003; 327(7421):951–953.
98. Moll E, Bossuyt PM, Korevaar JC, Lambalk CB, van der Veen, F. Effect of clomifene citrate plus metformin and clomifene citrate plus placebo on induction of ovulation in women with newly diagnosed polycystic ovary syndrome: randomised double blind clinical trial. BMJ 2006; 332(7556):1485.
99. Schwartz S, Fonseca V, Berner B, Cramer M, Chiang YK, Lewin A. Efficacy, tolerability, and safety of a novel once-daily extended-release metformin in patients with type 2 diabetes. Diabetes Care 2006; 29(4):759–764.
100. Legro RS, Barnhart HX, Schlaff WD, Carr BR, Diamond MP, Carson SA et al. Clomiphene, metformin, or both for infertility in the polycystic ovary syndrome. N Engl J Med 2007; 356(6):551–566.
101. Desilets AR, Dhakal-Karki S, Dunican KC. Role of metformin for weight management in patients without type 2 diabetes. Ann Pharmacother 2008; 42(6):817–826.
102. Rowan JA, Hague WM, Gao W, Battin MR, Moore MP. Metformin versus insulin for the treatment of gestational diabetes. N Engl J Med 2008; 358(19):2003–2015.
103. Bolton S, Cleary B, Walsh J, Dempsey E, Turner MJ. Continuation of metformin in the first trimester of women with polycystic ovarian syndrome is not associated with increased perinatal morbidity. Eur J Pediatr 2008; [Epub ahead of print].
104. Moore LE, Briery CM, Clokey D, Martin RW, Williford NJ, Bofill JA et al. Metformin and insulin in the management of gestational diabetes mellitus: preliminary results of a comparison. J Reprod Med 2007; 52(11):1011–1015.
105. Gilbert C, Valois M, Koren G. Pregnancy outcome after first-trimester exposure to metformin: A meta-analysis. Fertil Steril 2006; 86(3):658–663.
106. Glueck CJ, Goldenberg N, Pranikoff J, Loftspring M, Sieve L, Wang P. Height, weight, and motor-social development during the first 18 months of life in 126 infants born to 109 mothers with polycystic ovary syndrome who conceived on and continued metformin through pregnancy. Hum Reprod 2004; 19(6):1323–1330.
107. Vanky E, Salvesen KA, Heimstad R, Fougner KJ, Romundstad P, Carlsen SM. Metformin reduces pregnancy complications without affecting androgen levels in pregnant polycystic ovary syndrome women: results of a randomized study. Hum Reprod 2004; 19(8):1734–1740.
108. Gutzin SJ, Kozer E, Magee LA, Feig DS, Koren G. The safety of oral hypoglycemic agents in the first trimester of pregnancy: A meta-analysis. Can J Clin Pharmacol 2003; 10(4):179–183.
109. Coetzee EJ, Jackson WP. The management of non-insulin-dependent diabetes during pregnancy. Diabetes Res Clin Pract – Suppl 1985; 1(5):281–287.
110. Hellmuth E, Damm P, Molsted-Pedersen L. Oral hypoglycaemic agents in 118 diabetic pregnancies. Diabetic Medicine 2000; 17(7):507–511.
111. Karalliedde J, Buckingham RE. Thiazolidinediones and their fluid-related adverse effects: facts, fiction and putative management strategies. Drug Saf 2007; 30(9):741–753.
112. Hermansen K, Mortensen LS. Bodyweight changes associated with antihyperglycaemic agents in type 2 diabetes mellitus. Drug Saf 2007; 30(12):1127–1142.
113. Kahn SE, Haffner SM, Heise MA, Herman WH, Holman RR, Jones NP et al. Glycemic durability of rosiglitazone, metformin, or glyburide monotherapy. N Engl J Med 2006; 355(23):2427–2443.
114. Glintborg D, Andersen M, Hagen C, Heickendorff L, Hermann AP. Association of pioglitazone treatment with decreased bone mineral density in obese premenopausal patients with polycystic ovary syndrome: a randomized, placebo-controlled trial. J Clin Endocrinol Metab 2008; 93(5):1696–1701.
115. Demissie YN, Fiad TM, Klemm K, Twfeeg A, Al Amoudi A, Meer L et al. Spontaneous singleton and twin pregnancy in two patients with polycystic ovary syndrome and type 2 diabetes following treatment with metformin combined with rosiglitazone. Ann Saudi Med 2006; 26(4):296–299.
116. Choi JS, Han JY, Ahn HK, Shin JS, Yang JH, Koong MK et al. Exposure to rosiglitazone and fluoxetine in the first trimester of pregnancy. Diabetes Care 2006; 29(9):2176.
117. Ortega-Gonzalez C, Luna S, Hernandez L, Crespo G, Aguayo P, Arteaga-Troncoso G et al. Responses of Serum Androgen and Insulin Resistance to Metformin and Pioglitazone in Obese, Insulin-Resistant Women with Polycystic Ovary Syndrome. J Clin Endocrinol Metab 2005; 90(3):1360–1365.
118. Kalyoncu NI, Yaris F, Ulku C, Kadioglu M, Kesim M, Unsal M et al. A case of rosiglitazone exposure in the second trimester of pregnancy. Reprod Toxicol 2005; 19(4):563–564.
119. Yaris F, Yaris E, Kadioglu M, Ulku C, Kesim M, Kalyoncu NI. Normal pregnancy outcome following inadvertent exposure to rosiglitazone, gliclazide, and atorvastatin in a diabetic and hypertensive woman. Reprod Toxicol 2004; 18(4):619–621.

120. Ghazeeri G, Kutteh WH, Bryer-Ash M, Haas D, Ke RW. Effect of rosiglitazone on spontaneous and clomiphene citrate-induced ovulation in women with polycystic ovary syndrome. Fertil Steril 2003; 79(3):562–566.
121. Kashyap S, Wells GA, Rosenwaks Z. Insulin-sensitizing agents as primary therapy for patients with polycystic ovarian syndrome. Hum Reprod 2004; 19(11):2474–2483.
122. Palomba S, Orio F, Jr, Falbo A, Manguso F, Russo T, Cascella T et al. Prospective parallel randomized, double-blind, double-dummy controlled clinical trial comparing clomiphene citrate and metformin as the first-line treatment for ovulation induction in nonobese anovulatory women with polycystic ovary syndrome. J Clin Endocrinol Metab 2005; 90(7):4068–4074.
123. Palomba S, Orio F, Jr, Falbo A, Russo T, Tolino A, Zullo F. Clomiphene citrate versus metformin as first-line approach for the treatment of anovulation in infertile patients with polycystic ovary syndrome. J Clin Endocrinol Metab 2007; 92(9): 3498–3503.
124. Neveu N, Granger L, St Michel P, Lavoie HB. Comparison of clomiphene citrate, metformin, or the combination of both for first-line ovulation induction and achievement of pregnancy in 154 women with polycystic ovary syndrome. Fertil Steril 2007; 87(1):113–120.
125. Legro RS, Barnhart HX, Schlaff WD, Carr BR, Diamond MP, Carson SA et al. Ovulatory response to treatment of polycystic ovary syndrome is associated with a polymorphism in the STK11 gene. J Clin Endocrinol Metab 2008; 93(3):792–800.
126. Khattab S, Mohsen IA, Foutouh IA, Ramadan A, Moaz M, Al Inany H. Metformin reduces abortion in pregnant women with polycystic ovary syndrome. Gynecol Endocrinol 2006; 22(12):680–684.
127. Jakubowicz DJ, Iuorno MJ, Jakubowicz S, Roberts KA, Nestler JE. Effects of metformin on early pregnancy loss in the polycystic ovary syndrome. J Clin Endocrinol Metab 2002; 87(2):524–529.
128. Glueck CJ, Wang P, Goldenberg N, Sieve-Smith L. Pregnancy outcomes among women with polycystic ovary syndrome treated with metformin. Hum Reprod 2002; 17(11):2858–2864.
129. Palomba S, Orio F, Jr, Nardo LG, Falbo A, Russo T, Corea D et al. Metformin administration versus laparoscopic ovarian diathermy in clomiphene citrate-resistant women with polycystic ovary syndrome: A prospective parallel randomized double-blind placebo-controlled trial. J Clin Endocrinol Metab 2004; 89(10):4801–4809.
130. Balen AH, Tan SL, MacDougall J, Jacobs HS. Miscarriage rates following in-vitro fertilization are increased in women with polycystic ovaries and reduced by pituitary desensitization with buserelin. Hum Reprod 1993; 8(6):959–964.
131. Sagle M, Bishop K, Ridley N, Alexander FM, Michel M, Bonney RC et al. Recurrent early miscarriage and polycystic ovaries. BMJ 1988; 297(6655):1027–1028.
132. Jakubowicz DJ, Essah PA, Seppala M, Jakubowicz S, Baillargeon J-P, Koistinen R et al. Reduced serum glycodelin and insulin-like growth factor-binding protein-1 in women with polycystic ovary syndrome during first trimester of pregnancy. J Clin Endocrinol Metab 2004; 89(2):833–839.
133. Jakubowicz DJ, Seppala M, Jakubowicz S, Rodriguez-Armas O, Rivas-Santiago A, Koistinen H et al. Insulin reduction with metformin increases luteal phase serum glycodelin and insulin-like growth factor-binding protein 1 concentrations and enhances uterine vascularity and blood flow in the polycystic ovary syndrome. J Clin Endocrinol Metab 2001; 86(3): 1126–1133.
134. Ratts VS, Pauls RN, Pinto AB, Kraja A, Williams DB, Odem RR. Risk of multiple gestation after ovulation induction in polycystic ovary syndrome. J Reprod Med 2007; 52(10):896–900.
135. Azziz R, Ehrmann D, Legro RS, Whitcomb RW, Hanley R, Fereshetian AG et al. Troglitazone improves ovulation and hirsutism in the polycystic ovary syndrome: a multicenter, double blind, placebo-controlled trial. J Clin Endocrinol Metab 2001; 86(4):1626–1632.
136. Rautio K, Tapanainen JS, Ruokonen A, Morin-Papunen LC. Endocrine and metabolic effects of rosiglitazone in overweight women with PCOS: a randomized placebo-controlled study. Human reproduction (Oxford, England) 2006.
137. Brettenthaler N, De Geyter C, Huber PR, Keller U. Effect of the insulin sensitizer pioglitazone on insulin resistance, hyperandrogenism, and ovulatory dysfunction in women with polycystic ovary syndrome. J Clin Endocrinol Metab 2004; 89(8): 3835–3840.
138. Mitwally MF, Kuscu NK, Yalcinkaya TM. High ovulatory rates with use of troglitazone in clomiphene-resistant women with polycystic ovary syndrome. Hum Reprod 1999; 14(11):2700–2703.
139. Zhang CL, Gao HY, Zhao ZG, Jia P. Effect of rosiglitazone on ovulation induction in women with polycystic ovary syndrome. Chung Hua Fu Chan Ko Tsa Chih 2004; 39(3):173–175.
140. Shobokshi A, Shaarawy M. Correction of insulin resistance and hyperandrogenism in polycystic ovary syndrome by combined rosiglitazone and clomiphene citrate therapy. Journal of the Society for Gynecologic Investigation 2003; 10(2): 99–104.
141. Rouzi AA, Ardawi MS. A randomized controlled trial of the efficacy of rosiglitazone and clomiphene citrate versus metformin and clomiphene citrate in women with clomiphene citrate-resistant polycystic ovary syndrome. Fertil Steril 2006; 85(2): 428–435.
142. Kelly CJ, Gordon D. The effect of metformin on hirsutism in polycystic ovary syndrome. Eur J Endocrinol 2002; 147(2): 217–221.
143. Harborne L, Fleming R, Lyall H, Sattar N, Norman J. Metformin or Antiandrogen in the treatment of hirsutism in polycystic ovary syndrome. J Clin Endocrinol Metab 2003; 88(9):4116–4123.
144. Kolodziejczyk B, Duleba AJ, Spaczynski RZ, Pawelczyk L. Metformin therapy decreases hyperandrogenism and hyperinsulinemia in women with polycystic ovary syndrome. Fertil Steril 2000; 73(6):1149–1154.

145. Ibanez L, Valls C, Ferrer A, Marcos MV, Rodriguez-Hierro F, de Zegher F. Sensitization to insulin induces ovulation in nonobese adolescents with anovulatory hyperandrogenism. J Clin Endocrinol Metab 2001; 86(8):3595–3598.
146. Loverro G, Lorusso F, De Pergola G, Nicolardi V, Mei L, Selvaggi L. Clinical and endocrinological effects of 6 months of metformin treatment in young hyperinsulinemic patients affected by polycystic ovary syndrome. Gynecol Endocrinol 2002; 16(3):217–224.
147. Kazerooni T, Dehghan-Kooshkghazi M. Effects of metformin therapy on hyperandrogenism in women with polycystic ovarian syndrome. Gynecol Endocrinol 2003; 17(1):51–56.
148. Aruna J, Mittal S, Kumar S, Misra R, Dadhwal V, Vimala N. Metformin therapy in women with polycystic ovary syndrome. Int J Gynaecol Obstet 2004; 87(3):237–241.
149. Kriplani A, Agarwal N. Effects of metformin on clinical and biochemical parameters in polycystic ovary syndrome. J Reprod Med 2004; 49(5):361–367.
150. Marcondes JA, Yamashita SA, Maciel GA, Baracat EC, Halpern A. Metformin in normal-weight hirsute women with polycystic ovary syndrome with normal insulin sensitivity. Gynecol Endocrinol 2007; 23(5):273–278.
151. Cicek MN, Bala A, Celik C, Akyurek C. The comparison of clinical and hormonal parameters in PCOS patients treated with metformin and GnRH analogue. Archives of Gynecology & Obstetrics 2003; 268(2):107–112.
152. Gambineri A, Pelusi C, Genghini S, Morselli-Labate AM, Cacciari M, Pagotto U et al. Effect of flutamide and metformin administered alone or in combination in dieting obese women with polycystic ovary syndrome. Clin Endocrinol (Oxf) 2004; 60(2):241–249.
153. Ganie MA, Khurana ML, Eunice M, Gulati M, Dwivedi SN, Ammini AC. Comparison of efficacy of spironolactone with metformin in the management of polycystic ovary syndrome: An open-labeled study. J Clin Endocrinol Metab 2004; 89(6): 2756–2762.
154. Yilmaz M, Karakoc A, Toruner FB, Cakir N, Tiras B, Ayvaz G et al. The effects of rosiglitazone and metformin on menstrual cyclicity and hirsutism in polycystic ovary syndrome. Gynecol Endocrinol 2005; 21(3):154–160.
155. Meyer C, McGrath BP, Teede HJ. Effects of medical therapy on insulin resistance and the cardiovascular system in polycystic ovary syndrome. Diabetes Care 2007; 30(3):471–478.
156. Orio F, Jr, Palomba S, Cascella T, De Simone B, Manguso F, Savastano S et al. Improvement in endothelial structure and function after metformin treatment in young normal-weight women with polycystic ovary syndrome: Results of a 6-month study. J Clin Endocrinol Metab 2005; 90(11):6072–6076.
157. Morin-Papunen L, Vauhkonen I, Koivunen R, Ruokonen A, Martikainen H, Tapanainen JS. Metformin versus ethinyl estradiol-cyproterone acetate in the treatment of nonobese women with polycystic ovary syndrome: A randomized study. J Clin Endocrinol Metab 2003; 88(1):148–156.
158. Gambineri A, Patton L, Vaccina A, Cacciari M, Morselli-Labate AM, Cavazza C et al. Treatment with flutamide, metformin, and their combination added to a hypocaloric diet in overweight-obese women with polycystic ovary syndrome: A randomized, 12-month, placebo-controlled study. J Clin Endocrinol Metab 2006; 91(10):3970–3980.
159. Ibanez L, Valls C, Ferrer A, Ong K, Dunger DB, de Zegher F. Additive effects of insulin-sensitizing and anti-androgen treatment in young, nonobese women with hyperinsulinism, hyperandrogenism, dyslipidemia, and anovulation. J Clin Endocrinol Metab 2002; 87(6):2870–2874.
160. Romualdi D, Guido M, Ciampelli M, Giuliani M, Leoni F, Perri C et al. Selective effects of pioglitazone on insulin and androgen abnormalities in normo- and hyperinsulinaemic obese patients with polycystic ovary syndrome. Hum Reprod 2003; 18(6):1210–1218.
161. Dereli D, Dereli T, Bayraktar F, Ozgen AG, Yilmaz C. Endocrine and metabolic effects of rosiglitazone in non-obese women with polycystic ovary disease. Endocr J 2005; 52(3):299–308.
162. Tarkun I, Cetinarslan B, Turemen E, Sahin T, Canturk Z, Komsuoglu B. Effect of rosiglitazone on insulin resistance, C-reactive protein and endothelial function in non-obese young women with polycystic ovary syndrome. Eur J Endocrinol 2005; 153(1):115–121.
163. Lemay A, Dodin S, Turcot L, Dechene F, Forest JC. Rosiglitazone and ethinyl estradiol/cyproterone acetate as single and combined treatment of overweight women with polycystic ovary syndrome and insulin resistance. Hum Reprod 2006; 21(1): 121–128.
164. Sharma ST, Wickham EP, III, Nestler JE. Changes in glucose tolerance with metformin treatment in polycystic ovary syndrome: a retrospective analysis. Endocr Pract 2007; 13(4):373–379.
165. Luque-Ramirez M, Alvarez-Blasco F, Botella-Carretero JI, Martinez-Bermejo E, Lasuncion MA, Escobar-Morreale HF. Comparison of ethinyl-estradiol plus cyproterone acetate versus metformin effects on classic metabolic cardiovascular risk factors in women with the polycystic ovary syndrome. J Clin Endocrinol Metab 2007; 92(7):2453–2461.
166. Romualdi D, Costantini B, Selvaggi L, Giuliani M, Cristello F, Macri F et al. Metformin improves endothelial function in normoinsulinemic PCOS patients: a new prospective. Hum Reprod 2008.
167. Topcu S, Tok D, Caliskan M, Ozcimen EE, Gullu H, Uckuyu A et al. Metformin therapy improves coronary microvascular function in patients with polycystic ovary syndrome and insulin resistance. Clin Endocrinol (Oxf) 2006; 65(1): 75–80.
168. Luque-Ramirez M, Mendieta-Azcona C, Alvarez-Blasco F, Escobar-Morreale HF. Effects of metformin versus ethinyl-estradiol plus cyproterone acetate on ambulatory blood pressure monitoring and carotid intima media thickness in women with the polycystic ovary syndrome. Fertil Steril 2008.

169. Goldenberg N, Glueck CJ, Loftspring M, Sherman A, Wang P. Metformin-diet benefits in women with polycystic ovary syndrome in the bottom and top quintiles for insulin resistance. Metabolism 2005; 54(1):113–121.
170. Moghetti P, Castello R, Negri C, Tosi F, Perrone F, Caputo M et al. Metformin effects on clinical features, endocrine and metabolic profiles, and insulin sensitivity in polycystic ovary syndrome: a randomized, double-blind, placebo-controlled 6-month trial, followed by open, long-term clinical evaluation. J Clin Endocrinol Metab 2000; 85(1):139–146.
171. Fleming R, Hopkinson ZE, Wallace AM, Greer IA, Sattar N. Ovarian function and metabolic factors in women with oligomenorrhea treated with metformin in a randomized double blind placebo-controlled trial. J Clin Endocrinol Metab 2002; 87(2):569–574.
172. Morin-Papunen L, Rautio K, Ruokonen A, Hedberg P, Puukka M, Tapanainen JS. Metformin reduces serum C-reactive protein levels in women with polycystic ovary syndrome. J Clin Endocrinol Metab 2003; 88(10):4649–4654.
173. Diamanti-Kandarakis E, Spina G, Kouli C, Migdalis I. Increased endothelin-1 levels in women with polycystic ovary syndrome and the beneficial effect of metformin therapy. J Clin Endocrinol Metab 2001; 86(10):4666–4673.
174. Wu J, Zhu Y, Jiang Y, Cao Y. Effects of metformin and ethinyl estradiol-cyproterone acetate on clinical, endocrine and metabolic factors in women with polycystic ovary syndrome. Gynecol Endocrinol 2008; [Epub ahead of print]:1–7.
175. Ibanez L, de Zegher F. Ethinylestradiol-drospirenone, flutamide-metformin, or both for adolescents and women with hyperinsulinemic hyperandrogenism: opposite effects on adipocytokines and body adiposity. J Clin Endocrinol Metab 2004; 89(4):1592–1597.
176. Sahin Y, Unluhizarci K, Yilmazsoy A, Yikilmaz A, Aygen E, Kelestimur F. The effects of metformin on metabolic and cardiovascular risk factors in nonobese women with polycystic ovary syndrome. Clin Endocrinol (Oxf) 2007; 67(6): 904–908.
177. Tan S, Hahn S, Benson S, Dietz T, Lahner H, Moeller LC et al. Metformin improves polycystic ovary syndrome symptoms irrespective of pre-treatment insulin resistance. Eur J Endocrinol 2007; 157(5):669–676.
178. Nawrocka J, Starczewski A. Effects of metformin treatment in women with polycystic ovary syndrome depends on insulin resistance. Gynecol Endocrinol 2007; 23(4):231–237.
179. Salley KE, Wickham EP, Cheang KI, Essah PA, Karjane NW, Nestler JE. Glucose intolerance in polycystic ovary syndrome–a position statement of the Androgen Excess Society. J Clin Endocrinol Metab 2007; 92(12):4546–4556.
180. Gagnon C, Baillargeon JP. Suitability of recommended limits for fasting glucose tests in women with polycystic ovary syndrome. CMAJ 2007; 176(7):933–938.
181. Glueck CJ, Moreira A, Goldenberg N, Sieve L, Wang P. Pioglitazone and metformin in obese women with polycystic ovary syndrome not optimally responsive to metformin. Hum Reprod 2003; 18(8):1618–1625.
182. Glueck CJ, Aregawi D, Agloria M, Winiarska M, Sieve L, Wang P. Sustainability of 8% weight loss, reduction of insulin resistance, and amelioration of atherogenic-metabolic risk factors over 4 years by metformin-diet in women with polycystic ovary syndrome. Metabolism 2006; 55(12):1582–1589.
183. Lo JC, Feigenbaum SL, Escobar GJ, Yang J, Crites YM, Ferrara A. Increased prevalence of gestational diabetes mellitus among women with diagnosed polycystic ovary syndrome: a population-based study. Diabetes Care 2006; 29(8):1915–1917.
184. Standards of medical care in diabetes–2006. Diabetes Care 2006; 29 Suppl 1:S4–S42.
185. Turner MJ, Walsh J, Byrne KM, Murphy C, Langan H, Farah N. Outcome of clinical pregnancies after ovulation induction using metformin. J Obstet Gynaecol 2006; 26(3):233–235.
186. Glueck CJ, Bornovali S, Pranikoff J, Goldenberg N, Dharashivkar S, Wang P. Metformin, pre-eclampsia, and pregnancy outcomes in women with polycystic ovary syndrome. Diabetic Med 2004; 21(8):829–836.
187. Glueck CJ, Pranikoff J, Aregawi D, Wang P. Prevention of gestational diabetes by metformin plus diet in patients with polycystic ovary syndrome. Fertil Steril 2008; 89(3):625–634.
188. Siega-Riz AM, Laraia B. The implications of maternal overweight and obesity on the course of pregnancy and birth outcomes. Matern Child Health J 2006; 10(5 Suppl):S153-S156.
189. Chu SY, Kim SY, Schmid CH, Dietz PM, Callaghan WM, Lau J et al. Maternal obesity and risk of cesarean delivery: a meta-analysis. Obes Rev 2007; 8(5):385–394.
190. Chu SY, Kim SY, Lau J, Schmid CH, Dietz PM, Callaghan WM et al. Maternal obesity and risk of stillbirth: a metaanalysis. Am J Obstet Gynecol 2007; 197(3):223–228.
191. Chu SY, Callaghan WM, Kim SY, Schmid CH, Lau J, England LJ et al. Maternal obesity and risk of gestational diabetes mellitus. Diabetes Care 2007; 30(8):2070–2076.
192. Chu SY, Bachman DJ, Callaghan WM, Whitlock EP, Dietz PM, Berg CJ et al. Association between obesity during pregnancy and increased use of health care. N Engl J Med 2008; 358(14):1444–1453.
193. Harlass FE, Plymate SR, Fariss BL, Belts RP. Weight loss is associated with correction of gonadotropin and sex steroid abnormalities in the obese anovulatory female. Fertil Steril 1984; 42(4):649–652.
194. Pasquali R, Antenucci D, Casimirri F, Venturoli S, Paradisi R, Fabbri R et al. Clinical and hormonal characteristics of obese amenorrheic hyperandrogenic women before and after weight loss. J Clin Endocrinol Metab 1989; 68(1):173–179.
195. Kiddy DS, Hamilton-Fairley D, Bush A, Short F, Anyaoku V, Reed MJ et al. Improvement in endocrine and ovarian function during dietary treatment of obese women with polycystic ovary syndrome. Clin Endocrinol (Oxf) 1992; 36(1):105–111.
196. Hamilton-Fairley D, Kiddy D, Anyaoku V, Koistinen R, Seppala M, Franks S. Response of sex hormone binding globulin and insulin-like growth factor binding protein-1 to an oral glucose tolerance test in obese women with polycystic ovary syndrome before and after calorie restriction. Clin Endocrinol (Oxf) 1993; 39(3):363–367.

197. Guzick DS, Wing R, Smith D, Berga SL, Winters SJ. Endocrine consequences of weight loss in obese, hyperandrogenic, anovulatory women. Fertil Steril 1994; 61(4):598–604.
198. Holte J, Bergh T, Berne C, Wide L, Lithell H. Restored insulin sensitivity but persistently increased early insulin secretion after weight loss in obese women with polycystic ovary syndrome. J Clin Endocrinol Metab 1995; 80(9):2586–2593.
199. Andersen P, Seljeflot I, Abdelnoor M, Arnesen H, Dale PO, Lovik A et al. Increased insulin sensitivity and fibrinolytic capacity after dietary intervention in obese women with polycystic ovary syndrome. Metabolism 1995; 44(5):611–616.
200. Wahrenberg H, Ek I, Reynisdottir S, Carlstrom K, Bergqvist A, Arner P. Divergent effects of weight reduction and oral anticonception treatment on adrenergic lipolysis regulation in obese women with the polycystic ovary syndrome. J Clin Endocrinol Metab 1999; 84(6):2182–2187.
201. Pasquali R, Gambineri A, Biscotti D, Vicennati V, Gagliardi L, Colitta D et al. Effect of long-term treatment with metformin added to hypocaloric diet on body composition, fat distribution, and androgen and insulin levels in abdominally obese women with and without the polycystic ovary syndrome. J Clin Endocrinol Metab 2000; 85(8):2767–2774.
202. Randeva HS, Lewandowski KC, Drzewoski J, Brooke-Wavell K, O'Callaghan C, Czupryniak L et al. Exercise decreases plasma total homocysteine in overweight young women with polycystic ovary syndrome. J Clin Endocrinol Metab 2002; 87(10):4496–4501.
203. Moran LJ, Noakes M, Clifton PM, Tomlinson L, Norman RJ. Dietary composition in restoring reproductive and metabolic physiology in overweight women with polycystic ovary syndrome. J Clin Endocrinol Metab 2003; 88(2):812–819.
204. Hoeger KM, Kochman L, Wixom N, Craig K, Miller RK, Guzick DS. A randomized, 48-week, placebo-controlled trial of intensive lifestyle modification and/or metformin therapy in overweight women with polycystic ovary syndrome: a pilot study. Fertil Steril 2004; 82(2):421–429.
205. Jayagopal V, Kilpatrick ES, Holding S, Jennings PE, Atkin SL. Orlistat is as beneficial as metformin in the treatment of polycystic ovarian syndrome. J Clin Endocrinol Metab 2005; 90(2):729–733.
206. Eid GM, Cottam DR, Velcu LM, Mattar SG, Korytkowski MT, Gosman G et al. Effective treatment of polycystic ovarian syndrome with Roux-en-Y gastric bypass. Surg Obes Relat Dis 2005; 1(2):77–80.
207. Moran LJ, Noakes M, Clifton PM, Wittert GA, Williams G, Norman RJ. Short-term meal replacements followed by dietary macronutrient restriction enhance weight loss in polycystic ovary syndrome. Am J Clin Nutr 2006; 84(1):77–87.
208. Vigorito C, Giallauria F, Palomba S, Cascella T, Manguso F, Lucci R et al. Beneficial effects of a three-month structured exercise training program on cardiopulmonary functional capacity in young women with polycystic ovary syndrome. J Clin Endocrinol Metab 2007; 92(4):1379–1384.
209. Palomba S, Giallauria F, Falbo A, Russo T, Oppedisano R, Tolino A et al. Structured exercise training programme versus hypocaloric hyperproteic diet in obese polycystic ovary syndrome patients with anovulatory infertility: a 24-week pilot study. Hum Reprod 2008; 23(3):642–650.

Chapter 19
Therapy of Hirsutism

Salvatore Benvenga

There has been a great deal of scientific research on the therapeutic aspects of PCOS/hirsutism/acne, which has intensified more recently. A PubMed search on "Treatment of polycystic ovary syndrome" returned 3580 items published in the 51 years comprised between 1957 and March 04, 2008; of these, 607 (17%) were in the 2 years, between Jan 01, 2006 and March 04, 2008. A PubMed search on "Treatment of hirsutism" returned 2211 items published in the 57 years comprised between 1951 and March 04, 2008; of these, 192 (9%) were in the 2 years between Jan 01, 2006 and March 04, 2008. At the recent 13th World Congress on Gynecological Endocrinology (Florence, February 28-March 02, 2008), 15 oral presentations and 3 posters focused on treatment of PCOS.

As PCOS is so frequently accompanied by overweight/obesity and, regardless of body mass index (BMI), by insulin resistance, the physician has to illustrate to the patient the long-term consequences of PCOS in terms of development of type 2 diabetes mellitus and cardiovascular risk. Motivation of the patient is greater if the physician explains that the benefits of changes in lifestyle (hypocaloric diet, physical exercise) are not only long term, but also short term, as reduction of BMI per se favors improvement of hyperandrogenism. In a classic study [1], 24 obese women with PCOS (mean body weight = 91.5 ±14.7 Kg) were scheduled for treatment for 6–7 months with a 1000 kcal, low fat diet. Nineteen of the 24 women had menstrual disturbances, 12 had infertility and 19 were hirsute. Of the 24 patients, 13 lost more than 5% of their starting weight (range 5.9–22%). In this group, there were significant changes: a marked increase in concentrations of sex hormone-binding globulin and a reciprocal change in free testosterone levels, as well as a reduction in both fasting and OGTT-stimulated insulin levels. There were no significant changes in these indices in the group who lost less than 5% of their initial body weight. Of the 13 women who lost greater than 5% of their pretreatment weight, 11 had menstrual dysfunction. Of these 11 women, 9 showed an improvement in reproductive function, i.e., they either conceived (5) or experienced a more regular menstrual pattern. There was a reduction in hirsutism in 40% of the women in this group. By contrast, in the group who lost less than 5% of their initial weight, only one of the eight with menstrual disturbances noted an improvement in reproductive function and none had a significant reduction in hirsutism [1].

These benefits of weight loss were reinforced in a very recent review [2]. A significant reduction in hirsutism was found for flutamide, spironolactone, cyproterone acetate combined with an oral contraceptive, thiazolidinediones, oral contraceptive pills, finasteride, and metformin. Reduction in Ferriman–Gallwey score in response to treatment was negatively associated with BMI. It was concluded that *Obesity has a negative impact on the efficacy of treatments for hirsutism, thus appropriate lifestyle advice is necessary for a successful treatment programme* [2].

The corollary is that insulin sensitizers should not be used as substitutive of the hypocaloric diet and exercise but, rather, follow and complement such beneficial changes in weight-control programs. A recent consensus document released on March, 2008, mentioned avoiding smoking and alcohol consumption as additional changes in lifestyle [3]. Lifestyle modification is often referred to as the first-line therapy of PCOS.

S. Benvenga (✉)
Master on Childhood, Adolescent and Women's Endocrine Health, University of Messina, Programma di Endocrinologia Molecolare Clinica, A.O.U. Policlinico G. Martino, Padiglione H, 4 piano, 98125 Messina, Italy,
e-mail: s.benvenga@me.nettuno.it

N.R. Farid, E. Diamanti-Kandarakis (eds.), *Diagnosis and Management of Polycystic Ovary Syndrome*,
DOI 10.1007/978-0-387-09718-3_19,

19.1 Physical Methods of Hair Removal

Hirsutism, especially in visible areas such as face, is cause of embarrassment and emotional distress, thus reducing the quality of life. In a study on 45 women hirsute for PCOS or idiopathic hirsutism [4], patients with hirsutism displayed significantly higher social fears, and significantly more anxiety and psychotic symptoms than controls; however, there were no significant differences in depression, somatization, anger-hostility, and cognitive symptoms.

19.1.1 Depilation and Creams

Strictly speaking, bleaching is not a method of hair removal, as it simply masks hair by merging the new color with the skin tone (hair camouflage). Bleaching works best for hair that is dark in color and fine in texture. Bleaching is very fast, painless, and inexpensive. Hair removal includes depilation or epilation.

Depilation removes the hair above the skin surface, essentially by shaving, by threading, or by chemical means that dissolve the protein structure of hair (depilatories in the form of cream, gel, lotion, roll-on, aerosol). Most commonly, depilatories contain the highly alkaline thioglycollates. Results of all these methods are very transient (hours to days). The popular assumption that hair removed by shaving grows faster, and even becomes thicker and darker, is false.

19.1.2 Particular Creams

Because of their peculiarities, two creams are to be treated separately. For easy of exposure, we deal with these creams here, even though their effect is long-lasting. The active principles are eflornithine in one cream and spironolactone in the other cream.

Eflornithine (α-difluoromethylornithine or DFMO) was incidentally found to effectively treat sleeping sickness by killing *Trypanosoma brucei gambiense* through inhibition of ornithine decarboxylase, a key enzyme in polyamine biosynthesis. Eflornithine HCl 13.9% cream (11.5% weight/weight as eflornithine base) is the first topical prescription treatment to be approved by the Food and Drug Administration (FDA) for the reduction of unwanted facial hair in women. One 30-g tube of eflornithine hydrochloride monohydrate (Vaniqua® by Shire Pharmaceutical Ltd) in Italy costs about euro 40/00. One tube usually lasts 2 months if used as recommended (twice a day, every day).

Eflornithine irreversibly inhibits ornithine decarboxylase, an enzyme that catalyzes the rate-limiting step for follicular polyamine synthesis, which is necessary for hair growth. In clinical trials, eflornithine cream slowed the growth of unwanted facial hair in up to 60% of women. Improvement occurs gradually over a period of 4–8 weeks or longer. Most reported adverse reactions consisted of minor skin irritation [5]. Eflornithine cream is usually applied twice a day, waiting at least 8 hours between applications, and washing hands thoroughly. Cosmetics and sunscreens can be applied after eflornithine cream has dried, while the area can be washed after a minimum of 4 hours from eflornithine application.

Eflornithine cream slows hair growth but does not prevent it, so hirsutism returns upon stopping the topical treatment. Efficacy has only been demonstrated for affected areas of the face and under the chin, so that application should be limited to these areas. The woman should continue to use her current method of hair removal (e.g., shaving, plucking), but frequency of use is appreciably delayed. Improvement in the condition may be noticed within 8 weeks of starting treatment. Use should be discontinued if no beneficial effects are noticed within 4 months of commencing therapy. Approximately, one-third of women will experience an improvement in facial hair, with return to baseline conditions by 8 weeks after stopping application. Clinical studies have shown that eflornithine cream improves the effectiveness of laser hair removal (see below).

Side effects of eflornithine include stinging, burning, or tingling of the skin, skin rash, worsening of preexisting acne, or de novo appearance of acne. Women who are pregnant or planning pregnancy should use an alternative means to manage facial hair, as of 22 women who used Vaniqua®, 4 had a spontaneous abortion and a 35-yr-old woman had a baby with Down's syndrome [6]. Breast-feeding is discouraged, as it is not known if eflornithine is excreted in human milk [6].

Spironolactone (an aldosterone-antagonist diuretic provided of androgen-receptor competing activity as well as inhibition of 5-α-reductase activity) will be dealt with in more detail below. Spironolactone is used for the topical treatment of acne and hirsutism in the form of either 2% or 5% cream [7]. The inhibition of binding of dihydrotestosterone (DHT) to nuclear androgen receptors contained in human sebaceous gland was shown in a skin biopsy-based study conducted on six men with acne *vulgaris* who were treated with a 5% spironolactone cream twice a day for 1 month [8]. In Italy, both the 2% and 5% cream (Spiroderm®, Searle) were retired from the market once these creams were introduced in the list of the doping substances with a decree of the Ministry of Health in February 2006. One 30-g tube costed about euro 15.

19.1.3 Epilation

Epilation removes the part of the hair above the skin and that below the skin, thus giving more long-lasting results (weeks).

Mechanical means – Epilation can be done by plucking the hair shaft from the follicle with tweezers, by waking, electrolysis, photoepilation (also called phototricholysis, using laser or intense pulse light). When plucking, care must be taken to avoid folliculitis, pigmentation, and scarring [9]. With waxing (or "sugaring", if a sugar solution is used in lieu of melted wax to embed the hairs), groups of hairs are removed at one time. The treated area is covered with a linen strip which is quickly stripped off once the wax has cooled and hardened. Stripping occurs in the opposite direction of hair growth, while heated wax had been applied in the same direction of hair growth. In addition to hairs, also the wax-embedded (or sugar-embedded) dead skin is removed. Waxes are beeswax, paraffin, or oils, and are combined with a resin for permitting adherence to the skin. Both hot waxes and cold waxes are available. Wax should not be applied onto areas such eyelash, ears, genitals, and above varicose veins or warts. Tweezers epilators for personal use at home grasp the hair close to the skin, and applied current travels down the hair shaft to the root.

Electrical means – Electrolysis destroys the hair follicles by delivering electricity to a single hair root at a time, though the multiple-needle galvanic method permits a dozen hairs to be treated simultaneously. Electricity is delivered through a probe (a very fine wire) causing caustication by an electrochemical process (galvanic method), causing overheating (thermolysis method, also known as diathermy or electrocoagulation), or causing both (blend method). The blend method combines the high efficiency of the galvanic method (that is, destruction of about three-fourths of the treated hairs as opposed to about one-tenth of thermolysis) with the rapidity of thermolysis. Electrolysis is the only method for which FDA allows the claim "*permanent hair removal*" [10]. In contrast, FDA declared that laser and similar devices can only claim to reduce hair growth, not permanently remove it [10]. The major risks of electrolysis are electrical shock, which can occur if the needle is not properly insulated, infections (including those from poorly sterilized needles), and scarring.

The negative side of electrolysis and phototricholysis (see below) is cost and the limited amount of area that can be treated at a time (so-called *investment of time and money*). For best results, each hair is treated during its active growing stage. Because it is not possible to remove the hair permanently in one treatment, additional treatments (sessions) are necessary. The average cost for an-hour electrolysis session is generally between $100 and $200. The average cost of a complete treatment of large areas, like chest, back, and legs can approximate $5000, requiring one to 2 years or treatment.

Light-based means – Phototricholysis (also known as photoepilation) burns the hair follicle using controlled flashes of light. The two forms of photoepilation are laser hair removal and intense pulse light (IPL) hair removal.

The hair can be burnt because it contains the natural cromophore melanin, the dark pigment of the skin that absorbs light. To destroy the hair root, but prevent the skin from absorbing the energy from the machine's light, this light has to be of the same color (wavelength) of the hair. Laser has different wavelengths depending on the lasing medium used: 694 nm (red) for ruby laser, 755 nm (infrared) for alexandrite laser, 810 nm for pulsed diode array laser, and 1064 nm for Nd:YAG (neodymium-doped yttrium aluminum garnet) laser. Nd:YAG is a crystal that is used as a lasing medium for solid-state lasers. In addition to dermatology (hirsutism, spider veins), Nd:YAG lasers are used in ophthalmology (diabetic retinopathy, posterior cataract), dentistry (gingivectomy and other oral surgery), etc. Lasers work best with dark coarse hair in persons with light skin, however new lasers are now able to target dark black hair even in patients with dark skin. With either laser or IPL method, the treated skin has to be cooled, most often with a gel. The aim of the cooling skin gel is to make the darkly pigmented hair follicles heat up so they become destroyed, but skin beyond the hair follicles should not be affected.

In February 2000, the American FDA approved IPL as a valid technology for permanent hair reduction and for treatment in black persons. In contrast to the fixed wavelength of lasers light, IPL covers a range from 500 to 1200 nm and is emitted by a xenon flash lamp at pulses of a few milliseconds duration; longer wavelengths infiltrate deeper into the skin. IPL, which is converted to heat energy burning the hair shaft once the chromophore melanin has absorbed the light itself, is filtered to remove ultraviolet wavelengths that could damage the skin. Because wavelength can be changed over the said spectrum, IPL epilation allows treatment to be adapted (in intensity or the way the light pulses) individually to the type of skin and hair follicles to be removed in each individual.

The following information is taken from The Center for Devices and Radiological Health of the Food and Drug Administration (FDA) [10]. The popularity of laser hair removal has increasingly grown, prompting many laser manufacturers to conduct research and seek FDA clearance for their lasers for this indication. The market is growing so quickly that FDA cannot maintain an up-to-date list of all laser manufacturers whose devices have been cleared for hair removal, as this list continues to change. To learn if a specific manufacturer has received FDA clearance, one can check FDA's Website at http://www.fda.gov/cdrh/databases.html. Manufacturers should be aware that receiving an FDA clearance for general permission to market their devices does not permit them to advertise the lasers for either hair removal or wrinkle treatment, even though hair removal or wrinkle treatment may be a by-product of any cleared laser procedure. Furthermore, manufacturers may not claim that laser hair removal is either painless or permanent unless the FDA determines that there are sufficient data to demonstrate such results. Several manufacturers received FDA permission to claim, "*permanent reduction*," not "*permanent removal*" for their lasers. The specific claim granted is "*intended to effect stable, long-term, or permanent reduction*" through selective targeting of melanin in hair follicles. Permanent hair reduction is defined as the long-term, stable reduction in the number of hairs regrowing after a treatment regime, which may include several sessions. The number of hairs regrowing must be stable over time greater than the duration of the complete growth cycle of hair follicles, which varies from 4 to 12 months according to body location. Permanent hair reduction does not necessarily imply elimination of all hairs in the treatment area.

In a recent meta-analysis [11], a total of 9 randomized controlled (RCTs) and 21 controlled trials (CTs) were identified. The best available evidence was found for the alexandrite (three RCTs, eight CTs) and diode (three RCTs, four CTs) lasers, followed by the ruby (two RCTs, six CTs) and Nd:YAG (two RCTs, four CTs) lasers, whereas limited evidence was available for intense pulse light sources (one RCT, one CT). Based on the present best available evidence, it was concluded that (i) epilation with lasers and light sources induces a partial short-term hair reduction up to 6 months postoperatively, (ii) efficacy is improved when repeated treatments are given, (iii) efficacy is superior to conventional treatments (shaving, wax epilation, electrolysis), (iv) evidence exists for a partial long-term hair removal efficacy beyond 6 months postoperatively after repetitive treatments with alexandrite and diode lasers and probably after treatment with ruby and Nd:YAG lasers, whereas evidence is lacking for long-term hair removal after IPL. Another study concluded that diode laser is the most effective, and Nd:YAG has the least effect of hair removal [12]. Indeed, hair reduction at least 6 months after the last treatment and hair reductions were 57, 42, 55, and 53% after three sessions for diode, Nd:YAG, alexandrite, and ruby, respectively [12]. There is recent literature, essentially based on facial hirsutism, which shows a better quality of life after sessions of laser epilation [13–15].

It was very recently published a randomized, double-blind, placebo-controlled, right-left comparison study of alexandrite laser treatment combined with eflornithine cream versus laser alone for treating unwanted hair on the upper lip in women [16]. Laser treatments were performed every 4 weeks for up to 6 sessions. Each patient also applied either eflornithine or placebo cream twice daily to each side of the upper lip in a double-blinded manner. At the end of the 6 months of the study, complete or almost complete hair removal was achieved in 29 of 31 (93.5%) of the eflornithine-laser-treated sites versus 21 of 31 (67.9%) for the placebo cream-laser-treated sites.

19.2 Pharmacological Treatment

19.2.1 Inhibition of Ovarian Steroidogenesis

A short reminder on oral contraceptives – First-generation oral contraceptives contain $\geq$ 50 μg ethinyl estradiol. Second-generation oral contraceptives contain 30 or 35 μg ethinyl estradiol combined with levonorgestrel, norgestimate, or other progestins. Third-generation oral contraceptives contain 20 or 30 μg ethinyl estradiol combined with desogestrel or gestodene; a combined oral contraceptive (COC) containing $\leq$20 ethinyl estradiol in combination with a progestinic is referred to as an ultra low-dose pill. COCs are categorized as monophasic, biphasic, and triphasic. In monophasic pills, each pill of the pack contains the same amount of estrogen and progestin. In biphasic and triphasic pills, the amounts of the estrogenic component and progestin component in not fixed as in the monophasic type but variable, depending on the phase of the menstrual cycle; the change can interest either or both components. In biphasic pills, the first 7–10 pills have one composition while the next 11–14 pills have another composition (more progestin). In triphasic pills, the composition of the 7 pills taken at week one is different from that of the 7 pills taken at week two which, in turn, have a composition different from the 7 pills taken at week three (increase of estrogen at mid-cycle, and progressive increase of progestin). Regardless of the phasic type, the 7 pills of a 28-tab pack contain placebo. An exhaustive discussion of COCs, including side effects, is beyond the scope of this chapter.

Because of the metabolic aspects of PCOS, it is appropriate to remind, as appropriately underscored in a recent paper [17], that the increased insulin resistance given by oral contraceptives in both PCOS or non-PCOS populations is an inconsistent finding, with more adequate studies needed. In general, insulin resistance is related to the estrogen dose.

Use of COCs in hirsutism – The simplest method to inhibit ovarian steroidogenesis, which is LH dependent, is suppression of LH secretion using COCs.

Further to LH suppression given by the progestin component of COCs, the estrogen component increases the circulating levels of sex-hormone binding globulin (SHBG). SHBG levels are frequently low or low-normal in PCOS patients due to hyperinsulinemia. An increase in SHBG results in reduction of freely circulating testosterone and other androgens; consequently, less androgens will be available for action on the hairs and sebaceous glands. The progestin component adds to this benefit on the hair because progestins inhibit skin 5α-reductase activity. The progestins 17-hydroxyprogesterone acetate (cyproterone), chlormadinone acetate (6-chloro-Δ6-dehydro-17α-acetoxyprogesterone), and dienogest (17α-cyanomethyl-17ß-hydroxy-estra-4, 9-dien-3-one) have the further advantage of competing with testosterone and dihydrotestosterone (DHT) for binding to the androgen receptor.

Most of the progestins derived from 19-nortestosterone (e.g., the second-generation progestin levonorgestrel), in addition to their progestational effects, have some androgenic activity; hence, they are not indicated in hirsute women. However, desogestrel (13-ethyl-17-ethynyl-11-methylidene-1, 2, 3, 6, 7, 8, 9, 10, 12, 13, 14, 15, 16, 17- tetradecahydrocyclopenta[a] phenanthren-17-ol), which is contained in third-generation oral contraceptives such as Gracial® or Mercilon® (Organon), has no androgenic activity. In February 2007, the consumer advocacy group Public Citizens petitioned the FDA to ban oral contraceptives containing desogestrel, citing studies that suggest a 2-fold greater risk of venous thrombosis in women who use third-generation oral contraceptives containing desogestrel compared to women using second-generation oral contraceptives [18].

An oral contraceptive (not available in the United States and Japan) containing cyproterone acetate is Diane® (also known as Diane-35®, Diane-35 Diario®, Dianette®, depending on country, by Schering; Co-cyprindiol, non-proprietary); each tablet contains 2 mg of cyproterone acetate and 35 μg of ethinyl estradiol. Depending on the commercial product, the package contains 21 or 28 tablets. In the first case, the woman takes the first of the 21 tablets on day one (by convention, the first day of menstruation), the second on day two and so on until finishing the package on day 21, and having 7 days of break (during which a withdrawal bleed occurs) before starting the cycle again. In the second case, the package contains seven placebo tablets that are to be taken, one per day, during the days 22 through 28. Obviously, because of the potent antiandrogen activity of cyproterone acetate, the combination of cyproterone acetate plus ethinyl estradiol cannot be taken for purely contraception purposes. Its correct use is for treatment of hirsutism and/or acne.

In one open-label, 4-month duration Turkish trial, 40 nonobese women with PCOS were randomized to treatment with either Diane® or Diane® plus metformin 500 mg, 3 times daily for 4 months [19]. The Ferriman–Gallwey score was similarly improved in both treatment groups (–13 and –14%, respectively). In a very recent open-label 24-week duration Spanish trial [20], 34 PCOS women were randomized to treatment the Diane-35 Diario® pill or metformin (850 mg twice daily). Diane-35 Diario® resulted in higher reductions in hirsutism score and serum androgen levels compared with metformin. Menstrual regularity was restored in all the patients treated with Diane-35 Diario® compared with only 50% of those receiving metformin. Plasma apolipoprotein A-I and HDL-phospholipid levels increased with Diane-35 Diario®, whereas metformin did not induce any change in the lipid profile. In contrast, insulin sensitivity increased with metformin but did not change with Diane-35 Diario®.

In Italy, the cost one 21-tablet pack is approximately euro 7. Cyproterone acetate (Androcur®, Schering) can be administered at higher dosages (see below, Antiandrogens).

Use of gonadotropin releasing hormone (GnRH) analogs in hirsutism – LH suppression with monthly injections of a long-acting GnRH analog (e.g., buserelin, Suprefact® Depot; triptorelin, Trelstar® Depot, leuprolide acetate, Lupron® Depot) represents an expensive option (for instance, in Italy one vial of Suprefact® Depot costs euro 323). This option is commonly reserved for severe forms of androgenization, which is usually due to hyperthecosis, that have not responded to other therapies. Because of the resulting hypogonadism, an add-back estrogen-progestin treatment (in practical terms, a COC) has to be associated to the GnRH analog. Practically, the benefit given by this expensive therapy is comparable to other modalities, as illustratively shown by a 6-month duration trial on 35 PCOS women [21]. These women were randomly assigned to three groups: a long-acting GnRH analog alone, a long-acting GnRH analog combined with COCs or combined with flutamide. The three groups showed the same therapeutic efficacy, including comparable final hirsutism score [21].

19.2.2 Antagonism on Androgen Receptors

Antiandrogens used include cyproterone acetate (both generic and proprietary, Androcur®), spironolactone (both generic and proprietary, Aldactone®), and flutamide (both generic and proprietary, Drogenil®, Eulexin®).

While at low doses (e.g., 2 mg), cyproterone acetate is administered daily for 21 days (see above, Diane® and similars); at doses $\geq$10 mg, it has to be administered according to the reverse sequential regimen. In the reverse sequential regimen, the ethinylestradiol tablet ($\leq$30 μg) is taken from day 1 through 21 (or day 5 through 25), while the cyproterone acetate tablet is taken only from day 1 through 10 (or day 5 through 15). Cyproterone acetate is in tablets of 50 or 100 mg. In Italy, a pack containing 25 tablets of 50 mg costs euro 24, while a pack containing 30 tab of 100 mg costs euro 51.

The effect of cyproterone acetate is substantially the same on hirsutism and/or acne regardless of whether given at low doses (for 21 days combined with ethinylestradiol) or at high doses (for the first 10 days combined with ethinylestradiol). In a classic 12-month trial on 48 hyperandrogenic women with acne, the therapeutic effect on acne given by 2 mg cyproterone acetate +35 μg ethinylestradiol (combination for 21 days) or 50 mg cyproterone acetate +25 μg ethinylestradiol (reverse sequential regimen) was comparable [22]. Of the 48 women, a group received flutamide (250 mg daily) and another group received finasteride (5 mg daily), the latter turning out to be the least effective of the four modalities tested [22].

Unlike cyproterone acetate and spironolactone, flutamide is a nonsteoroidal inhibitor of the androgen receptor and it does not alter the periodicity of menstrual cycle. Flutamide must be associated with an effective contraception means, such as COCs, to avoid pregnancy. Indeed, blocking of the androgen receptor in the urogenital sinus and urogenital tubercle of a male fetus may lead to pseudohermafroditism.

Based on a very recent meta-analysis [23], spironolactone or finasteride in combination with contraceptives, or flutamide with metformin, appear superior to monotherapy with contraceptives and metformin, respectively. *In general, two to six women need to receive antiandrogens for one to experience any detectable benefit* [23] (for more details see below, inhibition of 5α-reductase).

In regard to the hepatotoxicity of flutamide, a study on 190 hyperandrogenic girls and young women receiving so-called low or ultra-low doses of flutamide (250–62.5 mg/day) for an average of 19 months (range 3–54) showed no changes in circulating levels of alanine aminotransferase (ALT) and aspartate aminotransferase (AST) that were used as markers of hepatotoxicity [24]. This Spanish group has reported on treating PCOS teenage girls or young women with low-dose or ultralow-dose flutamide combined with insulino-sensitizers [25, 26]. In one trial [25], flutamide (125 mg/day) was combined with metformin (1275 mg/day); in the other trial [26], flutamide (62.5 mg/day) was combined with both metformin (850 mg/day) and low-dose pioglitazone (7.5 mg/day) plus a trandermal estroprogestagen.

19.3 Inhibition of 5α-Reductase

The potent antiandrogen with inhibiting activity on the type 2 isoform of 5α-reductase is finasteride (non-proprietary and proprietary, Proscar®, Propecia®). Flutamide, cyproterone acetate, spironolactone, desogestrel, and drosperinone exert lesser inhibition of 5α-reductase.

Finasteride, which in Italy is marketed in 5-mg tablets with a cost of euro 56 for 1 pack of 28 tablets, is given at a daily dose of 2.5–5.0 mg. In Italy, finasteride is registered only for the treatment of benign prostatic hyperplasia (BPH) and androgenic alopecia in men, while minoxidil is registered only for the treatment of androgenic alopecia in both men and women. Thus, writing finasteride or flutamide for treating hirsutism/acne is an off-label prescription. Finasteride is somewhat less effective than flutamide. Finasteride does not alter the periodicity of menstrual cycle. Finasteride or flutamide (see above) must be associated with an effective contraception means, such as COCs, to avoid pregnancy. Indeed, inhibition of 5-alpha reductase or blocking of the androgen receptor in the urogenital sinus and urogenital tubercle of a male fetus may lead to pseudohermafroditism.

In a 12-month duration, 4-arm Italian trial, 66 hirsute women were randomized to finasteride (5 mg/day), flutamide (250 mg/day), ketoconazole (300 mg/day), or cyproterone acetate (12.5 mg/day for the first 10 days of the menstrual cycle) plus ethynil-estradiol (for the first 21 days of the menstrual cycle) [27] Considering the hirsutism score, the hierarchy of effectiveness was cyproterone acetate + ethynilestradiol (60% decrease in Ferriman–Gallwey score), flutamide (55% decrease), ketoconazole (53% decrease), and finasteride (44% decrease); the difference between finasteride and either cyproterone acetate plus ethynilestradiol or flutamide was statistically significant. In this study, ketoconazole and, to a lesser degree, cyproterone acetate plus ethynilestradiol gave the greatest number of side effects, while finasteride gave none [27]. In a 6-month duration, 4-arm Italian study on 40 hirsute women who were assigned to 5 mg/day 250 mg/day finasteride, 100 mg/day spironolactone or placebo, each drug was superior to placebo and the three drugs were equivalent in effectiveness (Ferriman–Gallwey score, hair diameter, cosmetic use). However, in terms of Ferriman–Gallwey score, some hierarchy was apparent, with finasteride, flutamide, or spironolactone having decreased this score by 32%, 39%, or 41% (reduction given by placebo = 5%) [28]. In a 12-month duration, 2-arm Turkish study that compared 70 hirsute patients assigned to either 5 mg/day finasteride or 250 mg/day flutamide, the latter was more effective [29].

The results of a very recent meta-analysis commissioned by The Endocrine Society Task Force on Hirsutism is now available [23]. Of 348 studies published through May, 2006, only 38 were potentially eligible for meta-analysis but only 12 (3 % !) satisfied the stringent criteria to be finally included in the systematic review; 26 of 38 (7% of 348) were not considered because no antiandrogen was under study in the trial. At one extreme, there were 5/12 studies evaluating antiandrogens vs. placebo, and at the other extreme there was a single study evaluating antiandrogens vs. oral contraceptives. Eligible randomized clinical trials had a treatment of at least 6-month duration, and measured hirsutism by patient's self-assessment, clinician assessment, or laboratory assessment of hair (hair diameter, hair length, or rate of hair growth). Outcomes collected were at the longest point of complete follow-up while women were still under interventions. The eligible trials assessed four antiandrogens (50–100 mg spironolactone, 100 mg cyproterone acetate, 250–500 mg flutamide, and 5.0–7.5 mg finasteride per day). Metformin (1000–1700 mg per day) was the only insulin sensitizer that these trials evaluated. Oral contraceptives contained either 35 μg ethinyl estradiol with 2 mg cyproterone acetate or 30 μg ethinyl estradiol with 150 μg desogestrel. Durations of treatments ranged 6–12 months. The overall quality of evidence across all comparisons was judged *low to very low*. The principal findings were that "... *antiandrogens are effective agents for the treatment of hirsutism. [...] antiandrogens are superior to placebo and metformin, and when spironolactone or finasteride are combined with OCPs, or when flutamide is combined with metformin, these regimens are superior to monotherapy with OCPs and metformin, respectively*". Basically, these conclusions [23] are consistent with those of two other systematic reviews [30, 31], and conclusions do not change upon taking into account three trials published when this meta-analysis was completed [17, 32, 33].

In the Italian study [32], 76 of the 80 enrolled overweight-obese PCOS women completed the randomized, placebo-controlled 4-arm trial. The trial consisted in placing the women (BMI > 28 Kg/m^2) on an hypocaloric diet for the first month and then on a hypocaloric diet plus placebo, metformin (850 mg, orally, twice a day), flutamide (250 mg, orally, twice a day), or metformin plus flutamide for the subsequent 12 months (20 subjects in each group). After 12 months, flutamide maintained the significant effects observed after 6 months on visceral/sc fat mass and androstenedione , whereas it produced an additional significant decrease in dehydroepiandrosterone sulfate and hirsutism score; metformin further and significantly improved the menstrual pattern. Concerning reduction of hirsutism score, after 12 months it was 14% (diet + placebo), 20% (diet + metformin), 61% (diet + flutamide), and 55% (diet + metformin + flutamide); in these four groups, the corresponding reduction in body weight after 12 months was 5.2%, 4.3%, 10.7%, and 11.2%. Moreover, after 12 months, flutamide improved significantly more than placebo the menstrual pattern, glucose-stimulated glucose level, insulin sensitivity, and low-density lipoprotein cholesterol levels, whereas metformin decreased significantly glucose-stimulated insulin levels. The combination of the two drugs maintained the specific effect of each of the compounds, without any additive or synergistic effect. The Spanish 12-month trial [33] evaluated efficacy and tolerability of three doses of flutamide (125, 250, and 375 mg) combined with a triphasic oral contraceptive (ethynylestradiol/levonorgestrel) for treating moderate to severe hirsutism in patients with (PCOS) or idiopathic hirsutism. Based on the intention-to-treat analysis of a total of 119 patients, all flutamide doses induced a significant decrease in hirsutism, acne, and seborrhea scores after 12 months compared with placebo without differences among dose levels. Similar related side effects were observed with placebo and 125 mg flutamide (12.5%), and slightly higher with 250 mg (17.3%) and 375 mg (21.2%). In the Australian open-label, 6-month study [17], 110 overweight PCOS women (MI > 27 Kg/m^2) were randomized to a control group (higher-dose oral contraceptive 35 μg ethinylestradio [EE] 1/2 mg cyproterone acetate, metformin (1 g twice a day) or low-dose oral contraceptive [20 μg [EE]/100 microg levonorgestrel + aldactone 50 mg twice a day]). In the 100/110 women who completed the study, all treatments similarly and significantly improved symptoms including hirsutism and menstrual cycle length. In regard to decrease in hirsutism score, it was 31% (both metformin group and high-dose contraceptive group), and 33% (low-dose oral contraceptive plus aldactone). Insulin resistance was improved by metformin and worsened by the high-dose oral contraceptive. Arterial stiffness worsened in the higher-dose oral contraceptive group, related primarily to the increased insulin resistance.

The Swiglo et al. meta-analysis [23] underlines the *extremely poor reporting of side effects in these trials*. Under the heading unanswered question, the meta-analysis underlines that "*needed are trials comparing antiandrogens with biological modifiers of hair growth (e.g., eflornithine) and with mechanical modifiers (e.g., shaving, depilation, electrolysis, and laser epilation)*".

Because PCOS is a heterogeneous syndrome, it is not surprising that therapy is multimodal. In circumstances like this, typically the physician takes into account and discusses with the patient her particular needs. In the case of PCOS, these needs include esthetics (acne and/or hirsutism), menstrual irregularities, anovulation and related infertility or contraception when fertility is not desired. Needs can change over time in the same patient.

The wide armamentariun consists of mechanical and medical means, the former to be used as complementary to the latter. Importantly, both the patient and the physician should not forget the so-called first-line therapy, that is change in lifestyle.

References

1. Kiddy DS, Hamilton-Fairley D, et al. Improvement in endocrine and ovarian function during dietary treatment of obese women with polycystic ovary syndrome. Clin Endocrinol (Oxf) 1992; 36:105–11
2. Koulouri O, Conway GS. A systematic review of commonly used medical treatments for hirsutism in women. Clin Endocrinol (Oxf). 2008 Feb 14 [Epub ahead of print]
3. Thessaloniki ESHRE/ASRM-Sponsored PCOS Consensus Workshop Group. Consensus on infertility treatment related to polycystic ovary syndrome. Hum Reprod 2008; 23: 462–77
4. Sonino N, Fava GA, Mani E et al. Quality of life of irsute women. Postgrad Med J 1993; 69:186–189
5. Shapiro J, Lui H. Vaniqa – eflornithine 13.9% cream. Skin Therapy Lett 2001; 6:1–3
6. http://emc.medicines.org.uk/emc/assets/c/html/DisplayDoc.asp?DocumentID=14852 (accessed March 04, 2008)
7. Califano L, Cannavò S, Siragusa M, et al. Experience in the therapy of acne with topical administration of spironolactone as an antiandrogen. Clin Ter 1990; 15;135:193–99
8. Berardesca E, Gabba P, Ucci G, et al. Topical spironolactone inhibits dihydrotestosterone receptors in human sebaceous glands: an autoradiographic study in subjects with acne vulgaris. Int J Tissue React 1988; 10:115–19.
9. Richards RN, Uy M, Meharg G. Temporary hair removal in patients with hirsutism: a clinical study. Cutis 1990; 45: 199–202.
10. (http://www.fda.gov/cdrh/consumer/laserfacts.html updated February 28, 2008) (accessed, March 04, 2008)
11. Haedersdal M, Wulf HC. Evidence-based review of hair removal using lasers and light sources. J Eur Acad Dermatol Venereol 2006; 20: 9–20
12. Sadighha A, Mohaghegh Zahed G. Meta-analysis of hair removal laser trials. Lasers Med Sci 2007 Nov 20 [Epub ahead of print]
13. Loo WJ, Lanigan SW. Laser treatment improves quality of life of hirsute females. Clin Exp Dermatol 2002; 27 :439–41
14. Clayton WJ, Lipton M, Elford J, et al. A randomized controlled trial of laser treatment among hirsute women with polycystic ovary syndrome. Br J Dermatol 2005; 152: 986–92
15. Conroy FJ, Venus M, Monk B. A qualitative study to assess the effectiveness of laser epilation using a qualify-of-life scoring system. Clin Exp Dermatol 2006; 31:753–56
16. Hamzavi I, Tan E, Shapiro J, et al. A randomized bilateral vehicle-controlled study of eflornithine cream combined with laser treatment versus laser treatment alone for facial hirsutism in women. J Am Acad Dermatol 2007; 57:54–9.
17. Meyer C, McGrath BP, Teede HJ. Effects of medical therapy on insulin resistance and the cardiovascular system in polycystic ovary syndrome. Diabetes Care 2007; 30: 471–78
18. http://www.notmypill.org/ (accessed March 04, 2008)
19. Elter K, Imir G, Durmusoglu F. Clinical endocrine and metabolic effects of metformin added to ethinyl estradiol-cyproterone acetate in non-obese women with polycystic ovary syndrome: a randomized controlled study. Human Reprod 2002; 17: 1729–37
20. Luque-Ramírez M, Alvarez-Blasco F, Botella-Carretero JI, et al. Comparison of ethinyl-estradiol plus cyproterone acetate versus metformin effects on classic metabolic cardiovascular risk factors in women with the polycystic ovary syndrome. J Clin Endocrinol Metab 2007; 92:2453–61
21. De Leo V, Fulghesu AM, La Marca A et al. Hormonal and clinical effects of GnRH agonist alone, or in combination with a combined oral contraceptive or flutamide in women with severe hirsutism. Gynecol Endocrinol. 2000; 14:411–16
22. Carmina E, Lobo RA. A comparison of the relative efficacy of antiandrogens for the treatment of acne in hyperandrogenic women. Clin Endocrinol (Oxf) 2002; 57:231–34.
23. Swiglo BA, Cosma M, Flynn DN, et al. Clinical review: Antiandrogens for the treatment of hirsutism: a systematic review and metaanalyses of randomized controlled trials. J Clin Endocrinol Metab. 2008 Apr;93(4):1153–60. Epub 2008 Feb 5.
24. Ibáñez L, Jaramillo A, Ferrer A, et al. Absence of hepatotoxicity after long-term, low-dose flutamide in hyperandrogenic girls and young women. Hum Reprod 2005; 20:1833–36.
25. Ibáñez L, Ong K, Ferrer A, et al. Low-dose flutamide-metformin therapy reverses insulin resistance and reduces fat mass in nonobese adolescents with ovarian hyperandrogenism. J Clin Endocrinol Metab 2003; 88:2600–06.
26. Ibáñez L, López-Bermejo A, del Rio L, et al. Combined low-dose pioglitazone, flutamide, and metformin for women with androgen excess. J Clin Endocrinol Metab 2007; 92:1710–14.
27. Venturoli S, Marescalchi O, Colombo FM, et al. A prospective randomized trial comparing low dose flutamide, finasteride, ketoconazole, and cyproterone acetate-estrogen regimens in the treatment of hirsutism J Clin Endocrinol Metab 1999; 84: 1304–10

28. Moghetti P, Tosi F, Tosti A, et al. Comparison of spironolactone, flutamide, and finasteride efficacy in the treatment of hirsutism: a randomized, double blind, placebo-controlled trial. J Clin Endocrinol Metab 2000; 85:89–94
29. Müderris II, Bayram F, Güven M. prospective, randomized trial comparing flutamide (250 mg/d) and finasteride (5 mg/d) in the treatment of hirsutism. Fertil Steril 2000; 73:984–87
30. Farquhar C, Lee O Toomath R, et al. Spironolactone versus placebo or in combination with steroids for hirsutism and/or acne Cochrane database Syst Rev 2003; 4:CD000194
31. Van der Spuy ZM, le Roux PA. Cyproterone acetate for hirsutism. Cochrane database Syst Rev 2003; 4:CD001125
32. Gambineri A, Patton L, Vaccina A, et al. Treatment with flutamide, metformin, and their combination added to a hypocaloric diet in overweight-obese women with polycystic ovary syndrome: a randomized, 12-month, placebo-controlled study J Clin Endocrinol 2006; 91:3970–80
33. Calaf J, Lopez E, Millet A, et al. Long-term efficacy and tolerability of flutamide combined with oral contraception in moderate to severe hirsutism: a 12-month, double-blind, parallel clinical trial. J Clin Endocrinol Metab 2007; 92:3446–52

Chapter 20
Ovulation Induction in PCOS

Evert J.P. van Santbrink

20.1 Introduction

In the general population, ovarian dysfunction is the most common reason of fertility problems. About 20% of couples consulting a fertility clinic present with oligo- or amenorrea [1,2]. Occasionally, ovulatory cycles may be observed in oligomenorreic women, but the frequency of ovulations appears to decrease as cycle length progresses. Unfortunately, well-designed longitudinal follow-up studies regarding this issue are lacking.

Classification of anovulation is performed usually with World Health Organisation (WHO) criteria [3] using anamnestic determination of oligomenorrea (menstrual cycle >35 days) or amenorrea (menstrual cycle > 6 months) in combination with serum concentrations of prolactin, follicle stimulating hormone (FSH) and estradiol (E_2). In case of a hyperprolactinemia, a macro-prolactinoma should be ruled out by a scan (CT or MRI) of the sella turcica, and hyperprolactinemia should be treated with a dopamine agonist. In case the oligo- or amenorrea persists after this intervention, these patients may be classified as follows: 1) ± 15% hypo-gonadotropic, hypo-estrogenic status (WHO_1), 2) ± 80% normo-gonadotropic, normo-estrogenic status (WHO_2) or 3) ± 5% hyper-gonadotropic, hypo-estrogenic status (WHO_3). The vast majority of these patients, the WHO_2 group, appears to be a very heterogeneous population in which – besides anovulation – obesity, biochemical or clinical hyperandrogenism (alopecia, acne or hirsutism) and insulin resistance play an important role. A large subgroup of the WHO_2 population fulfil the criteria for polycystic ovary syndrome (PCOS). The prevalence of PCOS depends on the criteria used (Fig. 20.1) [4]. The syndrome was formerly known as the Stein–Leventhal syndrome [5] and more recently, criteria of the National Institute of Health [6] were replaced by criteria of the Rotterdam consensus meeting on PCOS [7,8]. According to the latest consensus meeting, after exclusion of related disorders (Cushing's syndrome, CAH and hyperprolacinemia), PCOS is defined as having 2 out of 3 of the following disorders: (1) oligo- or anovulation, (2) clinical and/or biochemical signs of hyperandrogenemia, (3) polycystic ovaries on ultrasound. It has to be noticed that the Rotterdam criteria, rather than replacing the NIH criteria, just broadened the definition of PCOS. Now, patients with hyperandrogenemia and polycystic ovaries without ovulation disorders and patients with polycystic ovaries and ovulation disorders without hyperandrogenism are also included [9]. The primary goal of the WHO classification of anovulation was to provide a clinical useful tool for treatment of this important patient group. In recent years, there has been growing evidence supporting the importance of patient characteristics determining treatment outcome, rather than the medication dose regimen applied. As a result, a more relevant classification system would be based on specific organ dysfunction, enabling a more patient tailored treatment algorithm and also able to identify short- and long-term health risks [10]. The next step would be to replace individual phenotypical patient characteristics with specific genotypical characteristics to predict individual treatment response and outcome.

E.J.P. van Santbrink (✉)
Senior consultant in Reproductive Medicine, Division of Reproductive Medicine, Department of Obstetrics and Gynecology, Erasmus Medical Center, Rotterdam, The Netherlands
e-mail: e.vansantbrink@erasmusmc.nl

N.R. Farid, E. Diamanti-Kandarakis (eds.), *Diagnosis and Management of Polycystic Ovary Syndrome*,
DOI 10.1007/978-0-387-09718-3_20,

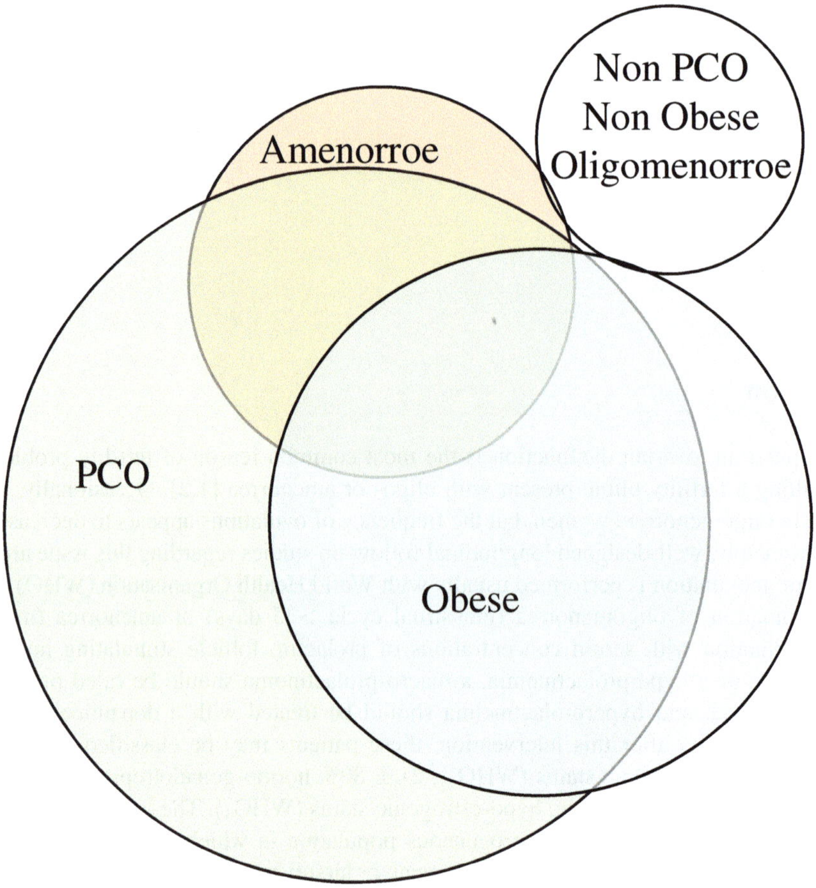

Fig. 20.1 Venn diagram showing distribution of initial patient characteristics (polycystic ovaries [pco] on ultrasound, amenorrea and obesity) in 240 normogonadotropic anovulatory fertility patients (WHO_2) before treatment (from van Santbrink, Fauser [10] by permission from Trends Endocrinol Metab)

20.2 Treatment of Anovulation

It should be well recognized that the treatment of chronic anovulation is aiming at restoration of the normal physiology and therefore the selection and growth of one single dominant follicle. This is the primary goal, in contrast with (mild) ovarian hyperstimulation used in intra-uterine insemination (IUI) or in vitro fertilisation (IVF).

From the beginning, treatment of chronic anovulation has been focussed on increasing the FSH serum concentration (increasing endogenous FSH production or exogenous FSH administration), but more recently also on improving the endocrine milieu and thereby improving ovarian responsiveness to FSH (weight reduction, insulin sensitizers, laparoscopic ovarian drilling). The traditional treatment sequence used in the majority ($\pm 80\%$) of patients presenting with chronic normogonadotropic normo-estrogenic anovulation (WHO_2) is the anti-oestrogen clomiphene citrate followed, in case of treatment failure, by gonadotropins (Fig. 20.2) [10]. Major complications of this effective sequential protocol are ovarian hyperstimulation and multiple pregnancies, as a result of the limited control of follicle growth [11]. In the patient group with hypogonadotropic hypo-estrogenic anovulation (WHO_1), treatment may consist of pulsatile GnRH administration or treatment with gonadotropins. Dependent on the underlying defect, administration of LH should be considered as well during the follicular as the luteal phase (luteal support), in this specific patient group. As far as the WHO_3 group (hypergonadotropic hypo-estrogenic anovulation) is concerned, this status represents ovarian failure and ovulation induction may

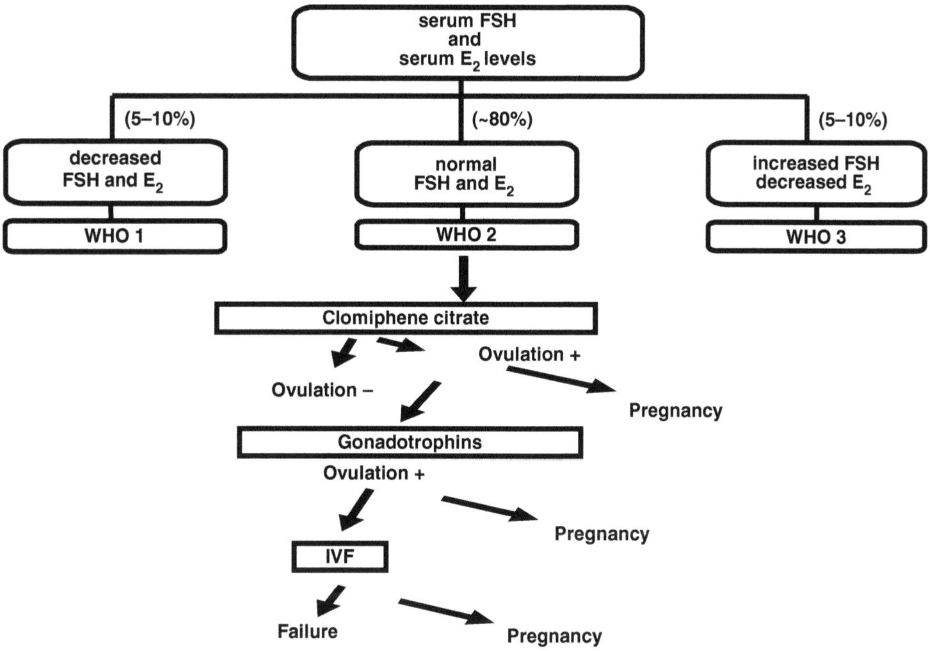

Fig. 20.2 Classification of anovulation according to the World Health Organisation (WHO) and conventional treatment algorithm of WHO class 2 anovulation: clomiphene citrate followed by gonadotropins and in vitro fertilisation (from van Santbrink and Fauser [10] by permission from Trends Endocrinol Metab)

not be considered a useful treatment option. For the remaining part of this chapter, we will restrict ourselves to the normo-gonadotropic, normo-estrogenic patient group (WHO_2) because this (sub)group encompasses the majority of anovulatory patients treated with ovulation induction (>80%).

20.3 Lifestyle Modification

Besides chronic anovulation, the WHO_2 patient group may be characterized by chemical (increased serum concentrations of testosterone and androstenedion) or/and clinical (hirsutism, acne and alopecia) hyperandrogenism, insulin resistance and obesity (Fig. 20.1). In particular, central obesity is correlated with insulin resistance and hyperandrogenism [12,13] and nearly 50% of PCOS patients have a body mass index (BMI = length/weight^2) above 25 m/kg^2.

With the rapidly increasing prevalence of obesity in all industrialized countries, this may be considered as a major and growing problem. Obesity has not only been correlated with diminished chances for both natural and assisted conception [14,15], but also with increased rates of miscarriage [16], congenital abnormalities, gestational diabetes, pregnancy-induced hypertension, stillbirth and maternal mortality [17,18]. Apart from this, long-term health risks like type 2 diabetes and cardiovascular disease may be increased [15,19].

Modification of lifestyle and weight reduction has been reported to normalize the endocrine milieu and may result in improvement of insulin sensitivity and decreased androgen excess. Therefore, a limited but permanent weight reduction may not only lead to a return of regular spontaneous ovulation and pregnancy [20,21], but also improve quality of life regarding long-term health risks.

In literature it is proposed that all obese women (BMI>35 kg/m^2) seeking pregnancy should be denied any form of fertility treatment until limited (5–10%) weight reduction has been achieved. Non-hormonal contraception may be advised during the weight-loss period until the critical weight has been reached because pregnancy would be unfavourable during this period [22,23].

20.4 Surgical Intervention

Ovarian wedge resection by laparotomy was the treatment modality for polycystic ovaries in the early days [24], and this shifted when ovulation inducing drugs, i.e. clomiphene and urinary gonadotropins, became available for clinical use during the 1960s [25,26]. As treatment results of ovulation induction with these drugs did not further improve, alternative treatment modalities were introduced. In the 1990s, this included a modern re-introduction of the wedge-resection: laparoscopic ovarian drilling of the ovarian surface (LOD). This is accomplished either by electrocautery or by laser treatment of the ovarian surface [27]. By drilling small holes in the ovarian cortex, the circulating serum androgen concentration is lowered; and this may result in restoration of ovulation. Although the technique is theoretically not fully understood, it may be rather effective [28]. Recently, unilateral drilling has been demonstrated to be as successful as bilateral drilling but less time consuming [29]. In clomiphene resistant PCOS patient's cumulative pregnancy rate, live birth rate and abortion rate with LOD are comparable with gonadotropin therapy, but multiple pregnancy rate was significantly decreased. Potential drawbacks regarding LOD are risks of laparoscopic surgery and general anaesthesia, formation of periadnexal adhesions [30] and potential accelerated decline of ovarian reserve [31].

20.5 Induction of Ovulation

20.5.1 Anti-estrogens (Clomiphene Citrate)

The anti-oestrogen clomiphene citrate (CC) has been the first-line treatment (Fig. 20.2) of normogonadotropic anovulation since the early 1960s [26]. It is a non-selective oestrogen receptor antagonist and interferes with the endogenous oestrogen feedback on the pituitary and hypothalamic level. This interference results in increased release of gonadotropins by the pituitary gland and hence increased ovarian stimulation. As an alternative anti-oestrogen to CC, tamoxifen can be used for ovulation induction and has been reported to result in similar pregnancy rates (22% with tamoxifen versus 15% with clomifene citrate; RR 1.45, 95% CI 0.58 to 3.63) and ovulation rates (44% with tamoxifen versus 45% with clomifene citrate) in normogonadotropic anovulation [32]. Clomiphene therapy is generally started on day 3 after a spontaneous or progestagen-induced withdrawal bleeding. It is continued for 5 days at a daily dosage of 50 mg. In case of anovulation, the daily dosage can be raised in two steps to a maximum of 150 mg in subsequent cycles. Further daily dose increase (above 150 mg/day) will not result in substantial additional ovulatory cycles and subsequent pregnancies [33]. The effect of the chosen starting day of CC is reported to influence ovulation and pregnancy rates: treatment initiation on day 1 was reported to be superior to day 5 [34]. In about 80% of CC-treated patients, menstrual cycle pattern and ovulation will be restored, and this may result in a 40% cumulative live birth rate [35]. Most pregnancies will occur within the first 6 ovulatory treatment cycles, and after 12 cycles additional pregnancies are unlikely to occur [36]. Multiple pregnancies and severe ovarian hyperstimulation are rare complications [35].

In a large cohort study ($n = 240$), initial patient characteristics predicting for CC-response failure (anovulation) are hyperandrogenemia, obesity, increased ovarian volume on ultrasound and amenorrea. These characteristics were combined in a nomogram (Fig. 20.3) predicting individual live birth chance after CC treatment in normogonadotropic anovulation [37].

20.5.2 Follicle Stimulating Hormone (FSH)

After CC treatment has failed, patients remaining anovulatory on the highest CC dose (CC-resistant) or failing to conceive although ovulatory on CC (CC-failure), are traditionally treated with exogenous FSH. Obviously, biological feedback mechanisms are surpassed, and this may contribute, next to the long FSH half-life (both for urinary and recombinant FSH about 40–44 hours), to the limited control of follicle growth using this treatment strategy. As a result, the variation in the daily FSH dose needed to induce dominant follicle selection and ongo-

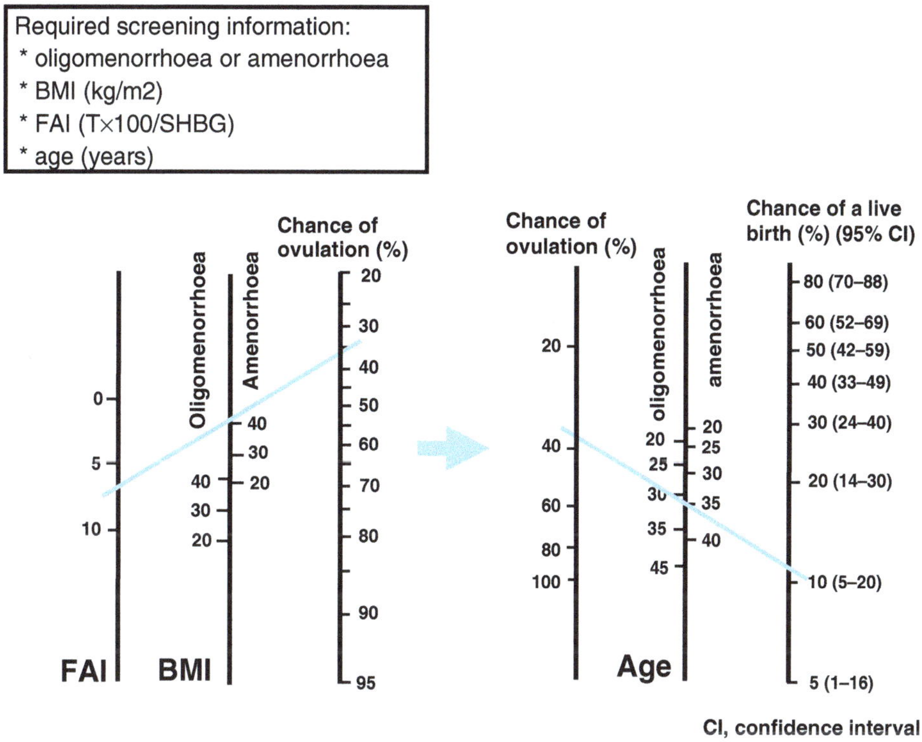

Fig. 20.3 A nomogram predicting chances for ovulation and live birth after CC treatment based on initial screening parameters. Sloping lines are examples how to use this nomogram: a patient with an FAI of 7, amenorrhea and BMI of 40 kg/m^2 has a chance of ovulation during CC treatment of 36%. This patient, age 35 years has an 11% chance of live birth during CC treatment (from Imani, Eijkemans, te Velde [37] by permission of The Endocrine Society)

ing growth (the 'FSH-response dose') may be considered the major complicating factor. The lack of possible anticipation may cause inadequate stimulation and results in multiple follicle growth, ovarian hyperstimulation and multiple pregnancies [38].

Over the years, attempts to improve treatment outcome and decrease complication chances included different FSH preparations (urinary, highly purified, recombinant and filled by mass) and different dose regimens (step-up, low-dose step-up and low-dose step-down). From the 1960s onwards, FSH was extracted from urine of postmenopausal women. In the 1990s recombinant DNA technology made it possible to produce recombinant human FSH in Chinese hamster ovary cells. This improved batch-to-batch variability and purity of the contents. Nevertheless, treatment results with urinary and recombinant FSH may be considered comparable [39]. Mainly two different treatment approaches using exogenous FSH have been developed, the 'step-up' and 'step-down' approach. The step-up protocol starts with an initial low daily FSH dose (37.5–50 IU), and this is increased by small steps (37.5–50 IU) at intervals of 7–14 days until ongoing follicle growth (the FSH response dose) has been reached. From that moment on, the daily dose is unchanged until ovulation can be triggered [40]. The step-down protocol is aiming at a starting dose equal to the FSH threshold. This may result in immediate ongoing follicle growth while the daily FSH dose can be decreased every 3 days by small amounts (37.5–50 IU) until a single pre-ovulatory follicle is present and ovulation can be triggered [41]. To determine the FSH response dose, a single 'dose-finding' step-up cycle is proposed, which may be followed by step-down cycles [10]. Although the step-down protocol may result in a more physiologic serum FSH profile and in general requires a shorter treatment period, it appears that for a substantial number of patients (30%) the starting dose of the step-up protocol equals the response dose. In those patients, a fixed dose regimen is more appropriate. It may be concluded that patients with a low FSH-threshold (i.e. the easy responders) are more suited for a step-up (or fixed-dose) protocol, while for patients with a high FSH-threshold (poor responders) a step-down approach may be more appropriate. In both protocols, frequent ultrasound monitoring of ovarian response is required to prevent multiple follicle development. When a pre-ovulatory follicle (>16 mm diameter) is present, human chorionic gonadotropin (hCG) is administered to induce ovulation and the couple is advised to have intercourse. Stimulation may be cancelled when more than 3 follicles >12 mm are present, and barrier contraceptives are recommended to prevent pregnancy.

Ovulation induction with FSH in normogonadotropic anovulation may result in 82% cumulative ovulation rate, 58% ongoing pregnancy rate and 43% single live birth rate [42]. Although complication rates are reported to be low (overall multiple pregnancy rates between 5 and 10%), a substantial part of all higher order multiple pregnancies origin from FSH ovulation induction. This may be due to the limited control of ovarian stimulation. (Fig. 20.4) [43]. The overall results of ovulation induction (CC followed by exogenous FSH, in case of treatment failure) may be considered rather effective. A prospectively followed cohort of 240 normogonadotropic anovulatory patients (WHO_2) resulted in an overall singleton live birth rate of 71% after 24 months follow-up [44].

Patient characteristics predicting for low response in FSH ovulation induction are more severe PCOS criteria such as obesity, hyperandrogenism and polycystic ovaries [42]. Also no difference was reported in FSH ovulation induction treatment outcome between patients after CC-failure and after CRA.

20.5.3 Insulin-Sensitizing Drugs (Metformin)

Insulin resistance and hyperinsulinemia are key symptoms in chronic anovulation (PCOS consensus). Ovarian androgen and E_2 synthesis may be stimulated by hyperinsulinemia, while androgen binding protein (SHBG) production in the liver is inhibited [45,46]. This will change the ovarian response on FSH stimulation not only

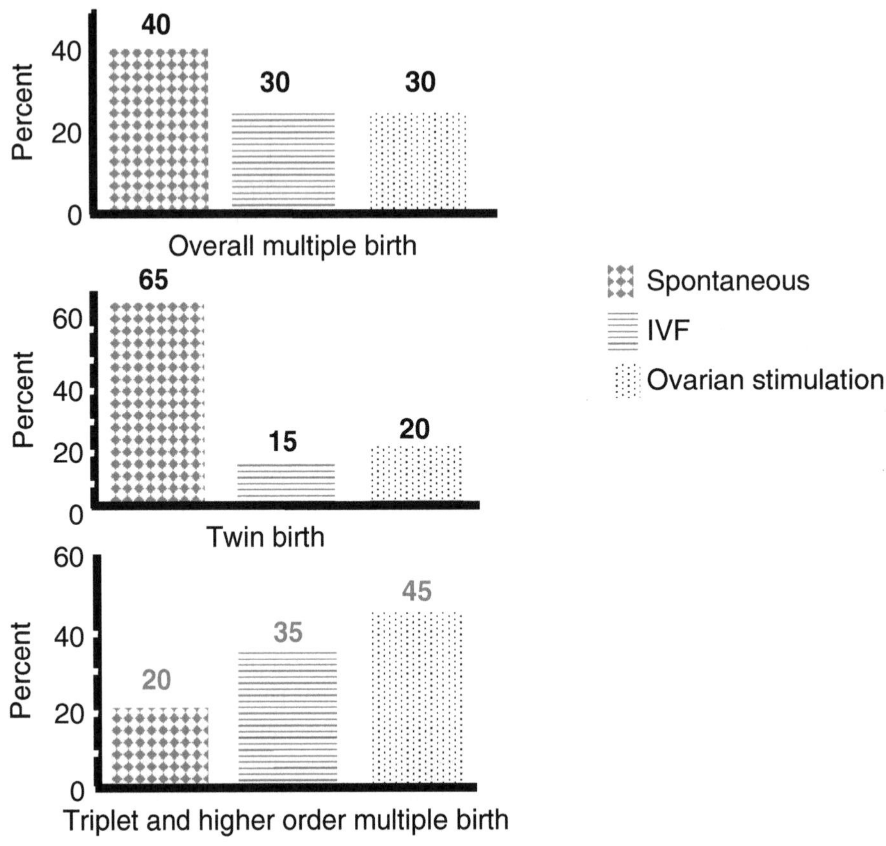

Fig. 20.4 Estimation of contribution of ovarian stimulation, in vitro fertilisation and spontaneous pregnancies to western world multiple pregnancies: Overall multiple birth (*upper panel*), twin birth (*middle panel*) and triplet or higher order pregnancies (*lower panel*)

by an increase of the fraction unbound androgens (and thereby hyperandrogenism), but also interfere with the FSH – E_2 feedback loop and may be responsible for the arrest in early antral follicle development (polycystic ovaries).

Insulin-sensitizing drugs, like the oral biguanide metformin, are reported to be capable of restoration of the endocrine milieu and may thus promote return of ovulation and regular menstrual cycles [47]. Within the group of obese patients with PCOS, about 10% may have undiagnosed diabetes and 35% impaired glucose intolerance [48]. The period of treatment needed to establish a substantial change in the endocrine milieu is still under debate, and randomized trials are lacking until now [49]. At first, systematic reviews of several small controlled trials suggested that metformin alone or combined with CC could achieve ovulation in normogonadotropic anovulation [50], although metformin resulted in less ovarian stimulation when directly compared to CC. In 2006, a large placebo controlled RCT [51] evaluated the effect of lifestyle modification and metformin in a group of morbid obese WHO_2 patients (mean BMI 38 kg/m^2). Patients who were able to accomplish weight reduction were equally divided to the placebo or metformin group, and this coincided with return of ovulation. From this study, it may be concluded that in severe obese patients metformin has no additional effect on return of ovulation but weight reduction does. Moreover, 2 other large multicentre RCTs concluded that metformin is significantly less effective than CC as first-line treatment and has little additional value when combined to CC in normogonadotropic anovulation [52,53]. Besides treatment results, metformin may cause serious side effects as nausea, vomiting and gastro-intestinal disturbances [50]. Another important issue concerning metformin may be that it is and will not be licensed for the indication ovulation induction. In conclusion, within the normogonadotropic anovulation group specific subgroups may be identified that will benefit the use of metformin alone or in combination with CC, but until now this is unclear. Therefore, application of metformin for this indication should be restricted [54].

20.5.4 Aromatase Inhibitors (Letrozole)

Although the main action of aromatase inhibitors and CC is equal – i.e. to reduce negative feedback of E_2 at the hypothalamus-pituitary level – their action is very different. While anti-estrogens are competitive oestrogen receptor modulators, aromatase inhibitors downregulate the conversion of androgens to estrogens in the granulose cells of the ovary. Both actions will result in increased FSH release in the pituitary and enhanced ovarian stimulation.

The application of aromatase inhibitors as ovulation induction agent instead of agent for advanced breast cancer has been introduced recently [55]. Important to notice is that aromatase inhibitors are not approved for the indication ovulation induction. Until now, a few small studies have been published suggesting superior, comparable or reduced ovarian stimulation to CC as first-line treatment modality in chronic anovulation [56–59]. A large prospective randomized trial should be undertaken to elucidate the value of aromatase inhibitors as first-line treatment in normogonadotropic ovulation induction.

There has also been discussion about the safety of aromatase inhibitors regarding the risk of congenital malformations. A relatively small study group treated with letrozole ($n = 150$) was compared to a large control group with spontaneous conceptions and suggested increased neonatal risk on bone and cardiac malformations in the former group [60]. This resulted in a warning of the pharmaceutical company not to use Letrozole for the indication ovulation induction. In reaction, two publications from the same research group followed, comparing neonatal outcome after CC and letrozole and concluded that there is no increased risk of congenital malformation after the application of aromatase inhibitors for ovulation induction [61,62]. Altogether, it may be concluded that there is insufficient evidence currently available to recommend the clinical use of aromatase inhibitors for routine ovulation induction.

20.6 Recommendations and Conclusions

- Patient characteristics rather than treatment protocols for ovulation induction may determine success and complication rates
- Most (80%) anovulatory patients can be classified as normogonadotropic normo-estrogenic (WHO_2)

- Patients with polycystic ovary syndrome (PCOS) are classified within the WHO_2 group
- Before treatment initiation, preconceptional counselling should be provided addressing potential life style modifications (i.e. overweight, smoking, alcohol consumption)
- Clomiphene citrate is the most effective first-line treatment in WHO_2 anovulation
- The traditional treatment sequence CC followed by FSH, in case failure to conceive, in WHO_2 anovulation is highly effective (cumulative single live birth rate of 71% after 2 years follow-up)
- Laparoscopic ovarian drilling (LOD) may be as effective as FSH second-line ovulation induction treatment in CC-resistant anovulation, both strategies have advantages and drawbacks.
- Use of metformin in ovulation induction should be restricted until beneficial patient groups can be identified
- There is insufficient evidence to apply aromatase inhibitors for ovulation induction
- More patient tailored approaches should be developed, based on initial patient characteristics, to improve treatment outcome and decrease complication rates

References

1. Hull MG. Epidemiology of infertility and polycystic ovarian disease: endocrinological and demographic studies. Gynaecol Endocrinol 1987; 235–245
2. Balen AH, Rutherford AJ. Managing anovulatory infertility and polycystic ovary syndrome. BMJ 2007. 335: 663–666
3. Rowe PJ, Combaire FH, Hargreave TB, et al. WHO manual for the standardized investigation and diagnosis of the infertile couple. Cambridge University Press, 2001
4. van Santbrink EJ, Hop WC, Fauser BC. Classification of nomogonadotrophic anovulatory infertility: Polycystic ovaries diagnosed by ultrasound versus endocrine characteristics of polycystic ovary syndrome. Fertil Steril 1997. 67: 453–458
5. Stein IF, Leventhal ML. Amenorrhea associated with bilateral polycystic ovaries. Am J Obstet Gynecol 1935. 29: 181–191
6. Zawadski JK, Dunaif A. Diagnostic criteria for polycystic ovary syndrome: towards a rational approach. In: Dunaif A, Givens JR, Haseltine F, eds. Polycystic Ovary Syndrome. Boston: Blackwell Scientific, 1992: 377–384
7. PCOS consensus. The Rotterdam ESHRE/ASRM-Sponsored PCOS consensus workshop group. Revised 2003 consensus on diagnostic criteria and long-term health risks related to polycystic ovary syndrome (PCOS). Hum Reprod 2004. 19: 41–47
8. PCOS consensus. The Rotterdam ESHRE/ASRM-Sponsored PCOS consensus workshop group. Revised 2003 consensus on diagnostic criteria and long-term health risks related to polycystic ovary syndrome (PCOS). Fertil Steril 2004. 81: 19–25
9. Azziz R. Diagnosis of polycystic ovarian syndrome: The Rotterdam criteria are premature. J Clin Endocrinol Metab 2007. 91: 781–785
10. van Santbrink EJ, Eijkemans MJ, Laven SJ, et al. Patient-tailored conventional ovulation induction algorithms in anovulatory infertility. Trends Endocrinol Metab 2005. 16: 381–389
11. Aboulghar MA, Mansour RT. Ovarian hyperstimulation syndrome: classifications and critical analysis of preventive measures. Hum Reprod Update 2003. 9: 275–289
12. Kiddy D, Sharp PS, White DM, et al. Differences in clinical and endocrine features between obese and non-obese subjects with PCOS: an analysis of 263 consecutive cases. Clin Endocrinol 1990; 213–220
13. Franks S, Kiddy D, Sharp P, et al. Obesity and polycystic ovary syndrome. Annals of the NY academy of Sciences 1991; 626:201–206
14. Rich-Edwards JW, Spiegelman D, Garland M, et al. Physical activity, body mass index, and ovulatory disorder infertility. Epidemiology 2002. 13: 184–190
15. Norman RJ, Davies MJ, Lord J, et al. The role of life-style modification in polycystic ovary syndrome. Trends Endocrinol Metab 2002. 13: 251–257
16. Wang JX, Davies MJ, Norman RJ. Obesity increases the risk of spontaneous abortion during infertility treatment. Obesity Research 2002. 10: 551–554
17. Dietl J. Maternal obesity and complications during pregnancy. J Perinat Med 2005. 33: 100–105
18. Boomsma CM, Fauser BC, Macklon NS. Pregnancy complications in women with PCOS. Semin Reprod Med 2008. 26: 72–84
19. Valkenburg O, Steegers-Theunissen RP, Smedts HP, et al. A more atherogenic serum lipoprotein profile is present in women with polycystic ovary syndrome: a case-control study. J Clin Endocrinol Metab 2007; epub ahead of print.
20. Clark AM, Thornley B, Tomlinson L, et al. Weight loss in obese infertile women results in improvement of reproductive outcome for all forms of fertility treatment. Hum Reprod 1998. 13: 1502–1505
21. Hoeger KM. Role of lifestyle modification in the management of polycystic ovary syndrome. Best Practice and research in Clin Endocrinol and Metab 2006. 20: 293–310
22. Balen AH, Dresner M, Scott EM, et al. Should obese women with polycystic ovary syndrome receive treatment for infertility? BMJ 2006. 332: 434–435
23. Nelson SM, Fleming RF. The preconceptual contraception paradigm: obesity and infertility. Hum Reprod 2007. 22: 912–915

24. Stein IF, Cohen MR, Elson R. Results of bilateral ovarian wedge resection in 47 cases of sterility; 20 year end results; 75 cases of bilateral polycystic ovaries. Am J Obstet Gynecol 1949. 58: 267–274
25. Mahesh VB and Greenblatt RB. Urinary steroid excretion patterns in hirsutism. II. Effect of ovarian stimulation with human pituitary FSH on urinary 17-ketosteroids. J Clin Endocrinol Metab 1964. 24: 1293–1302
26. Pildes RB. Induction of ovulation with clomiphene. Am J Obstet Gynecol 1965. 15: 466–479
27. Greenblatt EM, Casper RF. Laparoscopic ovarian drilling in women with polycystic ovarian syndrome. Prog Clin Biol Res 1993. 381: 129–138
28. Farquhar C, Lilford RJ, Marjoribanks J, et al. Laparoscopic 'drilling' by diathermy or laser for ovulation induction in anovulatory polycystic ovary syndrome. Cochrane Database Syst Rev 2007; 18: CD001122
29. Youssef H, Atallah MM. Unilateral ovarian drilling in polycystic ovarian syndrome: a prospective randomized study. Reprod Biomed Online 2007. 15: 457–462
30. Saleh AM, Khalil HS. Review of non-surgical and surgical treatment and the role of insulin-sensitizing agents in the management of infertile women with PCOS. Acta Obstet Gynecol Scand 2004. 83: 614–621
31. Seow KM, Juan CC, Hwang JL, et al. Laparoscopic surgery in polycystic ovary syndrome: reproductive and metabolic effects. Semin Reprod Med 2008. 26: 101–110
32. Boostanfar R. A prospective randomized trial comparing clomiphene citrate with tamoxifen citrate for ovulation induction. Fertil Steril 2001; 75:1024–1026
33. Imani B, Eijkemans MJ, te Velde ER, et al. Predictors of chances to conceive in ovulatory patients during clomiphene citrate induction of ovulation in normogonadotropic oligoamenorrheic infertility. J Clin Endocrinol Metab 1999. 84: 1617–1622
34. Dehbashi S, Vafaei H, Persanezhad M et al. Time of initiation of clomiphene citrate and pregnancy rate in polycystic ovary syndrome. Int J Gynaecol Obstet 2006. 93: 44–48
35. Imani B, Eijkemans MJ, te Velde ER, et al. Predictors of patients remaining anovulatory during clomiphene citrate induction of ovulation in normogonadotropic oligoamenorrheic infertility. J Clin Endocrinol Metab 1998. 83: 2361–2365
36. Koustra E, White DM, Franks S. Modern use of CC in induction of ovulation. Hum Reprod Update 1997. 3: 359–365
37. Imani B, Eijkemans MJ, te Velde ER, et al. A nomogram to predict the probability of live birth after clomiphene citrate induction of ovulation in normogonadotropic oligoamenorrheic infertility. Fertil Steril 2002. 77: 91–97
38. Fauser BC, van Heusden AM. Manipulation of human ovarian function: physiological concepts and clinical consequences. Endocr Rev 1997. 18: 71–106.
39. Bayram N, van Wely M, van Der Veen F. Recombinant FSH versus urinary gonadotrophins or recombinant FSH for ovulation induction in subfertility associated with polycystic ovary syndrome. Cochrane Database Syst Rev 2001; 2:CD002121
40. White DM, Polson DW, Kiddy D, et al. Induction of ovulation with low-dose gonadotropins in polycystic ovary syndrome: an analysis of 109 pregnancies in 225 women. J Clin Endocrinol Metab 1996. 81: 3821–3824
41. van Santbrink EJ, Fauser BC. Urinary follicle-stimulating hormone for normogonadotropic clomiphene-resistant anovulatory infertility: Prospective, randomized comparison between low-dose step-up and step-down dose regimens. J Clin Endocrinol Metab 1997. 82: 3597–3602
42. Mulders AG, Eijkemans MJ, Imani B, et al. Prediction of chances for success or complications in gonadotrophin ovulation induction in normogonadotrophic anovulatory infertility. Reprod BioMed Onl 2003. 7: 48–56
43. Fauser BC, Devroey P, Macklon NS. Multiple birth resulting from ovarian stimulation for subfertility treatment. Lancet 2005. 365: 1807–1816
44. Eijkemans MJ, Imani B, Mulders AG, et al. High singleton live birth rate following classical ovulation induction in normogonadotropic anovulatory infertility. Hum Reprod 2003. 18: 2357–2362
45. Dunaif A. Insulin resistance and the polycystic ovary syndrome: mechanisms and implications for pathogenesis. Endocr Rev 1997. 18: 774–800
46. Coffler MS, Patel K, Dahan MH, et al. Enhanced granulosa cell responsiveness to FSH during insulin infusion in women with PCOS treated with Pioglitazone. J Clin Endocrinol Metab 2003. 88: 5624–5631
47. Nestler JE, Jakubowicz DJ, Evans WS, et al. Effects of metformin on spontaneous and clomiphene-induced ovulation in the polycystic ovary syndrome. NEJM 1998. 338: 1876–1880
48. Ehrmann DA, Barnes RB, Rosenfield RL, et al. Prevalence of impaired glucose tolerance and diabetes in women with PCOS. Diabetes Care 1999. 22: 141–146
49. Sinawat S, Buppasiri P, Lumbiganon P, et al. Long versus short course treatment with Metformin and Clomiphene Citrate for ovulation induction in women with PCOS. Cochrane Database Syst Rev. 2008; Jan 23;(1):CD006226
50. Lord JM, Flight IH, Norman RJ. Metformin in polycystic ovary syndrome: systematic review and meta-analysis. Br Medical J 2003. 327: 951–953
51. Tang T, Glanville J, Hayden CJ, et al. Combined life-style modification and metformin in obese patients with PCOS. A randomized, placebo-controlled, double-blind, multi center study. Hum Reprod 2006. 21: 80–89
52. Moll E, Bossuyt PM, Korevaar JC, et al. Effect of clomiphene citrate plus metformin and clomiphene citrate plus placebo on induction of ovulation in women with newly diagnosed PCOS: randomised double-blind clinical trial. BMJ 2006. 332: 1485
53. Legro RS, Barnhart HX, Schlaff WD, et al. Clomiphene, Metformin, or both for Infertility in the PCOS. N Engl J Med 2007. 356: 551–566
54. The Thessaloniki ESHRE/ASRM-Sponsored PCOS Consensus Workshop Group March 2–3, 2007, Thessaloniki, Greece. Consensus on infertility treatment related to polycystic ovary syndrome. Fertil Steril. 2008 Feb 1 [Epub ahead of print]

55. Mitwally MF, Casper RF. Use of an aromatase inhibitor for induction of ovulation in patients with an inadequate response to clomiphene citrate. Fertil Steril 2001. 75: 305–309
56. Fisher SA, Reid RL, van Vught DA, et al. A randomized double blind comparison of the effects of CC and the aromatase inhitor Letrozole on the ovulatory function in normal women. Fertil Steril 2002. 78: 280–285
57. Mitwally MFM, Casper RF. Aromatase inhibitors for the treatment of infertility. Expert Opin Investig Drugs 2003. 12: 353–371
58. Fatemi HM, Kolibianakis E, Tournaye H, et al. Clomiphene citrate versus letrozole for ovarian stimulation: a pilot study. Reprod Biomed Online 2003. 7: 543–546
59. Bayar U, Basaran M, Kiran S, et al. Use of an aromatase inhibitor in patients with polycystic ovary syndrome: a prospective randomized trial. Fertil Steril 2006. 86: 1447–1451
60. Biljan MM, Hemmings R, Brassard N. The outcome of 150 babies following the treatment with letrozole or letrozole and gonadotropins. Fertil Steril 2005; 84 (supp. 1), O-231 Abstract 1033
61. Tulandi T, Martin J, Al-Fadhli R, et al. Congenital malformations among 911 newborns conceived after infertility treatment with letrozole or clomiphene citrate. Fertil Steril 2006; 85:1761–1765
62. Forman R, Gill S, Moretti M, et al. Fetal safety of letrozole and clomiphene citrate for ovulation induction. J Obstet Gynaecol Can 2007. 29: 668–671

Chapter 21
IVF in Polycystic Ovary Syndrome

Rehan Salim and Paul Serhal

21.1 Introduction

Polycystic ovary syndrome is recognised as the commonest cause of anovulatory infertility in women and may affect up to 80% of women with anovulatory infertility [1]. Although menstrual disturbance secondary to anovulation is the commonest presentation of PCOS, other factors including abnormal steroidogenesis, hyperinsulinaemia and abnormal gonadotrophin secretion, specifically hypersecretion of LH, will also contribute to the reduction of reproductive potential. Correction of anovulation using medicated ovulation induction regimes is a highly successful approach to establishing mono-follicular ovulatory cycles and achieving pregnancy [2]. However, a proportion of women will either fail to ovulate or achieve a multifollicular response or not achieve pregnancy with this approach, and this group of women may be considered for IVF. Ovarian stimulation in women with polycystic ovaries is approached with caution due to the propensity of the polycystic ovary to have an uncontrolled over response to stimulation. Additionally, the biochemical environment created that is a hallmark of the syndrome has an adverse impact on the development of oocytes and the early conceptus. In this chapter we will discuss the workup and management of IVF cycles in women with polycystic ovary syndrome.

21.2 Preconception Care in Women with PCOS

Along with the general consideration in optimising maternal health pre-conception, such as cessation of smoking, taking folic acid and reduction in alcohol intake, there are several specific factors to be addressed in women with PCOS. One of the most important factors to be considered is weight reduction in the obese or overweight patient [3]. Excess body fat, and especially central obesity, with a concomitant increased BMI (body mass index) are associated with insulin resistance, hyperinsulinaemia and hyperandrogenaemia. Indeed, up to 80% of women with PCOS will have evidence of biochemical insulin resistance [4]. Insulin has a trophic action on ovarian steroidogenesis and LH secretion and will cause a reduction in sex hormone binding globulin secretion. Furthermore, there is a direct correlation between the patient's weight, cycle disturbance and risk of infertility with even moderate obesity (i.e. BMI >27) being associated with an increased risk of anovulation [5,6]. Therefore, overweight women (i.e. BMI > 30) should be encouraged to loose weight prior to commencement of any fertility treatment. Obese women are also likely to respond less well to ovarian stimulation with a higher requirement for gonadotrophins, a greater risk of over response and a lower pregnancy rate with higher miscarriage rate. Furthermore, the risk to both mother and baby from obstetric complications is also considerable [7]. Therefore, weight loss should be the first-line treatment in obese women. Indeed, a loss of 5–10% of total body

R. Salim (✉)
Assisted Conception Unit, University College London, London, UK
e-mail: Rehan.Salim@uclh.nhs.uk

N.R. Farid, E. Diamanti-Kandarakis (eds.), *Diagnosis and Management of Polycystic Ovary Syndrome*,
DOI 10.1007/978-0-387-09718-3_21, © Springer Science+Business Media, LLC 2009

weight in obese women with PCOS has been shown to restore spontaneous reproductive function in 55–100% of women within 6 months of weight reduction [8]. Weight loss will cause an improvement of insulin sensitivity and a concomitant correction of hyperinsulinaemia and nearly every other biochemical abnormality seen within this group of women.

21.3 Pre-treatment with Metformin

Metformin is an oral biguanide that has been extensively used in diabetic patients; it causes a reduction in hyperglycaemia only in hyperglycaemic patients. Central to its action, it causes a reduction in total insulin level. In women with PCOS, metformin used in doses between 1500 and 2550 mg/day has been consistently shown to cause a reduction in circulating insulin levels, serum androgens, serum LH and increased SHBG levels. Velasquez et al. have shown that treatment with1500 mg/day of metformin for 8 weeks will show a measurable reduction on insulin levels and sensitivity. Furthermore, in the same study, treatment with metformin was shown to cause a significant reduction in LH levels and normalization of FSH:LH [9]. This leads to resumption of ovulatory cycles, and several studies have now shown that 78–96% of women will have restored ovulatory cycles [10,11]. In the largest placebo controlled randomised trail to date, Fleming et al. included 92 anovulatory women with PCOS and showed a significant improvement in ovulatory cycles in the metformin-treated group [12]. Thus, pre-treatment with metformin and restoration of ovulatory cycles may obviate the need for IVF and reduce the risk associated with fertility treatment with this group of women. The major advantage of metformin is that it is not inherently an ovulation induction agent and has no known direct ovarian stimulatory effect. Metformin functions at a more fundamental level and restores a more normal endocrinological milieu for monofollicular development, improved oocyte quality and chances of successful pregnancy.

In IVF cycles, co-administration of metformin has beneficial effects on clinical outcomes and biochemical markers of hyperinsulinaemia. Statdmauer et al compared the effects of co-administration of metformin 1000–1500 mg to 30 cycles in women undergoing an IVF cycle to matched controls [13]. In patients treated with metformin, the total number of follicles on the day of hCG treatment was decreased with no change in follicles14 mm in diameter. Metformin treatment did not affect the mean number of oocytes retrieved. However, the mean number of mature oocytes and embryos cleaved was higher after metformin treatment. Fertilization rates (64% vs. 43%) and clinical pregnancy rates (70% vs. 30%) were also increased after pre-treatment with metformin. In a subsequent study, Stadtmauer et al co-administered metformin in women with PCOS who were undergoing IVF cycles who required "coasting" to allow their oestradiol levels to fall prior to hCG administration (see below) [14]. In patients treated with metformin, follicular fluid concentrations of testosterone and insulin were significantly lower; however, the mean number of oocytes retrieved did not differ. The metformin group, however, showed an increase in the mean number of mature oocytes, oocytes fertilized and cleaving embryos (4-cell or greater by 72 h). Additionally, in the group of patients undergoing coasting, maximum oestradiol concentrations and number of days of coasting were all lower in the metformin-treated group with increased clinical pregnancy rates (71 vs. 30%, $P < 0.05$). In contrast, however, Kjotrod et al. conducted a randomised controlled trial to assess the impact of pre-treatment with metformin on outcome of IVF/ICSI in 72 oligomenorrhoeic women with PCOS [15]. No differences were found in the primary end-points: duration of FSH stimulation or estradiol on the day of HCG injection in the metformin and placebo groups, respectively. The secondary end-point's number of oocytes, fertilization rates, embryo quality, pregnancy rates and clinical pregnancy rates were equal. In the women with normal BMI (<28 kg/m^2), pregnancy rates following IVF were 71% vs. 23% in the metformin and placebo groups, respectively ($P = 0.04$). Overall clinical pregnancy rates were equal: 51% vs. 44% in the metformin and placebo groups, respectively. However, in the normal weight subgroup, clinical pregnancy rates were 67% and 33% ,respectively ($P = 0.06$). This would suggest that metformin may be most beneficial in anovulatory PCOS women who are of normal weight.

The fundamental dogma in women undergoing ovarian stimulation for IVF who have polycystic ovary syndrome is the control of excessive ovarian response and yet the achievement of sufficient mature oocytes to enable enough good quality embryos to be produced. The polycystic ovary is extremely sensitive to any ovarian stimulatory agent and as such polycystic ovary morphology alone on ultrasound is the single most important risk factor for the development of excessive response leading to ovarian hyperstimulation syndrome (OHSS) – a potentially life-threatening condition. Women with PCOS produce three times more follicles than women without PCOS when subjected to similar protocols [16]. Additionally, the biochemical environment of PCOS, namely elevation of LH and hyperandrogenism, are both independent risk factors for the development of OHSS [17,18]. The exact mechanism for ovarian responsiveness remains unknown in PCOS; however, it may be mediated via insulin- like growth factor (IGF) driven production of vascular endothelial growth factor (VEGF) in ovarian stroma, leading to increased delivery of ovarian stimulatory drugs to the ovary by improving overall blood flow [19].

The standard long protocol with the use of GnRH agonist starting in the preceding cycle to down regulate the hypothalamo-pituitary axis is a well-established regime as it leads to improved cycle control, higher pregnancy rates, lower cycle cancellation rates and improved yield of mature oocytes. However, there is usually a higher requirement for gonadotrophins with this approach as the GnRH agonist tends to suppress the ovarian responsiveness to gonadotrophins. In the context of PCOS, the GnRH agonist mediated suppression of ovarian response should in theory be expected to be a positive phenomenon as it would dampen the otherwise high sensitivity of the polycystic ovary for gonadotrophins with the added benefit of a reduction in cases of OHSS. However, several authors have reported that this expected reduction has not been seen in practice, and since the introduction of GnRH agonists into IVF cycles, there has been a six-fold increase in the incidence of OHSS in GnRH agonist cycles compared to non-GnRH agonist cycles [20]. In cycles using GnRH agonists in women with PCOS, there remains a higher yield of oocytes and higher peak oestradiol level. This paradoxical effect on oocyte yield and OHSS rates with GnRH agonists may be due to the abolition of the spontaneous LH surge that would otherwise occur and would in turn cause spontaneous luteinization and prevent excessive follicular growth [21]. This abolition of the LH surge would also explain the finding of an increased risk of OHSS in women with PCOS using GnRH agonist in a short protocol regime [22]. Similar effects on oocyte yield and the risk of OHSS have also been found in women with PCOS using GnRH antagonists during ovarian stimulation. In a systematic review and meta-analysis of five randomized trails, Al-Inany and Aboulghar have shown that the use of antagonists does not confer a statistically significant reduction in the risk of developing OHSS (RR 0.51; 95% CI 0.22–1.18) [23]. However, in practice most IVF centres would continue to use GnRH agonists in the management of cycles in women with PCOS, not least to prevent premature ovulation but also due to the improved outcomes in relation to pregnancy. GnRH antagonists do however offer potential option of triggering oocyte maturation with GnRH agonists rather than hCG, a strategy that may reduce the risk of developing OHSS [24].

The use of stimulation agent has undergone much scrutiny over the last decade. Clomiphene is no longer a standard stimulatory agent in IVF cycles and therefore a detailed discussion of its role in this context is not relevant. The mainstay of ovarian stimulation agent in contemporary practice is a gonadotrophin preparation. The choice of gonadotrophin preparation lies between the urinary derived or recombinant FSH. Daya et al. have shown in a meta-analysis of 18 randomised controlled trials that there is no difference in the oocyte yield or risk of OHSS in women with either product [25]. This is in contrast to the meta-analysis of the Cochrane database by Hughes et al., which showed a reduction in the risk of OHSS in clomiphene resistant PCOS when using purified forms of FSH compared to urinary FSH [26]. Rather than the type of FSH used, it is the polycystic ovary's sensitivity to FSH that remains the most significant factor with a higher peak oestradiol level attained with low doses of FSH or hMG and with a steeper slope of increment during stimulation [17,27]. Thus, stimulation regimes in women with PCOS have employed much lower doses of FSH with a stepwise increase if the response was inadequate (low-dose step-up protocol) with close ultrasound and serum oestradiol monitoring to ensure early identification of over response. With this approach, the incidence of OHSS and multiple pregnancy have been significantly reduced [20].

In general, women with PCOS have a higher yield of oocytes in response to ovarian stimulation compared to other groups of infertile women [28]. However, the quality of oocytes in women with PCOS seems to be less good with a lower overall fertilization rate and poorer embryo quality. The aetiology behind this remains unclear but may be reflective of the abnormal biochemical milieu in which the oocytes develop in PCOS [29]. As a result of the lower fertilization rate, most women with PCOS will undergo ICSI rather than conventional IVF in an attempt to improve fertilization rates.

21.4 Monitoring Response to Stimulation

Monitoring of the response and tailoring gonadotrophin dosage has also attracted much attention in an attempt to reduce the risk of OHSS. Several approaches have been proposed with the most popular being monitoring serum oestradiol levels, assessing size and number of developing follicles. Elevated oestradiol levels have been shown to correlate with the risk of OHSS, however, the cutoff used to define an "elevated" level does vary between studies. Asch et al. used a cutoff of 6000 pg/l to identify women with severe OHSS with a sensitivity of 83% and specificity of 99% [30]. Subsequent studies showed have variably confirmed or refuted this depending on the population included and criteria employed for definition of severity of OHSS [31,32]. Cross-sectional studies have shown a significant overlap between oestradiol levels in women who have OHSS suggesting that a single measurement is unlikely to be diagnostic but may contribute to overall risk analysis [17,33]. What is probably more significant is the rate at which the oestradiol rises, and sequential analysis of oestradiol levels are required for this; any rapid or exponential increase indicates a higher risk of over stimulation [34,35]. Ultrasound monitoring of IVF cycles has become a mainstay of management, and using this technique several authors have found a positive correlation between the number of intermediate-sized follicles (i.e. 12–16 mm) and risk of over response [34,36]. Additionally, the total number of follicles seen also correlates with risk of OHSS and, as this is a simpler observation and less prone to inter- and intra-observer variability than measuring size of follicles, is the most commonly used ultrasound marker, with a cutoff of 20 having a sensitivity of 83% and specificity of 67% [30,31].

21.5 Prevention of OHSS

It is conventional practice to induce ovulation using urinary derived hCG, as this has an LH-like effect. However, hCG has a longer half life, a higher receptor affinity and a longer duration of intracellular activity compared to LH, and as a consequence, the effect of hCG lasts for up to 6 days [37]. Additionally, hCG has been shown to have FSH-like effects and contributes to ovarian stimulation [38]. As a result, hCG administration has been recognised as a triggering factor for OHSS and as such a reduction in the dose or withholding of hCG given has been suggested as a strategy to reduce the risk of OHSS [22]. It should be clear from the outset that the development of OHSS requires an hCG trigger and without this the condition does not develop. Therefore, in women deemed to be at particular risk of the severest form, cancellation of the cycle and withholding of hCG could be considered. As nearly all cycles employ GnRH agonists, no endogenous LH surge would occur, and this would result in a complete prevention of OHSS. This is the only strategy that would completely prevent OHSS, all other approaches only reduce the risk. The most popular approach to reducing the risk of OHSS is "coasting". This involves withholding both hCG and exogenous gonadotrophins whilst maintaining GnRH agonists in women with high oestradiol levels. Once the oestradiol level has fallen to a more acceptable level, the hCG trigger is then given. The decline in oestradiol levels indicates atresia of granulosa cells; however, this atretic phase may also have an impact on the oocyte itself as coasting is associated with a lower yield of oocytes, poorer oocytes quality and fertilization and pregnancy rates [22,39]. The duration of coasting may also have an impact on endometrial function as women who require coasting for more than three days seem to have reduced implantation and pregnancy rates even in the presence of good quality oocytes [40]. Additionally, a rapid fall in oestradiol levels is also considered a poor prognostic indicator and in this situation the oocytes yield in low and quality poor.

References

1. Hull, M.G. Epidemiology of polycystic ovarian disease: endocrinological and demographic studies. Gynaecol Endocrinol 1987;1:235–359.
2. Adams, J., Franks, S. Mulitfollicular ovaries: clinical and endocrinological features and response to pulsatile gonadotrophin releasing hormone. Lancet 1985;ii:1375–1378.

3. Hamilton-Fairley, D., Kiddy, D., Watson, H. et al. Association of moderate obesity with a poor pregnancy outcome in women with polycystic ovary treated with low dose gonadotrophin. BJOG 1992;99:128–131.
4. Legro, R.S., Finegood, D. Dunaif, A. A fasting glucose to insulin ratio is a useful measure of insulin sensitivity in women with polycystic ovary syndrome. J Clin Endocrinol Metab 1998;83:2694–2698.
5. Balen, A.H. The pathogenesis of polycystic ovary syndrome: the enigma unravels. Lancet 1999;354:966–967.
6. Clarke, A.M., Ledger, W., Galletly C. et al. Weight loss results in significant improvement in pregnancy and ovulation rates in anovulatory obese women. Hum Reprod 1995;10:2705–2712.
7. Balen, A.H., Richardson, R.A. Impact of obesity on female reproductive health: British Fertility Society, Policy & Practice guidelines. Hum Fert 2007;10:195–206.
8. Pasquali, R., Antenucci, D., Casmirri, F. et al. Clinical and hormonal characteristics of obese amenorrhoiec hyperandrogenic women before and after weight loss. J Clin Endocrinol Metab 1989;68:173–179.
9. Velazquez, E.,M., Mendoza, S., Hamer, T. et al. Metformin therapy in polycystic ovary syndrome reduces hyperinsulinemia, insulin resistance, hyperandrogenemia and systolic blood pressure, while facilitating normal menses and pregnancy. Metabolism 1994;43:647–654.
10. Nestler, J.E., Jakubowicz, D.J., Evans, W.S. et al. Effects of metformin on spontaneous and clomiphene induced ovulation in the polycystic ovary syndrome. N Eng J Med 1998;338:1876–1880.
11. Nestler, J.E., Stovall., D., Akhter, N. et al. Strategies for the use of insulin sensitizing drugs to treat infertility in women with polycystic ovary syndrome. Fertil Steril 2002;77:209–215.
12. Fleming, R., Hopkinson, Z.E., Wallace, A.M. et al. Ovarian function and metabolic factors in women with oligomenorrhoea treated with metformin in a randomised double blind placebo controlled trial. J Clin Endocrinol Metab 2002;87:569–574.
13. Stadtmauer, L.A., Toma, S.K., Riehl, R.M. et al. Metformin treatment of patients with polycystic ovary syndrome undergoing in vitro fertilization improves outcomes and is associated with modulation of the insulin like growth factors. Fertil Steril 2001;75:505–509.
14. Stadtmauer, L.A., Toma, S.K., Riehl, R.M. et al. The impact of metformin on ovarian stimulation and outcome in coasted patients with polycystic ovary syndrome undergoing in-vitro fertilization. RBM Online 2002; 5:112–116.
15. Kjotrod, S.B., von During, V., Carlsen, S.M. Metformin treatment before IVF/ICSI in women with polycystic ovary syndrome; a prospective, randomized, double blind study. Hum Reprod 2004;19:1315–1322.
16. Shulman, A., Dor, J. In vitro fertilization treatment in patients with polycystic ovaries. J Assist Reprod Genet. 1997;14:7–10.
17. Delvigne, A., Demoulin, A., Smitz, J. et al. The ovarian hyperstimulation syndrome in in vitro fertilization: a Belgian multicentric study. II. Multiple discriminant analysis for risk prediction. Hum Reprod 1993;8:1361–1366.
18. Bodis, J., Torok, A., Tinneberg, H.R. LH/FSH ratio as a predictor of ovarian hyperstimulation syndrome. Hum Reprod 1997;12:869–870.
19. Kamat, K.S., Brown, L.F., Manseau, E.J. et al. Expression of vascular permeability factor/ vascular endothelial growth factor by human granulosa cells and theca lutein cells. Role in corpus luteum development. Am J Pathol 1995;146:157–165.
20. Delvigne, A., Rozenberg, S. A systematic review of coasting, a procedure to avoid ovarian hyperstimulation syndrome in in vitro fertilization patients. Hum Reprod Update 2002;8:291–296.
21. Rizk, B., Smitz, J. Ovarian hyperstimulation syndrome after superovulation using GnRH agonists for IVF and related procedures. Hum Reprod 1992;7:320–327.
22. Whelan, J.G. III, Vlahos, N.F. The ovarian hyperstimulation syndrome. Fertil Steril 2000;73:883–896.
23. Al-Inany, H., Aboulghar, M. GnRH antagonists in assisted reproduction: a Cochrane review. Hum Reprod 2002;17:874–885.
24. Griesinger, G., Diedrich, K., Devroey, P., Kolibianankis, E.M. GnRH agonist for triggering final oocyte maturation in the GnRH antagonist ovarian hyperstimulation protocol: a systematic review and meta-analysis. Hum Reprod Update 2006; 12:159–168.
25. Daya, S. Updated meta analysis of recombinant follicle-stimulating hormone (FSH) versus urinary FSH for ovarian stimulation in assisted reproduction. Fertil Steril 2002; 77:711–714.
26. Hughes, E., Collins, J., Vandekerckhove, P. Ovulation induction with urinary follicle stimulating hormone versus human menopausal gonadotrophin for clomiphene-resistant polycystic ovary syndrome. Cochrane Database Syst Rev 2000 (2), CD000087.
27. MacDougall, M.J., Tan, S.L., Balen, A.H. et al. A controlled study comparing patients with and without polycystic ovaries undergoing in-vitro fertilization. Hum Reprod 1993; 8:233–237.
28. Heijnen, E.M.E.W., Eikjemans, M.J.C., Devroey, P. et al. A meta-analysis of outcomes of conventional IVF in women with polycystic ovary syndrome Hum Reprod Update 2006;12:13–21.
29. Urman, B., Tiras, B., Yakin, K. Assisted reproduction in the treatment of polycystic ovarian syndrome. Reprod Biomed Online 2004;8:419–430.
30. Asch, R.H., Li, H.P., Balmaceda, J.P. et al. Severe ovarian hyperstimulation syndrome in assisted reproductive technology: definition of high risk groups. Hum Reprod 1991;6:1395–1399.
31. Morris, R.S., Wong, I.L., Kirkman, E. et al. Inhibition of ovarian-derived prorenin to angiotensin cascade in the treatment of ovarian hyperstimulation syndrome. Hum Reprod 1995;10:1355–1358.
32. Mathur, R.S., Akande, A.V., Keay, S.D. et al. Disctinction between early and late ovarian hypsretsimulation syndrome. Fertil Steril 2000;73:901–907.
33. Navot, D., Relou, A., Birkenfield, A. et al. Risk factors and prognostic variables in the ovarian hyperstimulation syndrome. Am J Obstet Gynecol 1988;159:210–215.

34. Enskog, A., Henriksson, M., Unander, M. et al. Prospective study of the clinical and laboratory parameters of patients in whom ovarian hyperstimulation developed during controlled ovarian hyperstimulation for in vitro fertilization. Fertil Steril 1999;71:808–814.
35. Fluker, M.R., Hooper, W.M., Yuzpe, A.A. Witholding gonadotrophins ("coasting") to minimize the risk of ovarian hysperstimulation during superovulation and in vitro fertilization-embryo transfer cycles. Fertil Steril 1999;71:294–301.
36. Engmann, L., Sladkevicius, P., Agrawal, R. et al. Value of ovarian stromal blood flow velocity measurement after pituitary suppression in the prediction of ovarian responsiveness and outcome of in vitro fertilization treatment. Fertil Steril 1999;71: 22–29.
37. Casper, R.F. Ovarian hyperstimulation: effects of GnRH analogues. Does triggering ovulation with gonadotrophin-releasing hormone analogue prevent severe ovarian hypsretsimulation syndrome? Hum Reprod 1996;11:1144–1146.
38. Gerris, J., De Vits, A. Joostensm, M. et al. Triggering of ovulation in human menopausal gonadotrophin stimulated cycles: comparison between intravenously administered gonadotrophin-releasing hormone (100 and 500 micrograms), GnRH agonist (buserelin, 500 micrograms) and human chorionic gonadotrophin (10 000 IU). Hum Reprod 1995;10:56–62.
39. Aboulghar, M.A., Mansour, R.T., Serour, G.I. et al. Oocyte quality in patients with severe ovarian hyperstimulation syndrome. Fertil Steril 1997;68:1017–1021.
40. Ulug, U., Bahceci, M., Erden, H.F. et al. The significance of coasting duration during ovarian stimulation for conception in assisted fertilization cycles. Hum Reprod 2002;17:310–313.

Chapter 22
The Surgical Management of Polycystic Ovarian Syndrome

Colin J. Davis

22.1 Introduction

Polycystic ovarian syndrome (PCOS) is defined by ultrasound appearance of polycystic ovaries (PCO), enlarged ovaries with at least 10 peripherally located follicles measuring between 2 and 10 mm, associated with symptoms of oligo-amenorrhoea, obesity and hyperandrogenism (acne and hirsutism) [1]. Stein–Leventhal syndrome was described in 1935 as a condition of obese women with amenorrhoea, signs of excess androgen production and bilateral enlarged, polycystic ovaries [2]. Many women with ultrasound detected PCO do not have the typical triad of symptoms and hence do not have PCOS. Raised serum luteinising hormone (LH) and raised androgens such as testosterone are the endocrine markers of PCOS and are associated with menstrual irregularity and infertility [3]. Increased androgen production in particular increased serum testosterone, LH and free androgen index, along with lower serum glucose/insulin ratios and lower sex hormone binding globulin (SHBG) are linked to disrupted folliculogenesis. Insulin resistance lies at the heart of the metabolic effects of PCOS. Women presenting with hirsutism and oligomenorrhea have the highest correlation with the metabolic markers of PCOS. These symptoms are markers of the underlying metabolic alterations possibly associated with increased health risks in later life. [4]. There is controversy surrounding hypersecretion of LH and infertility and miscarriage. The relation between pre-pregnancy follicular-phase serum luteinising hormone (LH) concentrations and outcome of pregnancy was investigated prospectively in 193 women with regular spontaneous menstrual cycles. The group of women with LH concentrations of less than 10 IU/l (normal LH group) had a lower miscarriage rate compared to the group of women with a higher early follicular phase LH level, more than 10 IU/l. This study concluded that there was an important association between hypersecretion of LH and miscarriage [5]. Other studies have examined the link between raised LH and miscarriage [6]. It has been proposed that treatments which decrease LH concentrations, such as gonadotrophin-releasing hormone analogues or laparoscopic ovarian diathermy, improve induction of ovulation and pregnancy rates and reduce miscarriage rates. Tonic hypersecretion of LH appears to induce premature oocyte maturation, causing the problems with fertilisation and miscarriage [7].

22.2 Obesity and PCOS

Obesity is defined as a body mass index (BMI) greater than 30 Kg/m^2 and is linked to hypersecretion of insulin which results in increased ovarian production of androgens. An important early study showed that obese women with polycystic ovary syndrome were more likely to present with hirsutism and menstrual disturbances compared to lean women with PCOS. The main biochemical differences between obese and lean women with PCOS were that SHBG concentrations were much lower in women with obesity. There was an inverse relationship

C.J. Davis (✉)
Consultant Obstetrician and Gynaecologist, St Bartholomews Hospital London, London, UK
e-mail: cdavisobgyn@aol.com

N.R. Farid, E. Diamanti-Kandarakis (eds.), *Diagnosis and Management of Polycystic Ovary Syndrome*,
DOI 10.1007/978-0-387-09718-3_22,

between SHBG levels and insulin concentrations, with insulin being shown to have a direct inhibitory action on SHBG secretion. Weight reduction of more than 5% was associated with an improved biochemical profile and, importantly, with restoration of fertility [8]. Women with PCOS are insulin resistant, have insulin secretory defects, and are at high risk for glucose intolerance. It was also suggested that PCOS may be a more important risk factor than ethnicity or race for glucose intolerance in young women [9]. It is therefore imperative that obese women undertake weight reducing measures before undergoing any other treatment for PCOS. There is evidence that weight loss alone is associated with a reduction in androgens, resumption of ovulation and increase spontaneous rate. The main objective is to adhere to a strict high-protein and low-carbohydrate diet for a minimum of 12 weeks. One randomised study compared the effects of this regime with a high-carbohydrate and low-protein diet followed by a 4-week weight maintenance diet. Greater weight loss resulted in greater improvement of insulin resistance, which led to enhancements of cardiovascular and reproductive parameters [10].

22.3 PCOS and Other Gynaecological Disorders

Amenorrhoea and oestrogen dominance are the normal endocrine environment for women with PCOS. As well as causing a proliferative effect on the endometrium, the oestrogen-dominant state will stimulate other common gynaecological conditions such as endometriosis and uterine fibroids. The endocrine changes can therefore be used to identify clinically effective hormonal treatments such as the oral contraceptive pill as well as pituitary downregulation with gonadotrophin releasing hormone (GnRH) agonists. In order to establish the correct treatment approach in gynaecological disorders, it is important to understand the endocrine pathophysiology. Surgical ablation of endometriosis and excision of uterine fibroids is the first-line treatment that will improve pelvic symptoms as well as enhance fertility.

22.4 Surgical Options for PCOS

Prior to the introduction of safe laparoscopy, ovarian wedge resection was performed for women with anovulatory PCOS. This involved a laparotomy and excision of a section of each ovary and was associated with morbidity, including long-term adhesion formation [11]. With the advent of new equipments and enhanced techniques, laparoscopic surgery has superseded open surgery for many gynaecological conditions, including ovarian diathermy. It is often performed as a day case and allows for a safe and effective assessment of the fallopian tubes, as well as the treatment of other common diseases such as endometriosis and pelvic adhesions. Laparoscopy is one of the commonest gynaecological procedures performed and should include ovarian diathermy for women with PCOS [12].

The technique of laparoscopic ovarian diathermy was described in a small study involving 21 nulliparous women with PCOS, oligoamenorhoea and infertility. The procedure involved introducing four 40 W diathermy burns to a depth of 4 mm to each ovary for 4 seconds. Regular menstrual cycles and regular ovulation ensued in 81% of women, and 52% of women conceived spontaneously. It was concluded that LOD was a useful option for women with PCOS [13]. Some authors have suggested that the benefits of LOD can be achieved when ovarian diathermy is performed to just one of the ovaries. Women with PCOS were randomised to either unilateral or bilateral laparoscopic ovarian diathermy as part of treatment in clomiphene resistant PCOS. The results showed that both unilateral and bilateral ovarian diathermy resulted in ovulation from both ovaries. The mechanism of action of laparoscopic ovarian diathermy is believed to be via a correction of disturbed ovarian-pituitary feedback. Unilateral ovarian diathermy was believed to be as effective as bilateral ovarian diathermy in the resumption of menstruation and pregnancy rates [14,15]. The risk of adhesion formation, bleeding and infection is extremely small following LOD although women should be counselled about these risks before undergoing surgery.

A new technique of transvaginal hydrolaparoscopy can be performed under local anaesthetic in an outpatient setting. Ovarian drilling by transvaginal fertiloscopy with bipolar electrosurgery appears to be an effective minimally invasive procedure in patients with PCOS resistant to clomiphene citrate [16]. It also allows for aqua assessment of the pelvis, fallopian tubes and ovaries. Subtle para-ovarian and peri-tubular adhesions are more readily seen and can be treated.

The presence of longstanding anovulation and amenorrhoea causes lengthy periods of unopposed oestrogen stimulation of the endometrium. This can result in endometrial hyperplasia. More often this is simple endometrial hyperplasia with no atypia [17]. If left untreated, it can ultimately result in endometrial carcinoma. The endometrium of reproductive aged women undergoes cyclical changes in preparation for implantation in response to oestrogen and progesterone. These steroids and their receptors are tightly regulated throughout the menstrual cycle, and their actions are facilitated by the presence of steroid receptor coactivators of the p160 family. A study compared coactivator expression patterns in fertile endometrium to the endometrium of anovulatory and clomiphene-induced ovulatory (secretory) women with PCOS. Compared with both fertile and infertile controls, PCOS women exhibited elevated levels of p160 coactivator expression, which may render the endometrium more sensitive to oestrogen [18]. It is essential therefore that hysteroscopy and endometrial curettage are performed at the same time as LOD for women with anovulatory PCOS. To prevent the long-term sequelae of unopposed oestrogen stimulation of the endometrium, regular menstruation should be induced with cyclical progestogens such as provera for 1 week every 3 months. This however may not be necessary if regular menstruation resumes following LOD.

There is evidence that LOD has long-term benefits for women with anovulation secondary to PCOS. In a long-term follow-up study, six to ten years after a randomised controlled study comparing LOD with gonadotrophin therapy, the LOD group of women had an increased number of ongoing spontaneous menstrual cycles and 79% had delivered live infants [19]. A large meta-analysis of nine studies compared the outcomes of women with clomiphene-resistant PCOS undergoing LOD or gonadotrophin stimulation [20]. It examined primary outcomes as ovulatory, pregnancy and live birth rates and secondary outcomes as miscarriage, multiple pregnancy and ovarian hyperstimulation syndrome (OHSS) rates. Whilst all the primary outcomes were similar, the LOD group had lower multiple pregnancy and ovarian OHSS rates compared to gonadotrophin treatment but similar pregnancy rates. There was no clear outcome data on the long-term effects of LOD on ovarian function.

It is believed that LOD may be beneficial in decreasing the risk of OHSS and improving the ongoing clinical pregnancy rate in women with PCOS undergoing in vitro fertilisation (IVF). Ovarian diathermy did not appear to have a deleterious effect on IVF outcomes, in terms of number of oocytes retrieved or embryos resulting [21].

22.5 Mechanisms by Which LOD Induces Ovulation

The mechanism by which ovarian diathermy induces ovulation remains unclear, but a number of theories have been proposed. Disruption of the ovarian cortex is thought to affect local paracrine factors leading to a reduction in androgen production. A prospective study examined the effects of LOD on 50 women with PCOS. Pre- and post-operative mean levels of Inhibin B were measured. There was an inverse correlation between body mass index (BMI) and Inhibin B serum levels. The study failed to show any significant changes in Inhibin B following LOD, and it makes it unlikely that this hormone has any direct role in the effects of LOD [22]. Another mechanism of action may result from a decrease in ovarian stromal blood flow velocity following laparoscopic ovarian diathermy. In one study, Colour Doppler blood flow within the ovarian stroma was recorded and serum concentrations of FSH, LH and testosterone were measured in 52 women with PCOS before and after laparoscopic ovarian diathermy. There was a significant correlation between hormonal and ovarian stromal blood-flow changes. Changes in the Doppler parameters were significantly higher in women who ovulated. The measurement of ovarian stromal blood flow correlated to changes in androgen markers of PCOS [23].

22.6 Effects of PCOS in Pregnancy

The direct link between PCOS and gestational diabetes has been well established. A screening glucose tolerance test (GTT) is mandatory at 26 weeks gestation. It is more common for women with PCOS to have larger babies and with that the obstetric risks are higher [24]. Pregnant women with PCOS experience a higher incidence of perinatal morbidity from gestational diabetes, pregnancy-induced hypertension and preeclampsia. Their babies are at an increased risk of neonatal complications, such as preterm birth and admission at a neonatal intensive care unit. Pre-pregnancy, antenatal and intrapartum care should be aimed at reducing these risks. Consequently, the risk of emergency lower segment caesarean section (LSCS) is much higher. For women with impaired glucose tolerance in pregnancy requiring insulin treatment, most obstetricians would recommend an elective caesarean section between 38 and 39 weeks gestation. This would avoid the risks of uteroplacental insufficiency as well as shoulder dystocia at the time of vaginal delivery. It should be noted that women with PCOS have a higher BMI compared to other pregnant women and are at increased risk of infection, bleeding, deep vein thrombosis (DVT), especially if they undergo LSCS.

22.7 Conclusion

In conclusion, the surgical management of PCOS has evolved with the introduction of new laparoscopic and minimally invasive techniques. There is good evidence from randomised studies to support the use of LOD for women with PCOS, especially those who are resistant to clomiphene treatment. The benefits of LOD include increased ovarian sensitivity as well as reduced circulating androgens and follicular phase LH levels. This results in more regular menstruation and ovulation and increased fertility. There is some evidence demonstrating a reduction in miscarriage rates along with a reduced risk of OHSS following IVF treatment. This approach allows for a full and complete inspection of the female pelvis along with the treatment of other conditions such as endometriosis, uterine fibroids and pelvic adhesions. The management of PCOS includes pregnancy care and may necessitate delivery by Caesarean section to avoid both maternal and fetal complications. Pre-pregnancy advice such as weight loss should be the first-line treatment when managing women with PCOS.

References

1. Broekmans, F, Fauser B. Diagnostic criteria for polycystic ovarian syndrome. Endocrine 2006;1:3–11.
2. Stein, I, Leventhal M. Amenorrhoea associated with bilateral polycystic ovaries. Am J Obstet Gynecol;1935;181–191.
3. Franks, S, Adams, J, Mason, H, Polson D. Ovulatory disorders in women with polycystic ovary syndrome. Clin Obstet Gynaecol. 1985;12:605–632.
4. Taponen, S, Martikainen, H, Järvelin M, et al. Hormonal profile of women with self-reported symptoms of oligomenorrhea and/or hirsutism: Northern Finland birth cohort 1966 study. J Clin Endocrinol Metab. 2003;88:141–147.
5. Regan, L, Owen, E, Jacobs H. Hypersecretion of LH, infertility and miscarriage. Lancet 1990;336:1141–1144.
6. Balen, A, Tan, S, Jacobs H. Hypersecretion of luteinising hormone-a significant cause of subfertility and miscarriage. Br J Obstet Gynaecol 1993;100:1082–1089.
7. Homburg R. Adverse effects of luteinizing hormone on fertility: fact or fantasy. *Baillieres* Clin Obstet Gynaecol 1998;12: 555–563.
8. Franks, S, Kiddy, D, Sharp, P, Singh, A, Reed, M, Seppälä, M et al. Obesity and polycystic ovary syndrome. Ann N Y Acad Sci 1991;626:201–206.
9. Legro RS, Kunselman AR, Dodson WC, Dunaif A. Prevalence and predictors of risk for type 2 diabetes mellitus and impaired glucose tolerance in polycystic ovary syndrome: a prospective, controlled study in 254 affected women. J Clin Endocrinol Metab 1999 Jan;84(1):165–169.
10. Moran, L, Noakes, M, Clifton, P, Tomlinson, L, Galletly, C, Norman R. Dietary composition in restoring reproductive and metabolic physiology in overweight women with polycystic ovary syndrome. J Clin Endocrinol Metab 2003;88:812–819.
11. Donesky, B, Adashi E. Surgically induced ovulation in the polycystic ovary syndrome: wedge resection revisited in the age of laparoscopy. Fertil Steril 1995;63:439–463.
12. Bosteels, J, Van Herendael, B, Weyers, S, D'Hooghe, T. The position of diagnostic laparoscopy in current fertility practice. Hum Reprod Update 2007;13:477–485.

13. Armar, N, McGarringle, H, Honour, J, Holownia, P, Jacobs, H, Lachelin, G. Laparoscopic ovarian diathermy in the management of anovulatory infertility in women with polycystic ovaries: endocrine changes and clinical outcome. Fertil Steril 1990;53:45–49.
14. Balen, A, Jacobs H. A prospective study comparing unilateral and bilateral laparoscopic ovarian diathermy in women with the polycystic ovary syndrome. Fertil Steril 1994;62:921–925.
15. Al-Mizyen, E, Grudzinskas, J. Unilateral laparoscopic ovarian diathermy in infertile women with clomiphene citrate-resistant polycystic ovary syndrome. Fertil Steril 2007;88:1678–1680.
16. Fernandez, H, Watrelot, A, Alby, J, Kadoch, J, Gervaise, A, deTayrac, R, et al. Fertility after ovarian drilling by transvaginal fertiloscopy for treatment of polycystic ovary syndrome. J Am Assoc Gynecol Laparosc 2004;11:374–378.
17. Tingthanatikul, Y, Choktanasiri, W, Rochanawutanon, M, Weerakeit, S. Prevalence and clinical predictors of endometrial hyperplasia in anovulatory women presenting with amenorrhea. Gynecol Endocrinol. 2006;22:101–105.
18. Gregory, C, Wilson, E, Apparao, K, Lininger, R, Meyer, W, Kowalik, A et al. Steroid receptor coactivator expression throughout the menstrual cycle in normal and abnormal endometrium. J Clin Endocrinol Metab 2002;87:2960–2966.
19. Mohiuddin, S, Besselink, D, Farquhar C. Long-term follow up with laparoscopic ovarian diathermy for women with clomiphene-resistant polycystic ovarian syndrome. Aust N Z J Obstet Gynaecol 2007;47:508–511.
20. Farquhar, C, Lilford, R, Marjoribanks J. Laparoscopic 'drilling' by diathermy or laser for ovulation induction in anovulatory polycystic ovarian syndrome. Cochrane Database Syst Rev 2005;3:CD001122.
21. Tozer, A, Al-Shawaf, T, Zosmer, A, Hussain, S, Wilson, C, Lower, A et al. Does laparoscopic ovarian diathermy affect the outcome of IVF-embryo transfer in women with polycystic ovarian syndrome? A retrospective comparative study. Hum Reprod 216:2001;91–95.
22. Amer, S, Laird, S, Ledger, W, Li T. Effect of laparoscopic ovarian diathermy on circulating inhibin B in women with anovulatory polycystic ovarian syndrome. Hum Reprod 2007;22:389–394.
23. Parsanezhad, M, Bagheri, M, Alborzi, S, Schmidt, E. Ovarian stromal blood flow changes after laparoscopic ovarian cauterization in women with polycystic ovary syndrome. Hum Reprod 2003;18:1432–1437.
24. Boomsma, C, Eijkemans, M, Hughes, E, Visser, G, Fauser, B, Macklon, N. A meta-analysis of pregnancy outcomes in women with polycystic ovary syndrome. Hum Reprod Update 2006;12:673–683.

Chapter 23
When Periods Stop: Long-Term Consequences of PCOS

Enrico Carmina, Ettore Guastella and Manfredi Rizzo

23.1 Introduction

Every year, many studies are dedicated to analyze the clinical and endocrine-metabolic problems of women with polycystic ovary syndrome (PCOS) [1]. However, almost all these studies interest patients during their fertile age. Yet, what happens after the menopause is largely unknown. In this short review, we will report the few data that are available about the continuing influence of PCOS after the menopause.

23.2 Menopausal Age in Women with Polycystic Ovary Syndrome

Initial reports suggest that PCOS women develop menopause later than control women [2]. However, more recent studies show that the menopausal age is the same in women with or without PCOS [3]. Instead, it has been reported that, at least in the United States, there is a greater frequency of surgical menopause, because of bilateral oopherectomy, in women with clinical features of PCOS (35.0% vs. 24.7% for non-PCOS women, $p = 0.052$) [3]. While the causes of this phenomenon are unclear (uterine problems such as endometrial hyperplasia or fibroids), an anticipated menopause may play a role in the future of these women (earlier appearance of cardiovascular disease, bone loss).

23.3 Increased Cardiovascular Risk in Women with PCOS

It is well known that fertile women with PCOS have increased cardiovascular risk, and this finding has been consistently confirmed across several geographic areas and ethnic groups [4–8]. Women with PCOS are more likely than normally cycling women to have insulin resistance, central adiposity and hypertension [1]; in addition, several markers of clinical and subclinical atherosclerosis, including serum markers (such as C-reactive protein and homocysteine), carotid intima-media thickness, coronary artery calcium and echocardiographic patterns have been found to be altered too [1, 4–8]. Dyslipidemia is very common in women with PCOS and include low HDL-cholesterol levels and elevated triglyceride concentrations [9]. Increased LDL and total cholesterol have been also found but with a lower prevalence and, beyond plasma lipids, women with PCOS have lower LDL size due to increased levels of atherogenic small, dense LDL [10].

In consideration of the high prevalence of metabolic and cardiovascular risk factors in young women with PCOS, we should expect increased cardiovascular diseases in postmenopausal women who were affected by PCOS. However, there is no clear evidence for this, and, although new studies are showing increased

E. Carmina (✉)
Professor of Medicine, Professor of Endocrinology and Head of Endocrine Unit, Department of Clinical Medicine, University of Palermo, Via delle Croci 47, 90139 Palermo, Italy
e-mail: enricocarmina@libero.it

N.R. Farid, E. Diamanti-Kandarakis (eds.), *Diagnosis and Management of Polycystic Ovary Syndrome*, DOI 10.1007/978-0-387-09718-3_23, cardiovascular morbidity, most available data suggest that the prevalence of cardiovascular consequences in women who were affected by PCOS is smaller than that expected on the basis of the risk calculation during fertile age [11].

23.4 Cardiovascular Disease in Postmenopausal PCOS Women

Initial studies on the prevalence of cardiovascular diseases in postmenopausal women, who were probably affected by PCOS during their fertile age, indicated an increased risk for developing myocardial infarction [11]. It was calculated that women with PCOS have 7.1 times higher risk than non-PCOS women to develop myocardial infarction [12] (Table 23.1). However, the number of studied subjects was small (only 33 patients), and the study did not demonstrate increased cardiovascular morbidity but only the increased risk [12].

Table 23.1 Long-term studies examining the prevalence of cardiovascular diseases in women with PCOS

Authors (year)	Study design	No. of PCOS	Mean age, years	PCOS definition	Results	Cardiovascular end points
Dahlgren (1992)	Population study	33	50 (40–59)	Histopathology typical of PCOS at wedge resection	Positive	Increased risk (relative risk of 7.4) of developing myocardial infarction in PCOS compared to age-matched women
Pierpoint (1998)	Population study	786	>45 at the time of follow-up	Histological evidence of PCOS or macroscopic evidence of ovarian dysfunction or clinical diagnosis	Negative	No difference in cardiovascular deaths between PCOS rates and national rates in a mean follow-up period of 30 years
Wild (2000)	Population study	309	<75 at the time of follow-up	Histological evidence of PCOS or macroscopic evidence of ovarian dysfunction or clinical diagnosis	Negative	No difference in cardiovascular morbidity and mortality compared to age-matched women
Cibula (2000)	Cross-sectional	28	52±5	Wedge resection for typical clinical symptoms and ovarian morphology of PCOS	Positive	Increased coronary artery diseases in PCOS in relation to age- and BMI-matched women
Krentz (2007)	Cross-sectional	64	78±8	Irregular menses, hyperandrogenism, infertility, central obesity, insulin resistance	Positive	Association between PCOS and cardiovascular diseases in non-diabetic post-menopausal women
Shaw (2008)	Prospective, multi-center	104	63±10	Premenopausal history of irregular menses and current biochemical evidence of hyperandrogenemia	Positive	Association between clinical features of PCOS and cardiovascular outcomes in a 5-year follow-up

A large successive study (786 postmenopausal women) did not demonstrate any difference in cardiovascular morbidity and mortality between women with PCOS and the general population [13]. On the basis of the observed alterations in several markers of clinical and subclinical atherosclerosis, these results were somehow unexpected and suggested that probably there are no long-term cardiovascular consequences of PCOS. However, this study has been criticized because the diagnosis of PCOS was based on the historical data during a very large period (hospital records between 1930 and 1979) and was not supported by hormonal studies or ovarian morphology.

In a successive report, the same authors [14] have studied a more restricted but more carefully selected cohort of patients (309 postmenopausal women who were diagnosed as affected by PCOS, before 1979, in the United Kingdom). The authors did not observe any increase in coronary heart disease (odd ratio 1.5) but noted a higher prevalence of cerebrovascular accidents (odd ratio 2.8). Interestingly, in the Framingham study, the reported presence of oligomenorrhea during fertile years was not associated to cardiac events but to increased number of cerebrovascular accidents [15].

A recent study has shown that women with PCOS may, indeed, also present an increased prevalence of some cardiac events. In fact, studying a large group of postmenopausal women who underwent an angiographic study because of the suspect of myocardial ischemia, an adverse association between clinical and hormonal features of PCOS and cardiovascular outcomes in a 6-year follow-up has been recently demonstrated [3]. In this study, multivessel cardiovascular disease was observed in 32% of PCOS women compared to 25% of non-PCOS women (odd ratio 1.7) and it correlated with several factors, including increased free testosterone. The survival rate from cardiovascular (CV) death was slightly lower in PCOS women (90.4 versus 94.8% in non-PCOS) with an odd ratio of 2.1 but the difference was not significant, probably because the relatively low number of CV deaths (25 totally). However, the event free survival (including fatal and non-fatal events) was significantly lower in PCOS (78.9%) compared to 88.7% of non-PCOS women ($p < 0.006$). The difference between the two groups was higher when cerebro-vascular accidents were considered too, confirming the association of PCOS with stroke. Interestingly, there was a big difference in risk of CV events between PCOS patients with increased C-reactive protein (CRP) and PCOS patients with low-normal CRP levels. In fact, the risk of CV death was 12.2 times higher in PCOS patients with high CRP levels [3]. While other studies are needed to confirm and expand this study, it is clear that PCOS is associated to an increased risk for cerebrovascular events (stroke) and probably also for fatal and nonfatal coronary heart disease. In addition, this risk is more severe in patients having higher androgens but mostly presenting higher inflammatory factors in the blood.

These findings are somewhat similar to those found in a cross-sectional study on old non-diabetic postmenopausal women where atherosclerotic cardiovascular events were associated with features of a putative PCOS phenotype [16]. Thus, data on cardiovascular outcome of postmenopausal women with PCOS are not conclusive, but evidence is accumulating that indeed these women have an increase in cerebrovascular accidents and probably also in cardiovascular morbidity.

However, the available evidence suggests that the increased morbidity and mortality for cardiovascular disease in PCOS women is smaller than that expected on the basis of the simple calculation of the risk in young age. It opens an important question. Why the increased risk does not translate in increased morbidity? Is the initial atherosclerosis that has been observed in many young PCOS women reversible? The answer to these questions may be relevant not only for PCOS women but also for the general population.

23.5 Changes in Polycystic Ovaries and Androgens with Age

The reduction of the risk and the reversibility of atherosclerotic lesions may be the consequence of the hormonal changes that happen in PCOS women after 35–40 years of age. In fact, several studies have shown that androgen secretion spontaneously decreases after the age of 35 in normal women [17] and in PCOS women [18], and that in the general population, the prevalence of polycystic ovaries appears to decrease with the age [19]. In a study, the prevalence of polycystic ovaries was only 7.8% in women older than 35 years, compared to 21.6% in women younger than this age [19]. In addition, women with polycystic ovaries may regain normal menses with age [20] and in some instances may get spontaneous fertility [21]. Therefore, not only the diagnosis of PCOS becomes less common with the age but also the syndrome presents with less alterations including lower androgen levels.

The progressive decrease of circulating androgens in PCOS women during their late fertile age may play a role in the reduction of their cardiovascular risk. Interestingly, in the recent study that demonstrated an increased number of cardiovascular events in postmenopausal PCOS women, a significant association was found between postmenopausal androgen levels and cardiovascular events [3]. It suggests not only that androgens may play an important role in cardiovascular disease but also that the development of cardiac events are influenced by the androgen excess that may persist also after the menopause.

23.6 Body Weight and Diabetes in Postmenopausal PCOS Women

As expected, postmenopausal women with PCOS present a higher prevalence of obesity and type II diabetes than postmenopausal controls [2, 3]. Both disorders may contribute to the increase of cerebro-vascular and cardio-vascular events in postmenopausal PCOS [3]. As previously reported, the factor that contributes more to the increase of cardiovascular events in postmenopausal PCOS is the increase of the circulating inflammatory factors [3] and it is well known that visceral adipose factor is the major contributor to the increase of such actors in blood [22]. It confirms that the maintenance of a regular body weight is one of the major targets of the long-term treatment of PCOS [23].

23.7 Cancer in Postmenopausal PCOS

Several studies have reported an increased prevalence of some forms of cancer in postmenopausal PCOS. The most established relation regards endometrial cancer. Probably because of the contemporaneous presence of hyperestrogenism, obesity and infertility, PCOS patients present an increased risk of developing endometrial cancer [24, 25]. However, this risk is higher in younger women because of unopposed estrogen action [25, 26] and no sufficient data have been reported to support an increased prevalence of endometrial cancer in postmenopausal women with PCOS [27].

Conflicting data have been presented regarding breast cancer and ovarian cancer in postmenopausal PCOS [13, 28–30]. Some studies have reported an increased risk such high as 3.6 for breast cancer in postmenopausal PCOS [28], while in other studies, the risk for breast cancer was absent ranging from 1 to 1.2 [29]. Finally, some studies have reported a reduced risk for ovarian carcinoma in PCOS women [13], while in others, a 2.5-fold increased risk was observed [30].

It is difficult to explain these big differences in results. Probably, the increased risk is relatively small and may be influenced by previous treatments or by environmental components such as diet and body weight.

23.8 Therapeutic Approaches in Postmenopausal PCOS

Lifestyle modification should constitute a first-line therapy [23]. It consists a long-life strategy that has to include not only diet but also regular physical exercise and avoidance of smoking, alcohol and drugs. The main objective is to reduce fat excess and fat altered distribution that may be present not only in obese and overweight women with PCOS but also in 30–40% of PCOS patients with normal body weight [31].

However, the dropout rate from lifestyle program is very high and, in addiction, in some patients, particularly during postmenopausal age, the reduction or the redistribution of fat mass is not sufficient to significantly improve the cardiovascular or metabolic risk factors.

This is further complicated by the fact that PCOS women may show alterations in plasma lipids even in the absence of insulin resistance or of fat excess [4].

Postmenopausal women with PCOS who present dyslipidemia, metabolic syndrome or signs of atherosclerosis and do not respond to lifestyle modification have to be treated to reduce their metabolic and cardiovascular risk [32]. Although no specific data exist on treatment of postmenopausal women with PCOS, the use of statins may represent an important therapeutic option because these drugs not only improve serum lipids but also are able to reduce endothelial intima-media thickness and atherosclerotic plaques [32]. In addition, it has been shown that in women with PCOS, statins may decrease insulin resistance and lower testosterone levels [33], an effect that may be important in reducing cardiovascular events [30]. Other lipid-lowering drugs, in particular nicotinic acid and fibrates, are indicated in PCOS patients who present severe dyslipidemia and do not respond to statins [32]. Finally, insulin-sensitizing medications [34] (generally metformin but in some instances also pioglitazone) may represent an important therapeutic option, but the long-term effects on dyslipidemia are often unsatisfactory [32].

23.9 Conclusions

We need many more studies on long-term consequences of PCOS. The data are few and often conflicting. However, the available data suggest that there is an increased number of cerebrovascular and cardiovascular events in postmenopausal PCOS. These events are partially related to the persisting hyperandrogenism but are mostly correlated to the excessive body weight (probably to the visceral obesity). It suggests that our best long-term strategy is the information. We need to convince women with PCOS that they are at higher risk for metabolic and cardiovascular problems, also that they may reduce their risk just maintaining a correct lifestyle.

References

1. Lobo RA, Carmina E. The importance of diagnosing the polycystic ovary syndrome. Ann Intern Med 2000; 132:989–93.
2. Dahlgren E, Johansson S, Lindstet G, Knutsson F, Oden A, Janson PO, Mattsson LA, Crona N, Lundberg PA. Women with Polycystic Ovary Syndrome wedge resected in 1956–1965: a long-term follow-up focusing on natural history and circulating hormones. Fertil Steril 1992; 57:505–13.
3. Shaw LJ, Merz CN, Azziz R, Stanczyk FZ, Sopko G, Braunstein GD, Kelsey SF, Kip KE, Cooper-Dehoff RM, Johnson BD, Vaccarino V, Reis SE, Bittner V, Hodgson TK, Rogers W, Pepine CJ. Post-Menopausal Women with a History of Irregular Menses and Elevated Androgen Measurements at High Risk for Worsening Cardiovascular Event-Free Survival: Results from the National Institutes of Health National Heart, Lung, and Blood Institute (NHLBI) Sponsored Women's Ischemia Syndrome Evaluation (WISE). J Clin Endocrinol Metab 2008 Jan 8; 93:1276–1284.
4. Guzick DS. Cardiovascular risk in PCOS. J Clin Endocrinol Metab 2004; 89:3694–5.
5. Talbott EO, Guzick DS, Sutton-Tyrrell K, McHugh-Pemu K, Zborowski J, Remsberg K, Kuller L. Evidence for association between polycystic ovary syndrome and premature carotid atherosclerosis in middle-aged women. Arterioscler Thromb Vasc Biol 2000; 20:2414–2421.
6. Christian RC, Dumesic DA, Behrenbeck T, Oberg A, Sheedy PF, Fitzpatrick L. Prevalence and predictors of coronary artery calcification in women with polycystic ovary syndrome. J Clin Endocrinol Metab 2003; 88:2562–2568.
7. Carmina E, Orio F, Palomba S, Longo RA, Cascella T, Colao A, Lombardi G, Rini GB, Lobo RA. Endothelial dysfunction in PCOS: role of obesity and adipose hormones. Am J Med 2006; 119(4):356.e1–6.
8. Orio F, Palomba S, Spinellli L, Cascella T, Tauchmanova L, Zullo F, Lombardi G, Colao A. The cardiovascular risk of young women with polycystic ovary syndrome: an observational, analytical, prospective case-control study. J Clin Endocrinol Metab 2004; 89:3696–3701.
9. Carmina E, Chu MC, Longo RA, Rini GB, Lobo RA. Phenotypic variation in hyperandrogenic women influences the findings of abnormal metabolic and cardiovascular risk parameters. J Clin Endocrinol Metab 2005; 90(5):2545–9.
10. Berneis K, Rizzo M, Fruzzetti F, Lazzaroni V, Carmina E. Atherogenic lipoprotein phenotype and LDL size and subclasses in women with polycystic ovary syndrome. J Clin Endocrinol Metab 2007; 92:186–189.
11. Legro RS. Polycystic ovary syndrome and cardiovascular disease: a premature association? Endocr Rev 2003; 24:302–12.
12. Dahlgren E, Janson PO, Johansson S, Lapidus L, Oden A. Polycystic ovary syndrome and risk for myocardial infarction. Evaluated from a risk factor model based on a prospective population study of women. Acta Obstet Gynecol Scand 1992; 71:599–604.
13. Pierpoint T, McKeigue PM, Isaacs AJ, Wild SH, Jacobs HS. Mortality of woman with polycystic ovary syndrome at long term follow up. J Clin Epidemiol 1998; 51:581–86.

14. Wild SH, Pierpoint T, Mckeigue PM, Jacobs HS. Cardiovascular disease in women with polycystic ovary syndrome at long-term follow-up: a retrospective cohort study. Clin Endocrinol 2000; 52:595–600.
15. Dawber TR, Meadors GF, Moore FE Jr. Epidemiological approaches to heart disease: the Framingham Study. Am J Public Health 1951; 41:279–81.
16. Cibula D, Cifkova R, Fanta M, Poledne R, Zivny J, Skibova J. Increased risk of non-insulin dependent diabetes mellitus, arterial hypertension and coronary artery disease in perimenopausal women with a history of the polycystic ovary syndrome. Hum Reprod 2000; 15:785–789.
17. Labrie F, Belanger A, Cusan L, Gomez J, Candas B. Marked decline in serum concentrations of adrenal C19 sex steroid precursors and conjugated androgen metabolites during aging. J Clin Endocrinol Metab 1997; 82:2396–2402.
18. Bili H, Laven J, Imani B, Eijkemans MJ, Fauser BC. Age-related differences in features associated with polycystic ovary syndrome in normogonadotrophic oligo-amenhorroeic infertile women of reproductive years. Eur J Endocrinol 2001; 145: 749–55.
19. Koivunen R, Laatikainen T, Tomas C, Huhtaniemi I, Tapanainen J, Martikainen H. The prevalence of polycystic ovaries in healthy women. Acta Obstet Gynecol Scand 1999; 78:137–41.
20. Elting MW, Korsen TJ, Rekers-Mombarg LT, Schoemaker J. Women with polycystic ovary syndrome gain regular menstrual cycles when ageing. Hum Reprod. 2000; 15:24–8.
21. Vulpoi C, Lecomte C, Guilloteau D L, Lecomte P. Ageing and reproduction: is polycystic ovary syndrome an exception? Ann. Endocrinol (Paris) 2007; 68:45–50.
22. Carmina E. Fat distribution and adipose products in Polycystic Ovary Syndrome. In: Diamanti-Kandarakis E, Nestler JE, Panidis D, Pasquali R (eds.) Insulin Resistance and the Polycystic Ovary Syndrome. Humana Press ed., Totowa, N. J., 2007; 235–244.
23. Moran LJ, Noakes M, Clifton PM, Tomlinson L, Norman RJ. Dietary composition in restoring reproductive and metabolic physiology in overweight women with Polycystic Ovary Syndrome. J Clin Endocrinol Metab 2003; 88:812–819.
24. Balen A. Polycystic Ovary Syndrome and cancer. Hum Reprod Update 2001; 7:522–525.
25. Dahlgren E, Friberg LG, Johansson S, Lindstrom B, Oden A, Samsioe G, Janson PO. Endometrial carcinoma: ovarian dysfunction- a risk factor in young women. J Obstet Gynecol Reprod Biol 2001; 41:143–150.
26. Hendersen BE, Casagrande JT, Pike MC, Mack T, Rosario I, Duke A. The epidemiology of endometrial cancer in young women. Br J Cancer 1983; 47:749–756.
27. Wagley A, Hardiman P. Menstrual dysfunction and endometrial neoplasia in the Polycystic Ovary Syndrome and other androgen excess disorders. In: Azziz R, Nestler JE, Dewailly D (eds.) Androgen Excess Disorders in Women, 2nd edition, Humana Press ed., Totowa, NJ, 2006; 303–318.
28. Moseson M, Koenig KL, Shore RA, Paternack BS. The influence of medical conditions associated with hormones to the risk of breast cancer. It J Epidemiol 1993; 22:1000–1009.
29. Anderson KE, Sellers TA, Chen PL, Rich SS, Hong CP, Folsom AR. Association of Stein-Leventhal syndrome with the incidence of postmenopausal breast carcinoma in a large prospective study of women in Iowa. Cancer 1997; 79:494–499.
30. Schildkraut JM, Schwingl PJ, Bastos E, Evanoff A, Hughes C. Epithelia ovarian cancer risk among women with polycystic ovary syndrome. Obstet Gynecol 1996; 88:554–559.
31. Carmina E, Bucchieri S, Esposito A, Del Puente A, Mansueto P, Di Fede G, Rini GB. Abdominal fat quantity and distribution in women with Polycystic Ovary Syndrome and extent of its relation to insulin resistance. J Clin Endocrinol Metab 2007; 92:2500–5.
32. Rizzo M, Berneis K, Carmina E, Rini GB. How should we manage atherogenic dyslipidemia in women with polycystic ovary syndrome? Am J Obstet Gynecol 2008; 198:28.e1–5.
33. Duleba AJ, Banaszewska B, Spaczynski RZ, Pawelczyk L. Simvastatin improves biochemical parameters in women with polycystic ovary syndrome: results of a prospective randomized trial. Fertil Steril 2006; 85:996–1001.
34. Pasquali R, Gambineri A. Insulin-sensitizing agents in polycystic ovary syndrome. Eur J Endocrinol 2006; 154:763–775.

Index

B

C

N

O

P

MIX
Papier aus verantwortungsvollen Quellen
Paper from responsible sources
FSC® C105338

If you have any concerns about our products,
you can contact us on
ProductSafety@springernature.com

In case Publisher is established outside the EU,
the EU authorized representative is:
Springer Nature Customer Service Center GmbH
Europaplatz 3, 69115 Heidelberg, Germany

Printed by Libri Plureos GmbH
in Hamburg, Germany